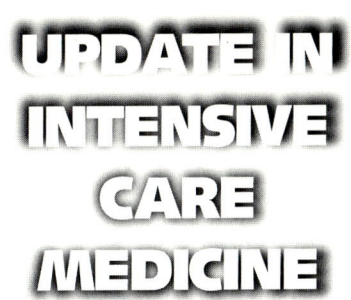

UPDATE IN INTENSIVE CARE MEDICINE

Series Editor: Jean-Louis Vincent

Springer
New York
Berlin
Heidelberg
Barcelona
Hong Kong
London
Milan
Paris
Tokyo

CEREBRAL BLOOD FLOW
Mechanisms of Ischemia, Diagnosis, and Therapy

Volume Editor:

Michael R. Pinsky, MD
Professor of Anesthesiology
Director of Research, Division of Critical Care Medicine
Department of Anesthesiology and Critical Care Medicine
University of Pittsburgh
Pittsburgh, Pennsylvania, USA

Series Editor:

Jean-Louis Vincent, MD, PhD, FCCM, FCCP
Head, Department of Intensive Care
Erasme University Hospital
Brussels, Belgium

With 57 Figures and 17 Tables

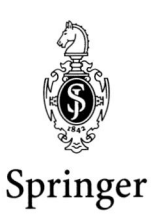

Springer

Michael R. Pinsky, MD
Professor of Anesthesiology
Director of Research, Division of Critical Care Medicine
Department of Anesthesiology and Critical Care Medicine
University of Pittsburgh
Pittsburgh, PA 15261
USA

Series Editor:
Jean-Louis Vincent, MD, PhD, FCCM, FCCP
Head, Department of Intensive Care
Erasme University Hospital
Route de Lennik 808
B-1070 Brussels
Belgium

Library of Congress Cataloging-in-Publication Data
Cerebral blood flow: mechanisms of ischemia, diagnosis, and therapy/M. Pinsky (ed.). p. ; cm. —
(Update in intensive care medicine, ISSN 0933-6788; 37) "Proceedings of the 5th Annual Symposium on
Applied Physiology of the Peripheral Circulation, June 9–11, 2000, Pittsburgh Hilton and tower,
Pittsburgh, PA" — Contents p. Includes bibliographical references and index.
    ISBN 3540426841 (softcover: alk. paper)
1. Cerebral ischemia—Congresses. 2. Cerebral circulation—Congresses. I. Pinsky, Michael R.
II. Symposium on Applied Physiology of the Peripheral Circulation (5th: 2000: Pittsburgh, Pa.)
III. Series. [DNLM: 1. Cerebrovascular Circulation—Congresses. 2. Brain—blood supply—Congresses.
3. Ischemia—Congresses. WI UP66H v.37 2002]

Printed on acid-free paper.

Production managed by PRO EDIT GmbH, Heidelberg, Germany.
Typeset by TBS, Sandhausen, Germany.
Printed and bound by Mercedes-Druck, Berlin, Germany.
Printed in Germany.

9 8 7 6 5 4 3 2 1

ISSN 0933-6788
ISBN 3-540-42684-1   SPIN 10851568

Springer-Verlag New York Berlin Heidelberg
A member of BertelsmannSpringer Science+Business Media GmbH

Preface

Cerebral Blood Flow: Quantifying Consciousness

Although the heart may be the source of energy needed to generate blood flow, and other organs absolutely essential for normal living, the brain is the reason we are alive. The collected book chapters are aimed at addressing this most fundamental organ and its blood flow. These papers reflect detailed descriptions of similar topics presented over a two-day period as part of the 5th International Symposium on Applied Physiology of the Peripheral Circulation held in Pittsburgh, Pennsylvania, in June 2000. The symposium and this volume were organized into four distinct groupings that follow in a logical fashion.

The initial papers focus on the basic unique physiology and pathophysiology of the cerebral circulation, including a historical review of the means to measure cerebral blood flow and its implications of the past 30 years. Dr. Walter D. Obrist was one of the original investigators to use radiolabeled markers to assess cerebral blood flow. His equations and initial studies form an impressive introduction to where we are now. As with much of the body's special organs, the brain too has many circulatory features unique to itself. These include the unique blood-brain barrier function of the endothelium, local neural regulation control, and intracranial pressure effects. These special issues, plus genetic factors that may predispose individuals to developing cerebral aneurysm, make up the initial section of the monograph.

The brain is unique in its response to ischemia. Since neurons contain vasoactive neurotransmitters, secondary vasospasm may occur, increasing the zone of ischemia to a greater extent than the original ischemia or traumatic process induced. Furthermore, assessment of neuronal function during ischemia and its potential for recovery is problematic. In this regard, the pioneering work by Drs. Siesjö, Kochanek, and Gjedde has led to exciting new insights and potential diagnostic tools and therapeutic options that should have measurable impact on future care. Genetic control of the fundamental aspects of neuronal cell death is described in the works from the Stroke Institute of the University of Pittsburgh. Dr. Safar develops the impressive history of cerebral resuscitation from temporary global brain ischemia seen in cardiac arrest. This discussion chronicles the history of the Safar Center for resuscitation and Dr. Safar's own work in cerebral cardiopulmonary resuscitation over the past 40 years. These topics logically lead to the concept of ischemic penumbra: that portion of the brain rendered dysfunctional but not yet irreversibly injured. The chapter by Dr. Hossmann describes a fundamental aspect of cerebral ischemia and infarction.

Once the processes of blood flow and ischemia/reperfusion are understood, what remain are diagnostic techniques and therapeutic options. These issues comprise the final two sections of the book and give the volume its decidedly clinical flavor. Clearly, if one is to diagnose and treat cerebral ischemia, it is essential to quantify the degree of cerebral ischemia and its evolution over time. Otherwise, only superficial inferences on the efficacy of clinical trials can be made. These areas are of the greatest interest to the practicing physician, but require an understanding of the fundamental aspects of physiology and pathophysiology from the preceding sections to put into context.

Measures of cerebral blood flow are problematic. What may be interesting to a perfusionist and one focusing on intravascular pathology may be the structural vascular changes induced by thrombosis or embolism, hemorrhage or trauma. However, functional imaging of neuronal function, tissue oxygenation, and potential for neuronal recovery represent the new imaging techniques available to the clinician. These and better methods of structural imaging are described in the third section by the worker who developed these technologies and are positioned in such a sequence that they proceed from structural to functional imaging.

Presently, many large multicentered clinical trials of stroke prevention and treatment have been completed and some new trials proposed. In the final section, we gather the principal investigators for several of these clinical trials. They present the results for thrombolysis, interventional neuroradiology, therapeutic hypothermia, and revascularization surgery. This is clearly the bleeding edge of clinical studies on cerebral ischemia management.

The clinical challenges in cerebral ischemia and stroke research remain the rapid and accurate diagnosis of ischemic injury in a timely fashion and the institution and titration of effective therapies. Data presented therein suggest that different imaging techniques describe different aspects of cerebral ischemia and that each technique has its specific strengths and weaknesses. Importantly, based on our present-day knowledge of ischemic stroke and its natural history, therapies to reverse ischemia and prevent subsequent injury may be quite different. This suggests that combination therapy with differing goals early on and then into active therapy is a realistic option. Regrettably, the large multicentered clinical trials described in this book are all of single therapies. Though each has a clear efficacy in specific patients, combination therapy will likely emerge and will be the most cost-effective approach to treatment. Our challenge will be defining the specific combination or group of combinations needed at each point in the treatment regimen and the diagnostic tests or clinical framework that will identify these specific patient groups and their subsequent response to therapy. This challenge is daunting, but our understanding of the pathophysiology of cerebral injury is increasing rapidly, our tools not only powerful but becoming more specific and noninvasive, and our treatment options more process-specific. Thus, we can feel optimistic that morbidity and mortality from ischemic stroke will continue to decline. Potentially, our ease in diagnosis and rapidity of effective treatment of ischemic brain injury will become well described and practiced as is our present-day diagnosis and treatment for acute myocardial ischemia.

Pittsburgh, Pennsylvania, USA   *Michael R. Pinsky, MD*
Autumn 2001

Contents

Contributors

Viken Babikian, MD
Professor of Neurology
Department of Neurology
Boston University School of Medicine
Boston, Massachusetts
USA

G.J. Bouma, MD, PhD
Department of Neurosurgery
Academic Medical Center
University of Amsterdam
Amsterdam
The Netherlands

Alastair M. Buchan, MD
Professor of Neurology
Department of Clinical Neurosciences
University of Calgary
Calgary, Alberta
Canada

Robert S.B. Clark, MD
Assistant Professor
Department of Anesthesiology and
    Critical Care
University of Pittsburgh School of Medicine
Pittsburgh, Pennsylvania
USA

Christopher F. Dowd, MD
Associate Clinical Professor
Department of Radiology and
    Neurological Surgery
University of California, San Francisco
San Francisco, California
USA

Frank M. Faraci, MD
Departments of Internal Medicine and
    Pharmacology
University of Iowa College of Medicine
Iowa City, Iowa
USA

Marc Fisher, MD
Vice Chairman
Department of Neurology
University of Massachusetts Memorial
    Healthcare
Worcester, Massachusetts
USA

Albert Gjedde, MD, DM, FAAAS
The Pathophysiology and Experimental
    Tomography Center
Aarhus University Hospital
Aarhus
Denmark

Joao Gomes, MD
Chief Resident
Department of Neurology
Boston University School of Medicine
Boston, Massachusetts
USA

Ramon Gilberto Gonzáles, MD, PhD
Associate Professor of Radiology
Department of Radiology
Harvard Medical School
Boston, Massachusetts
USA

Steven H. Graham, MD, PhD
Associate Professor
Department of Neurology
University of Pittsburgh School of Medicine
and
Associate Director for Research
Geriatric Research Educational and
    Clinical Center
Veterans Affairs Pittsburgh Health System
Pittsburgh, Pennsylvania
USA

Robert L. Grubb, Jr., MD
Professor of Neurological Surgery
Department of Neurosurgery
Washington University School of Medicine
St. Louis, Missouri
USA

Van V. Halbach, MD
Clinical Professor
Department of Radiology and
    Neurological Surgery
University of California, San Francisco
San Francisco, California
USA

Leena M. Hamberg, PhD
Assistant Professor of Radiology
Department of Radiology
Harvard Medical School
Boston, Massachusetts
USA

Kristy S. Hendrich, BS
Research Associate
Pittsburgh NMR Center for
    Biomedical Research
Carnegie Mellon University
Pittsburgh, Pennsylvania
USA

Robert W. Hickey, MD
Assistant Professor
Department of Pediatrics
University of Pittsburgh School of Medicine
Pittsburgh, Pennsylvania
USA

Randall T. Higashida, MD
Clinical Professor
Department of Radiology and
    Neurological Surgery
University of California, San Francisco
San Francisco, California
USA

Chien Ho, PhD
Alumni Professor of Biological Sciences
Department of Biological Sciences
Carnegie Mellon University
Pittsburgh, Pennsylvania
USA

Michael B. Horowitz, MD
Associate Professor of Neurosurgery and
    Radiology
Associate Director for Cranial Nerve
    Disorders
and
Center for Endovascular Surgery
University of Pittsburgh
Pittsburgh, Pennsylvania
USA

Konstantin-Alexander Hossmann, MD
Department of Experimental Neurology
Max Planck Institute of
    Neurological Research
Cologne
Germany

George Hunter, MD
Assistant Professor of Radiology
Department of Radiology
Harvard Medical School
Boston, Massachusetts
USA

Costantino Iadecola, MD
Professor
Department of Neurology
University of Minnesota
Minneapolis, Minnesota
USA

Can Ince, PhD
Professor of Anesthesiology
Department of Anesthesiology
Academic Medical Center
Amsterdam
The Netherlands

Larry W. Jenkins, PhD
Professor of Neurological Surgery
Department of Neurological Surgery
University of Pittsburgh School of Medicine
Pittsburgh, Pennsylvania
USA

Amin B. Kassam, MD, FRCS
Assistant Professor of Neurological Surgery
Otolaryngology/Head and Neck Surgery
Director, Center for Cranial Nerve Disorders
Co-Director, Center for Cranial Base
    Surgery
Departments of Neurological Surgery
    and Human Genetics
University of Pittsburgh
Pittsburgh, Pennsylvania
USA

Patrick M. Kochanek, MD
Director, The Safar Center for
    Resuscitation Research
Departments of Anesthesiology and
    Critical Care Medicine
University of Pittsburgh School of Medicine
Pittsburgh, Pennsylvania
USA

Jaroslaw Krejza, MD, PhD
Department of Radiology
Bialystok Medical Academy
Bialystok
Poland

Tibor Kristián, MD
Senior Researcher
The Neuroscience Institute
The Queen's Medical Center
Honolulu, Hawaii
USA

Michael H. Lev, MD
Instructor in Radiology
Department of Radiology
Harvard Medical School
Boston, Massachusetts
USA

Adel M. Malek, MD, PhD
Director
Cerebrovascular and Endovascular
    Neurosurgery
Department of Neurosurgery
Beth Israel Deaconess Medical Center
Boston, Massachusetts
USA

Donald W. Marion, MD
Director
Brain Trauma Research Center
UPMC Presbyterian Hospital
Pittsburgh, Pennsylvania
USA

Majaz Moonis, MD, MRCP, DM
Assistant Professor
Director, Stroke Prevention Clinic
Department of Neurology
University of Massachusetts
Worcester, Massachusetts
USA

Kiyoshi Niwa, MD, PhD
Research Associate
Department of Neurology
University of Minnesota
Minneapolis, Minnesota
USA

Walter D. Obrist, PhD
Professor Emeritus
University of Pittsburgh
Pittsburgh, Pennsylvania
USA

F.A. Pennings, MD
Department of Neurosurgery
Academic Medical Center
Amsterdam
The Netherlands

David G. Peters, PhD
Assistant Professor
Department of Human Genetics
Graduate School of Public Health
University of Pittsburgh
Pittsburgh, Pennsylvania
USA

Constantine C. Phatouros, FRACR
Department of Radiology
Division of Interventional Neurovascular
    Radiology
University of California, San Francisco
San Francisco, California
USA

Michael R. Pinsky, MD
Professor of Anesthesiology
Director of Research, Division of
    Critical Care Medicine
Department of Anesthesiology and
    Critical Care Medicine
University of Pittsburgh
Pittsburgh, Pennsylvania
USA

William J. Powers, MD
Professor of Neurology and Radiology
Department of Neurology and
    Neurological Surgery
Washington University School of Medicine
St. Louis, Missouri
USA

Peter Safar, MD, DRHC, FCCM, FCCP
Distinguished Professor of
    Resuscitation Medicine
University of Pittsburgh
Safar Center for Resuscitation Research
    (SCRR)
Pittsburgh, Pennsylvania
USA

Bo K. Siesjö, MD, PhD
Research Professor
John A Burns School of Medicine
University of Hawaii, Honolulu
Director of Research
The Neuroscience Institute
The Queen's Medical Center
Honolulu, Hawaii
USA

Kimberly D. Statler, MD
Department of Pediatric Critical Care
    Medicine
University of Pittsburgh School of
    Medicine
Pittsburgh, Pennsylvania
USA

Hiroyuki Uchino, MD
Senior Researcher
The Neuroscience Institute
The Queen's Medical Center
Honolulu, Hawaii
USA

Lawrence R. Wechsler, MD
Professor of Neurology and Neurosurgery
Director, Stroke Institute
University of Pittsburgh Medical Center
Pittsburgh, Pennsylvania
USA

Donald S. Williams, PhD
Assistant Director
Pittsburgh NMR Center for
    Biomedical Research
Carnegie Mellon University
Pittsburgh, Pennsylvania
USA

Howard Yonas, MD
Professor and Vice Chairman
Department of Neurosurgery
University of Pittsburgh
Pittsburgh, Pennsylvania
USA

Section I:
Physiology and Pathophysiology

History of Cerebral Blood Flow Assessment

W.D. Obrist

Over 100 years have passed since Adolf Fick [1] introduced in 1870 the now well-established principle that bears his name. Based on the conservation of mass, this principle simply states that the quantity of a substance taken up by an organ per unit of time is equal to the blood flow through that organ multiplied by the difference between its arterial and venous concentrations.

Fick had proposed this as a means of measuring cardiac output, using the total oxygen uptake of the body and the arteriovenous oxygen difference across the heart. However, it was not until cardiac catheterization became available in the 1940s that the technique could be applied to humans. The values so obtained compared favorably with those of the indicator dilution method.

In 1945, Kety and Schmidt [2] applied the Fick principle to CBF measurements in humans, using the exogenous substance, nitrous oxide (N_2O), an inert diffusible gas. Whole brain blood flow was estimated from repeated sampling of arterial and jugular venous blood during inhalation of 15% N_2O. In order to get a valid estimate of brain tissue concentration from jugular blood, it was necessary to inhale the gas for 10 minutes or more; i.e., to approach tissue saturation. This was the first quantitative CBF method in humans, and contributed greatly to our understanding of cerebral hemodynamics.

In 1951, Kety [3] extended the Fick principle to account for the exchange of inert diffusible gases in the lungs and tissues. He started with a differential expression of the Fick equation:

$$dCi(t)/dt = f(Ca(t) - Ci(t)/\lambda)$$

where $Ci(t)$ = tissue concentration of the substance at time t (quantity per unit weight of tissue), f = blood flow per unit weight of tissue, $Ca(t)$ = arterial concentration at time t, $Ci(t)/\lambda = Cv(t)$, the venous concentration, assuming instantaneous equilibrium between tissue and its venous blood, and λ = the tissue-blood partition coefficient for the substance.

The solution of this differential equation is the familiar *convolution integral*, proposed by Kety, and used in both the radioactive (Xe-133) and stable xenon methods:

$$Ci(t) = f\int_0^t Ca(u)e^{-k(t-u)}du$$

where $k=f/\lambda$, the exponential clearance rate of the tracer.

In the above equation, blood flow is obtained by least squares curve fitting of the uptake and /or clearance of the tracer, which yields solutions for two unknowns, f and k. The partition coefficient is calculated separately from the relationship: $f=\lambda/k$.

It should be noted that the convolution integral is not the same as the earlier Kety-Schmidt equation, which was based on simple integration of the differential equation. Unlike the Kety-Schmidt method that required saturation of the tissue, the convolution integral yields tissue concentration at any time t, so that it is not necessary to extend observations until saturation is achieved.

The first application of the convolution integral to CBF was the autoradiographic method in animals, carried out in Kety's laboratory during the 1950s. A diffusible radioactive gas (trifluoroiodomethane) was inhaled or intravenously infused over a one-minute period, and cerebral uptake was determined from postmortem brain slices. This provided, for the first time, highly localized CBF measurements in various brain regions. It clearly established differences in blood flow between gray and white matter.

Recognizing that radioisotopes could provide estimates of *regional* cerebral blood flow, Lassen and Ingvar [4] in 1961 introduced the intracarotid injection method. A bolus of Xe-133, a highly diffusible gas, was rapidly injected into one internal carotid artery. Gamma radiation was then monitored for 10 minutes over the ipsilateral hemisphere by multiple extracranial detectors. A simple Height /Area analysis of the clearance curves was performed, based on mean transit time concepts formulated by Zierler (1965) [5], which assumes that all of the isotope enters the brain before any of it leaves. This was the first quantitative regional method in humans, which greatly enhanced our understanding of focal blood flow changes.

Because of the invasiveness of intracarotid injection, Veall and Mallett [6] in1963 proposed a five-minute *inhalation* of trace amounts of Xe-133 and extracranial recording. Since this route of isotope administration produces a distributed input and considerable recirculation, they proposed correcting the clearance curves with estimates of arterial concentration derived from expired end-tidal air. The complete noninvasiveness of this approach made it especially suitable for human use.

In 1967, Obrist and coworkers [7] applied the convolution integral to Xe-133 clearance curves, based on a one-minute inhalation and monitoring of end-tidal air. This was the first application of Kety's equation to human studies. A two-compartment deconvolution, which involved least squares curve fitting, provided separate estimates of gray and white matter flow. Because of its noninvasiveness, Xe-133 inhalation became the most widely used CBF method in the 1970s and 80s. Intravenous injection of the isotope, also widely used, permitted easier administration in intensive care and operating room environments.

A limitation of the above Xe-133 techniques is the lack of three dimensional tomographic reconstruction. Although excellent cortical topography can be achieved with multiple, fixed external detectors, blood flow measurements in deeper structures of the brain are not obtainable. During the late 1970s and early 1980s several tomographic CBF methods were developed; specifically, PET, SPECT and stable Xe/CT. The PET method also provided valuable information on cerebral metabolism and blood volume[8]. Because of its complexity and expense, however, it has been limited primarily to research investigations. Although SPECT studies are more easily performed, they provide only semi-quantitative information; i.e., relative CBF values. An exception is Xe-133 SPECT, but this suffers from poor spatial resolution. The Xe/CT method is currently one of the more promising approaches, yielding quantitative data that can be correlated directly with morphologic CT scans.

Development of the Xe/CT method came shortly after the introduction of CT scanning when it was realized that xenon, with its high atomic number, could significantly attenuate x-rays when inhaled at 30% concentrations. In 1978, Kelcz and coworkers [9] proposed a method for determining the solubility of xenon in both tissues and blood, the latter being derived from the relationship between xenon solubility and hematocrit. This important contribution formed the basis for converting end-tidal xenon values to arterial concentration (in Hounsfield units), a procedure subsequently adopted in most Xe/CT studies. Kelcz et al. also emphasized the necessity of correcting the recorded brain curves for recirculation. Without such a correction, CBF would be underestimated relative to Xe-133 findings.

The first reports of Xe/CT CBF measurements involving a correction for recirculation were by Drayer et al. [10] and Meyer et al. [11] in 1980. In accordance with the Xe-133 inhalation model of Obrist and coworkers [7], they employed the convolution integral, using end-tidal air to estimate arterial input. This model was soon employed by British and Japanese investigators, and has become the standard for Xe/CT measurements of blood flow.

The early studies cited above performed CBF analyses on fairly large regions of interest (ROI). Although raw xenon enhancement images were obtained, pixel-by-pixel blood flow images were not available. It remained for Gur and coworkers [12] in 1982 to construct such CBF images. Instead of averaging enhancement values across pixels prior to computing blood flow, CBF was calculated separately for each pixel. In order to obtain meaningful images, however, both pre- and post-computation smoothing were necessary to reduce noise.

As documented by Gur et al. [12], CT noise introduces large errors in computed CBF values, there being a relatively poor signal-to-noise ratio for this method. Even with smoothing, CBF values for individual pixels are unreliable. As these authors demonstrated, statistically stable results (coefficient of variation <15%) require an ROI size of 100 mm^2 (10×10 pixels) or more. Nevertheless, an ROI of that size is adequate for most clinical studies, and is comparable or superior to that of other current methods.

A recent development has been the use of intravascular bolus techniques, first proposed by Axel (1983) [13] for CT estimates of mean transit time, and now employed by both CT [14] and MRI [15] for cerebral blood flow determinations. An iodinated or paramagnetic contrast agent is injected into a peripheral vein, followed by rapid sequential scanning. Because the bolus is no longer a brief impulse (delta function) by the time it reaches the brain, it is necessary to deconvolute the cerebral curves with an arterial input function obtained by scanning a nearby vessel.

In contrast to diffusible tracers, a nondiffusible intravascular bolus requires an intact blood brain barrier, not always present in diseased states. Due to variations in vascular topography, the bolus may undergo variable delays and dispersion between the monitored artery and tissue ROI, so that selection of an appropriate arterial input becomes critical. These techniques are still in the developmental phase. Their reliability and validity, particularly in pathological conditions, remain to be determined.

This brief historical review has attempted to trace the origin of concepts underlying the development of several CBF methods, starting with the Fick principle and ending with recent tomographic techniques. For historical accuracy, dates given in the text refer to an author's initial publication on the subject, not necessarily to the particular article cited.

References

1. Fick A. Ueber die Messung des Blutquantums in den Herzventrikeln. Sitz Physik-Med Ges Wurzburg 1870; 2:16–28.
2. Kety SS, Schmidt CF. The nitrous oxide method for the quantitative determination of cerebral blood flow in man: theory, procedure and normal values. J Clin Invest 1948; 27: 476–483.
3. Kety SS. The theory and applications of the exchange of inert gas at the lungs and tissues. Pharmacol Rev 1951; 3: 1–41.
4. Lassen NA, Ingvar DH. Radioisotopic assessment of regional cerebral blood flow. Prog Nucl Med 1972; 1: 376–409.
5. Zierler KL. Equations for measuring blood flow by external monitoring of radioisotopes. Circ Res 1965; 16: 309–321.
6. Veall N, Mallett BL. Regional cerebral blood flow determination by ^{133}Xe inhalation and external recording: the effect of arterial recirculation. Clin Sci 1966; 30: 353–369.
7. Obrist WD, Thompson HK, Wang HS, Wilkinson WE. Regional cerebral blood flow estimated by ^{133}xenon inhalation. Stroke 1975; 6: 245–256.
8. Baron JC, Frackowiak RSJ, Herholz K, Jones T, Lammertsma AA, Mazoyer B, Weinhard K. Use of PET methods for measurement of cerebral energy metabolism and hemodynamics in cerebrovascular disease. J Cereb Blood Flow Metab 1989; 9: 723–742.
9. Kelcz F, Hilal SK, Hartwell P, Joseph PM. Computed tomographic measurement of the xenon brain-blood partition coefficient and implications for regional cerebral blood flow: a preliminary report. Radiology 1978; 127: 385–392.
10. Drayer BP, Gur D, Wolfson SK, Cook EE. Experimental xenon enhancement with CT imaging: cerebral applications. AJR 1980; 134: 39–44.
11. Meyer JS, Hayman LA, Yamamoto M, Sakai F, Nakajima S. Local cerebral blood flow measured by CT after stable xenon inhalation. AJNR 1980; 1: 213–225.
12. Gur D, Yonas H, Good WF. Local cerebral blood flow by xenon-enhanced CT: current status, potential improvements, and future directions. Cerebrovasc Brain Metab Rev 1989; 1: 68–86.
13. Axel L. Tissue mean transit time from dynamic computed tomography by a simple deconvolution technique. Invest Radiol 1983; 18: 94–99.
14. Cenic A, Nabavi DG, Craen RA, Gelb AW, Lee T-Y. Dynamic CT measurement of cerebral blood flow: a validation study. Am J Neuroradiol 1999; 20: 63–73.
15. Calamante F, Thomas DL, Pell GS, Weirsma J, Turner R. Measuring cerebral blood flow using magnetic resonance imaging techniques. J Cereb Blood Flow Metab 1999; 19: 701–735.

Neural Regulation of the Cerebral Circulation

C. Iadecola and K. Niwa

Introduction

It was once believed that cerebral blood vessels could not dilate and constrict independently and that the cerebral circulation was entirely under the control of the systemic circulation [see ref. 1 for a historical review]. However, evidence accumulated over the past 100 years indicates that cerebral blood vessels are in a dynamic state. Thus, the cerebral vasculature is endowed with complex regulatory systems that allow the brain to finely regulate its own blood supply. One of the major factors that regulates cerebral blood flow (CBF) is neuronal activity. In this chapter, we will focus on the mechanisms governing the relationship between neural activity and blood flow with emphasis on the role of nitric oxide (NO) and cyclooxygenase-2 (COX-2).

Neural Activity Is One of the Major Factors Controlling Cerebral Blood Flow

The brain functional and structural integrity depends on a constant supply of oxygen and substrates through blood flow. Interruption of the blood supply to the brain alters neuronal function and, if the lack of flow is sustained, produces permanent damage to brain cells [2]. It has been known for more than a century that increases in brain activity are associated with increases in CBF restricted to the activated areas [see refs. 3, 4 for a review]. The functional significance of the flow increase is to assure that the increased energy requirements of the activated brain are adequately met. Furthermore, the increase in flow is also needed to remove heat and metabolic waste generated by brain activity. Early work in the late 1800-early 1900 provided indirect but highly suggestive evidence that increased brain activity is accompanied by concomitant increases in flow [e.g., 5–7]. The introduction of techniques for the measurement of regional CBF and/or neural activity both in the animal and human brain made possible a detailed study of the changes in CBF evoked by functional activity [8–10; see ref. 4 for a review].

The principle that the activity of local neurons is a major factor regulating CBF is supported by two lines of evidence. First, in the resting brain, there is a general correspondence between the flow of a given brain region and its rate of cerebral glucose utilization (CGU), a variable reflecting neural activity [3, 11]. Thus, regions with a relatively low glucose utilization, such as the corpus callosum, have low flow, whereas regions with high glucose use, such as the auditory cortex, have high flow [11]. Second, when the activity of the brain is enhanced, either focally or globally, local blood flow increases in proportion to the intensity of the activation [10, 12, 13]. Conversely, if brain activity is reduced, CBF decreases proportionally [14, 15]. Although dissociation between flow and CGU may occur in selected stages of brain development or during activation of autonomic pathways [16–18], the concept of coupling between neural activity and blood flow remains generally valid [19].

While there is a close correspondence between CBF and CGU during activation, the relationship between CBF and cerebral oxygen consumption is less straightforward. Somatosensory or visual stimuli increase CBF and CGU out of proportion to the increase in oxygen consumption [20, 21]. The uncoupling between glucose and oxygen consumption is surprising because the brain is believed to generate energy by aerobic metabolism [22]. The basis for the discrepancy between the magnitude of the increase in CBF and that in oxygen consumption are not entirely clear. One hypothesis is that brain energy metabolism is partly anaerobic, so that glucose is metabolized to lactic acid via anaerobic glycolysis, possibly, in astrocytes [see ref. 23 for a review]. In support of this hypothesis, some studies have showed that neural activity increases lactic acid in brain [15, 24]. On the other hand, Buxton and Frank have suggested that, due to limitations in the transfer of oxygen across the blood-brain barrier, a disproportionately large increase in CBF is required to provide the increase in oxygen needed to support oxidative metabolism during activation [25]. To date these issues remain unresolved and further studies are required.

Mechanisms Responsible for Coupling Neural Activity to Local Blood Flow

The mechanisms mediating the changes in blood flow initiated by neural activity remain to be clearly elucidated. One widely accepted hypothesis, stemming from the work of Roy and Sherrington, is that active neurons release "vasoactive factors" that reach local blood vessels and mediate smooth muscle relaxation [see ref. 26 for a review]. According to this view, the ideal mediator would be a vasoactive agent that: (a) is released in the extracellular space, or depleted from it, in proportion to the intensity of synaptic activity, (b) is highly diffusible and, (c) is rapidly inactivated.

A number of vasoactive agents have been identified that are either released by depolarizing neurons, e.g., neurotransmitters or K^+ and H^+ ions, or that are depleted from the extracellular and perivascular environment during brain activity, e.g., O_2, Ca^{++} [see ref. 26 for a review] (Fig. 1). Paulson and Newman have hypothesized that astrocytes could control microvascular flow during brain activity by "siphoning" extracellular K+ to the perivascular space through their endfeet [27] (Fig. 1). This attractive hypothesis, however, needs to be tested experimentally. The role of K+ ions was recently re-examined in two models of cerebellar activation [28]. It was found that during activation of the cerebellar climbing

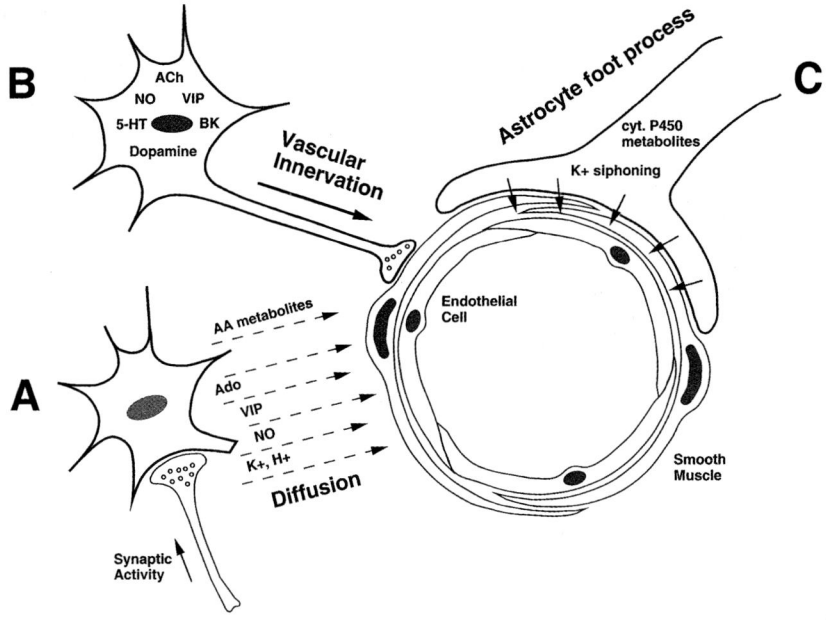

Fig. 1A–C. Potential mechanisms regulating the cerebral circulation during neural activity. **A** Increased neural activity releases vasoactive agents, such as adenosine (Ado), nitric oxide (NO), vasoactive intestinal polypeptide (VIP), arachidonic acid (AA) metabolites (prostanoids, superoxide), and the vasoactive ions potassium and hydrogen. These agents are thought to reach local vessels by simple diffusion and produce relaxation of vascular smooth muscles, which, in turn, leads to an increase in flow to the activated region. The involvement of these vasoactive agents is supported by a large number of studies using pharmacological inhibitors or "knockout mice" (see text for details). **B** Cerebral blood vessels receive nerve fibers from central and peripheral neurons. These nerve fibers contain several neurotransmitters and neuropeptides, such as, for example, acetylcholine (ACh), VIP, bradykinin (BK), catecholamines including dopamine, as well as serotonin (5-HT) and NO. Although vascular innervation can potentially influence vascular tone and regulate flow, its role in neurovascular coupling remains to be defined. The innervation could be involved in the initiation of the vascular response or in its propagation to larger upstream vessels (retrograde vasodilation; see text and Fig. 2 for details). **C** Astrocyte foot processes are in close contact with cerebral arterioles and capillaries and have long been postulated to play a role in cerebrovascular regulation. Astrocytes could contribute to control blood flow by siphoning potassium ions, generated by neural activity, into the perivascular space. Furthermore, astrocytes contain cytochrome P450 enzymes that synthesize epoxygenated products of arachidonic acid that are vasoactive and could play a role in coupling neural activity to CBF. These hypotheses, however, remain to be tested experimentally

fibers the evoked increases in K+ was not sufficient to account in full for the increase in CBF [28]. However, during activation of the parallel fibers the increase in K+ concentration could account for the vasodilation [28]. It is, therefore, likely that at least in some instances, K+ can act as a mediator of vasodilation during neural activation. In models of activity-dependent CBF increases in cerebral cortex and cerebellum, adenosine, a nucleoside that has long been implicated in vascular regulation [see 29 for a review], mediates a component of the vascular response [30, 31]. Neurotransmitters and neuropeptides, such as catecholamines and the vasoactive intestinal peptide (VIP), have also been proposed to participate in activity-induced CBF changes [32, 33]. In addition, it has been proposed that epoxygenated products of arachidonic acid, formed by P450 enzymes, participate in coupling neural activity to blood flow. These arachidonic acid metabolites are epoxyeicosatrienoic acid (EETs). One of these P450 enzymes is present in astrocytes [see ref. 34 for a review]. Therefore, EETs released by astrocytes could play a role in coupling neural activity to CBF. Recent data from our laboratory indicate that NO and COX-2 products are involved in flow-metabolism coupling. These mediators are presented in more detail below.

Nitric Oxide

NO is a short-lived and diffusible molecular mediator that has been implicated in a wide variety of biological functions in many organ systems [see refs. 35, 36 for a review]. NO is synthesized from one of the guanidino nitrogens of L-arginine (L-arg) by the enzyme NO synthase (NOS). The reaction leads to the formation of citrulline and NO in equimolar amounts [see ref. 36]. There are at least three isoforms of NOS one of which, neuronal NOS, is present in a restricted population of central and peripheral neurons [35]. Neuronal NOS requires calcium and calmodulin for its activation [see ref. 35 for a review]. It has been proposed that the rise in intracellular calcium associated with neuronal depolarization activates NOS leading to NO production [37; see ref. 36 for a review]. This agent then diffuses out of the cells in which is synthesized and exerts its actions by stimulating soluble guanylyl cyclase in neighboring cells. Therefore, NO may act as an intercellular messenger and, as such, has been implicated in a wide variety of neurobiological processes [see ref. 36 for a review]. Furthermore, because NO is a potent relaxant of cerebral arteries, it has also been proposed that this agent participates in the regulation of the cerebral circulation during neural activity [38].

A number of studies using models of activation in cerebral cortex and cerebellum have provided evidence that inhibition of NOS attenuates activation-induced increases in CBF, usually, by 50% [39–42; see ref. 43 for a review]. Furthermore, NOS inhibition attenuates the vasodilation elicited by local activation of glutamate receptors in neocortex or cerebellum [44, 45]. These findings have provided evidence that NO is one of the factors linking synaptic activity to blood flow [see ref. 26 for a review]. It must be noted, however, that some studies have failed to find a relationship between NO and the vasodilation evoked by neural activity [46, 47].

Recent data suggest that the role of NO in functional hyperemia is more complex than previously believed. In cerebral cortex, NO seems to act as a "permissive" factor that facilitates the vasodilation initiated by other mechanisms [see ref. 43 for a review]. Although inhibition of NO synthesis attenuates the increase in somatosensory cortex blood flow produced by stimulation of the facial vibrissae, the attenuation is completely reversed by administration of NO donors [48]. The idea that NO is not the final mediator of vasodilation during neural activity is also supported by the finding that the CBF response produced by vibrissal stimulation is not reduced in mice lacking neuronal NOS [49]. These observations suggest that in cerebral cortex NO acts more as a modulator of the response than the final mediator of vasodilation.

In cerebellum, however, the evidence suggests that NO is an obligatory mediator in the vasodilation produced by neural activity. Activation of cerebellar parallel fibers increases synaptic activity and elevates CBF, an effect associated with increased CGU [50]. Administration of NOS inhibitors attenuates the increase in CBF by approximately 50%, without attenuating the intensity of the synaptic activity produced by the stimulation [41, 51]. However, at variance with the cerebral cortex, administration of NO donors does not reverse the attenuation [52]. In a more "physiological" model of cerebellar activation, in which a region of the cerebellar hemisphere termed crus II is activated by stimulation of the ipsilateral upper lip, NOS inhibition virtually abolishes the increase in CBF, suggesting that NO is the major mediator of the vascular response [53]. Furthermore, the increase in CBF produced by crus II activation is markedly attenuated in nNOS null mice [Yang and Iadecola, Soc. Neurosci. Abstract, 2000] Therefore, in contrast to the somatosensory cortex where activation produces a normal CBF increase in nNOS null mice, in cerebellum the lack of neuron-derived NO cannot be adequately compensated for. These observations suggest that, in cerebellum, NO produced by synaptic activity is absolutely required for the vasodilation to occur. The difference in the role of NO in the response to activation in cerebral cortex and cerebellum, suggests that the participation of NO in the mechanisms of functional hyperemia varies from brain region to brain region.

Cyclooxygenase-2

COX-2 is an enzyme involved in the synthesis of prostaglandins and thromboxanes from arachidonic acid [see ref. 54 for a review]. In some organs, COX-2 is not present in the normal state, but its expression is induced by inflammatory stimuli or mitogens [54]. In brain, however, COX-2 is constitutively expressed, and is localized to dendritic arborizations and spines of excitatory neurons [55, 56]. In the adult cerebral cortex, neuronal COX-2 expression is upregulated by synaptic activity [56] and, in the developing nervous system of the rat, COX-2 expression increases at a time when activity-dependent synaptic remodeling occurs [55]. These observations, in concert with its synaptic localization, have suggested that COX-2 is involved in activity-dependent processes and synaptic signaling [55].

Because of this link between synaptic activity and COX-2, we recently investigated whether COX-2 is involved in the increases in CBF that accompany neural activity. Using activation of the rodent whisker-barrel cortex as a model of functional hyperemia [10, 57], we found that the selective COX-2 inhibitor NS-398 attenuates the increase in neocortical blood flow produced by vibrissal stimulation. Furthermore, the hyperemic response is impaired in mutant mice lacking COX-2, whereas the associated increase in CGU, a variable that reflects neural activity, is not affected [58]. Interestingly, COX-2 inhibition with NS398 or COX-2 deletion in null mice does not affect cerebrovascular responses elicited by systemic hypercapnia or by topical application of endothelium-dependent vasodila-tors, such as acetylcholine, bradykinin or the calcium ionophore A23187 [58]. Therefore, the evidence suggests that COX-2 contributes to the vasodilation initi-ated by neural activity but not by endothelial factors.

The findings presented above indicate that COX-2 participates in the mecha-nisms linking synaptic activity to local blood flow in the somatosensory cortex. However, the COX-2 reaction products that are responsible for the vasodilation remain to be identified. Reaction products of COX-2 include prostaglandin H2, which is the precursor of other prostanoids, and superoxide [54]. While some prostaglandins, such as PGE2, are vasodilators [59], superoxide is also a potent smooth muscle relaxant [60]. Further studies will have to determine the specific products of the COX-2 pathways that are responsible for the vasodilation.

Retrograde Vasodilation: Intrinsic Vascular Mechanisms vs. Vascular Innervation

As discussed in detail elsewhere [26, 61], the neural release of vasoactive agents cannot account entirely for the vascular changes initiated by synaptic activity. Hemodynamic considerations suggest that the pial arteries and arterioles that feed the activated tissue must also dilate in order to increase tissue flow effective-ly (Fig. 2). During activation, in cerebral or cerebellar cortex, vasodilation occurs also in arterioles remote from the site of activation [61, 62]. The mechanisms responsible for these complex and coordinated vascular events have not been elu-cidated. One possibility is that vasodilator signals provided by active neurons ini-tiate a local vascular response that is then propagated retrogradely to the pial arterioles via intrinsic vascular mechanisms, such as the retrograde vasodilation

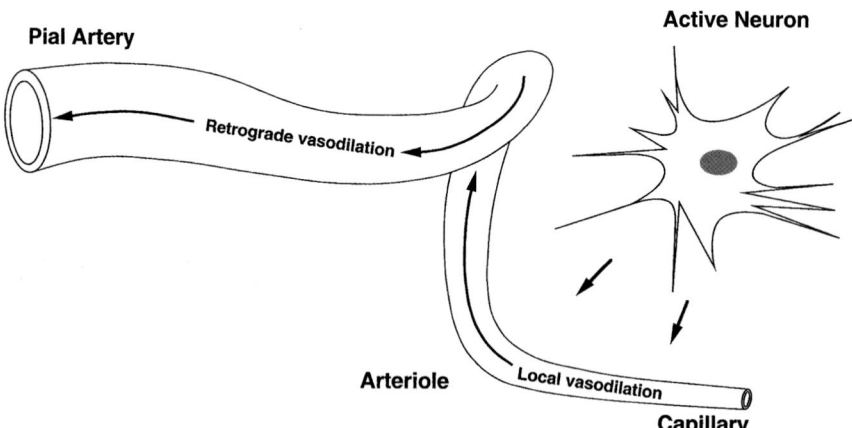

Fig. 2. Neural activation produces dilatation of arterioles located at the activated site (local vasodilation), as well as of larger arterioles located upstream (retrograde vasodilation). The vasodilation of upstream arterioles is needed to prevent a "steal" of blood flow from adjacent non-activated regions. The mechanisms responsible for the propagation of the vasodilation upstream are not well understood and may include mechanisms intrinsic and extrinsic to the vessel wall (see text for details)

of Duling and Berne [63, 64] and/or flow-mediated vasodilation [65, 66]. The observation that conducted vasodilation occurs in isolated cerebral vessels supports the hypothesis that the mechanisms of propagation are intrinsic to the vascular wall [67], perhaps, through intercellular gap junctions [68]. Another possibility is that the coordination between parenchymal neural activity and upstream vessels is controlled by perivascular nerves innervating pial arteries [69]. It is well known that cerebral blood vessels are innervated by nerve fibers intrinsic or extrinsic to the brain [see ref. 70 for a review]. Extrinsic nerves originate from cranial autonomic ganglia [70]. The intrinsic innervation originates from central neurons. Both intrinsic and extrinsic nerve terminals contain neurotransmitters and neuropeptides, including NO, acetylcholine, VIP, neuropeptide Y, catecholamines, bradykinin, substance P, serotonin, and calcitonin gene-related peptide [70] (Fig. 1). However, direct experimental evidence supporting a role for vascular innervation in this process is thus far lacking.

In summary, there is substantial evidence that neural activity is a major factor controlling CBF. However, the neurovascular mechanisms mediating the changes in flow have not been elucidated in full. Although recent evidence supports contributions by NO and cyclooxygenase products in the response, multiple mediators, including, neurotransmitters, neuropeptides and, perhaps, ions and cytochrome P450 metabolites, are also likely to play a role. Furthermore, the mechanisms regulating CBF are likely to vary regionally, depending on the neuronal circuitry and chemical anatomy of each brain region.

Acknowledgements. Supported by NIH grants NS31318 and NS38252. C. I. is the recipient of a Javits Award from NIH/NINDS.

References

1. Friedland, R. P. and C. Iadecola. Roy and Sherrington (1890): a centennial reexamination of "On the regulation of the blood-supply of the brain". Neurology 1991;41: 10–4.
2. Hossmann, K.-A. Viability thresholds and the penumbra of focal ischemia. Ann Neurol 1994;36: 557–565.
3. Reivich, M. Blood flow metabolism couple in brain. Res. Publ. Assoc. Res. Nerv. Ment. Dis. 1974;53: 125–140.
4. Raichle, M. E. Behind the scenes of functional brain imaging: a historical and physiological perspective. Proc Natl Acad Sci U S A 1998;95: 765–72.
5. Fulton, J. F. Observations upon the vascularity of the human occipital lobe during visual activity. Brain 1928;LI: 310–320.
6. Mosso, A. Ueber den Kreislauf des Blutes im menschlichen Gehirn. Leipzig: Viet; 1881: 203.
7. Schmidt, C. and J. Hendrix. Action of chemical substances on cerebral blood vessels. Res. Publ. Assoc. Res. Nerv. Ment. Dis. 1938;18: 229–276.
8. Freygang, W. H. and L. Sokoloff. Quantitative measurement of regional circulation in the central nervous system by the use of radioactive inert gas. Adv. Biol. Med. Phys. 1958;6: 263–279.
9. Olesen, J. Contralateral focal increase of cerebral blood flow in man during arm work. Brain 1971;94: 635–646.
10. Greenberg, J., P. Hand, A. Sylvestro and M. Reivich. Localized metabolic-flow couple during functional activity. Acta Neurol. Scand. 1979;72: 12–13.
11. Kuschinsky, W. Coupling of function metabolism and blood flow in the brain. NIPS 1987;2: 217–220.

12. Fox, P. T. and M. E. Raichle. Stimulus rate dependence of regional cerebral blood flow in human striate cortex, demonstrated by positron emission tomography. J. Neurophysiol. 1984;51: 1109–20.

13. Iadecola, C., M. Nakai, S. Mraovitch, D. A. Ruggiero, L. W. Tucker and D. J. Reis. Global increase in cerebral metabolism and blood flow produced by focal electrical stimulation of dorsal medullary reticular formation in rat. Brain Res 1983;272: 101–114.

14. Nilsson, B., S. Rehncrona and B. K. Siesjö. Coupling of cerebral metabolism and blood flow in epileptic seizures, hypoxia and hypoglycaemia. In: Elliot, K. and O'Connor, M., ed. Cerebral Vascular Smooth Muscle and its Control. New York: Elsevier; 1978: 199–218.

15. Ueki, M., F. Linn and K.-A. Hossmann. Functional activation of cerebral blood flow and metabolism before and after global ischemia of rat brain. J. Cereb. Blood Flow Metab. 1988;8: 486–494.

16. Nakai, M., C. Iadecola, D. Ruggiero, L. Tucker and D. Reis. Electrical stimulation of cerebellar fastigial nucleus increases cerebrocortical blood flow without change in local metabolism: evidence for an intrinsic system in brain for primary vasodilation. Brain Res. 1983;260: 35–49.

17. Ohata, M., U. Sundaram, W. R. Fredricks, E. London and S. I. Rapoport. Regional cerebral blood flow during development and aging in the rat brain. Brain 1981;104: 319–332.

18. Nakai, M. and M. Maeda. Vasodilatation and enhanced oxidative metabolism of the cerebral cortex provoked by the periaqueductal gray matter in anaesthetized rats. Neuroscience 1996;72: 1133–40.

19. Lou, H. C., L. Edvinsson and E. T. MacKenzie. The concept of coupling blood flow to brain function: Revision required? Ann. Neurol 1987; 22: 289–297.

20. Fox, P. T. and M. E. Raichle. Focal physiological uncoupling of cerebral blood flow and oxidative metabolism during somatosensory stimulation in human subjects. Proc. Natl. Acad. Sci. USA 1986;83: 1140–4.

21. Fox, P. T., M. E. Raichle, M. A. Mintun and C. Dence. Nonoxidative glucose consumption during focal physiological neural activity. Science 1988;241: 462–464.

22. Siesjo, B. K. Brain energy metabolism. New York: Wiley & Sons; 1978: 607.

23. Magistretti, P. J., L. Pellerin, D. L. Rothman and R. G. Shulman. Energy on demand. Science 1999;283: 496–7.

24. Prichard, J. W., D. L. Rothman, E. J. Novotny, O. A. C. Petroff, T. Kuwabara, M. Avison, A. Howseman, C. Hanstock and R. G. Shulman. Lactate rise detected by 1H NMR in human visual cortex during physiologic stimulation. Proc. Natl. Acad. Sci. USA 1991;88: 5829–5831.

25. Buxton, R. B. and L. R. Frank. A model for the coupling between cerebral blood flow and oxygen metabolism during neural stimulation. J. Cereb. Blood Flow Metab. 1997;17: 64–72.

26. Iadecola, C. Regulation of the cerebral microcirculation during neural activity: Is nitric oxide the missing link? Trends Neurosci 1993;16: 206–214.

27. Paulson, O. B. and E. A. Newman. Does the release of potassium from astrocyte endfeet regulate cerebral blood flow? Science 1987;237: 896–898.

28. Caesar, K., N. Akgoren, C. Mathiesen and M. Lauritzen. Modification of activity-dependent increases in cerebellar blood flow by extracellular potassium in anaesthetized rats. J Physiol (Lond) 1999;520 Pt 1: 281–92.

29. Phillis, J. W. Adenosine in the control of the cerebral circulation. Cerebrovasc Brain Metab Rev 1989;1: 26–54.

30. Ko, K. R., A. C. Ngai and R. H. Winn. Role of adenosine in regulation of regional cerebral blood flow in sensory cortex. Am J. Physiol 1990;259: H1703-H1708.

31. Li, J. and C. Iadecola. Nitric oxide and adenosine mediate vasodilation during functional activation in cerebellar cortex. Neuropharmacology 1994;33: 1453–1461.

32. Yaksh, T. L., J.-Y. Wang, V. L. G. Go and G. J. Harty. Cortical vasodilatation produced by vasoactive intestinal polypeptide (VIP) and by physiological stimuli in the cat. J. Cereb. Blood Flow Metab. 1987;7: 315–326.

33. Hartman, B., D. Zide and S. Udenfriend. The use of dopamine-betahydroxylase as a marker for the central noradrenergic nervous system in rat brain. Proc. Natl. Acad. Sci. USA 1972;69: 2722–2726.

34. Harder, D. R., R. J. Roman and D. Gebremedhin. Molecular mechanisms controlling nutritive blood flow: role of cytochrome P450 enzymes. Acta Physiol Scand 2000;168: 543–9.
35. Bredt, D. and S. A. Snyder. Nitric oxide: a physiologic messenger molecule. Annu Rev Biochem 1994;63: 175–195.
36. Garthwaite, J. and C. L. Boulton. Nitric oxide signaling in the central nervous system. Ann Rev Physiol 1995;57: 683–706.
37. Garthwaite, J., S. L. Charles and R. Chess-Williams. Endothelium-derived relaxing factor release on activation of NMDA receptors suggests role as intercellular messenger in the brain. Nature 1988;336: 385–388.
38. Gally, J. A., P. R. Montague, G. N. J. Reeke and G. M. Edelman. The NO hypothesis: possible effects of a short-lived, rapidly diffusible signal in the development and function of the nervous system. Proc Natl Acad Sci U S A 1990;87: 3547–51.
39. Northington, F. J., G. P. Matherne and R. M. Berne. Competitive inhibition of nitric oxide synthase prevents the cortical hyperemia associated with peripheral nerve stimulation. Proc. Natl. Acad. Sci. USA 1992;89: 6649–6652.
40. Dirnagl, U., U. Lindauer and A. Villringer. Role of nitric oxide in the coupling of cerebral blood flow to neural activation in rats. Neurosci. Lett. 1993;149: 43–46.
41. Iadecola, C., J. Li, T. J. Ebner and S. Xu. Nitric oxide contributes to functional hyperemia in cerebellar cortex. Am. J. Physiol. 1995;268 (Regulatory Integrative Comp. Physiol. 37): R1153-R1162.
42. Ngai, A. C., J. R. Meno and H. R. Winn. L-NNA suppresses cerebrovascular response and evoked potentials during somatosensory stimulation in rats. Am J Physiol 1995;H1803–10.
43. Iadecola, C. The role of NO in cerebrovascular regulation and stroke. In: Mathie, R. T. and Griffith, T. M., ed. London: Imperial College Press; 1999: 202–225.
44. Faraci, F. M. and K. R. Breese. Nitric oxide mediates vasodilation in response to activation of N-methyl-D-aspartate receptors in brain. Circ. Res. 1993;72: 476–480.
45. Yang, G. and C. Iadecola. Glutamate microinjections in cerebellar cortex reproduce cerebral vascular effects of parallel fiber stimulation. Am. J. Physiol. 1996;271 (Regulatory Integrative Comp. Physiol. 40): R1568-R1575.
46. Adachi, K., S. Takahashi, P. Melzer, K. L. Campos, T. Nelson, C. Kennedy and L. Sokoloff. Increases in local cerebral blood flow associated with somatosensory activation are not mediated by NO. Am J Physiol 1994;H2155–62.
47. Wang, Q., T. Kjaer, M. B. Jorgensen, O. B. Paulson, N. A. Lassen, N. H. Diemer and H. C. Lou. Nitric oxide does not act as a mediator coupling cerebral blood flow to neural activity following somatosensory stimuli in rats. Neurol Res 1993;15: 33–36.
48. Lindauer, U., D. Megow, H. Matsuda and U. Dirnagl. Nitric oxide: a modulator, but not a mediator, of neurovascular coupling in rat somatosensory cortex. Am J Physiol 1999;277: H799-H811.
49. Ma, J., C. Ayata, P. L. Huang, M. C. Fishman and M. A. Moskowitz. Regional cerebral blood flow response to vibrissal stimulation in mice lacking type I NOS gene expression. Am J Physiol 1996;270 (Heart Circ Physiol 39): H1085–90.
50. Iadecola, C., J. Li, G. Yang and S. Xu. Neural mechanisms of blood flow regulation during synaptic activity in cerebellar cortex. J. Neurophysiol. 1996;75: 940–950.
51. Akgören, N., M. Fabricius and M. Lauritzen. Importance of nitric oxide for local increases of blood flow in rat cerebellar cortex during electrical stimulation. Proc. Natl. Acad. Sci. USA 1994;91: 5903–5907.
52. Yang, G. and C. Iadecola. Obligatory role of NO in glutamate-dependent hyperemia evoked from cerebellar parallel fibers. Am. J. Physiol 1997;272 (Regulatory Integrative Comp. Physiol. 41): R1155-R1161.
53. Yang, G., G. Chen, T. J. Ebner and C. Iadecola. Nitric oxide is the predominant mediator of cerebellar hyperemia during somatosensory activation in rat. Am. J. Physiol. 1999;277 (Regulatory Integrative Comp. Physiol. 46): R1760-R1770.
54. Vane, J. R., Y. S. Bakhle and R. M. Botting. Cyclooxygenases 1 and 2. Annu Rev Pharmacol Toxicol 1998;38: 97–120.

55. Kaufmann, W. E., P. F. Worley, J. Pegg, M. Bremer and P. Isakson. COX-2, a synaptically induced enzyme, is expressed by excitatory neurons at postsynaptic sites in rat cerebral cortex. Proc Natl Acad Sci U S A 1996;93: 2317–21.
56. Yamagata, K., K. I. Andreasson, W. E. Kaufmann, C. A. Barnes and P. F. Worley. Expression of a mitogen-inducible cyclooxygenase in brain neurons: regulation by synaptic activity and glucocorticoids. Neuron 1993;11: 371–86.
57. Woolsey, T. A. and C. M. Rovainen. Wisker barrels: A model for direct observation of changes in the cerebral microcirculation with neural activity. In: Lassen, N. A., Ingvar, D. H. and Raichle, M. E., ed. Brain Work and Mental Activity. Copenhagen: Munksgaard; 1991: 189–200.
58. Niwa, K., E. Araki, S. G. Morham, M. E. Ross and C. Iadecola. Cyclooxygenase-2 Contributes to Functional Hyperemia in Whisker-Barrel Cortex. J Neurosci 2000;20: 763–770.
59. Ellis, E. F., E. P. Wei and H. A. Kontos. Vasodilation of cat cerebral arterioles by prostaglandins D2, E2, G2, and I2. Am J Physiol 1979;237: H381–5.
60. Wei, E. P., H. A. Kontos and J. S. Beckman. Mechanisms of cerebral vasodilation by superoxide, hydrogen peroxide, and peroxynitrite. Am J Physiol 1996;271: H1262–6.
61. Iadecola, C., G. Yang, T. Ebner and G. Cheng. Local and propagated vascular responses evoked by focal synaptic activity in cerebellar cortex. J. Neurophysiol. 1997;78: 651–659.
62. Ngai, A. C., K. R. Ko, S. Morii and H. R. Winn. Effect of sciatic nerve stimulation on pial arterioles in rats. Am. J Physiol 1988;254: H133-H139.
63. Duling, B. R. and R. M. Berne. Propagated vasodilation in the microcirculation of the hamster cheek pouch. Circ. Res. 1970;26: 163–170.
64. Segal, S. S. and B. R. Duling. Flow control among microvessels coordinated by intercellular conduction. Science 1986;234: 868–870.
65. Fujii, K., F. Faraci and D. D. Heistad. Flow-mediated vasodilation of the basilar artery in vivo. Circ. Res. 1991;69: 697–705.
66. Gaw, A. J. and J. A. Bevan. Flow-induced relaxation of the rabbit middle cerebral artery is composed of both endothelium-dependent and -independent componenets. Stroke 1993;24: 105–110.
67. Dietrich, H. H., T. Kajita and R. G. Dacey. Local and conducted vasomotor responses in isolated rat cerebral arterioles. Am . J. Physiol. 1996;271 (Heart Circ. Physiology 40): H1109-H1116.
68. Segal, S. S. Communication among endothelial and smooth muscle cells coordinates blood flow control during exercise. News Physiol. Sci. 1992;7: 152–156.
69. Iadecola, C. Neurogenic control of the cerebral microcirculation: Is dopamine minding the store? Nature Neurosci 1998;1: 263–265.
70. Iadecola, C. Intrinsic and extrinsic neural regulation of the cerebral circulation. In: Schmiedek, P., Einhäupl, K. and Kirsch, C.-M., ed. Stimulated Cerebral Blood Flow. Heidelberg: Springer-Verlag; 1992: 19–36.

Role of Endothelium in Regulation of the Brain Microcirculation

F.M. Faraci

Introduction

Endothelium is a major regulator of vascular tone. The primary mechanism by which endothelium regulates tone of underlying vascular muscle under normal conditions is by the release endothelium-derived relaxing factor(s) (EDRFs). These factors include nitric oxide, endothelium-derived hyperpolarizing factor(s) and prostacyclin [19, 69]. Although there are a few exceptions [see 19 and 20 for detailed reviews, 79], the vast majority of available evidence suggests that under normal conditions, nitric oxide is the predominant EDRF in both large arteries and microvessels of the cerebral circulation. For this reason, the present review will focus on the functional importance of endothelium-derived nitric oxide in regulation of cerebral vascular tone. In addition, mechanisms of nitric oxide mediated signaling, the interaction of nitric oxide and superoxide, and examples of changes in the functional importance of endothelium-derived nitric oxide in disease states will be summarized.

Nitric Oxide Synthase Is Expressed in Cerebral Endothelium

Expression of the endothelial isoform of nitric oxide synthase (also known as eNOS or NOS III) is controlled by expression of a single gene [22]. Studies using genetically-altered mice have demonstrated that the promoter for the eNOS gene directs expression of eNOS to vascular endothelium in many regions including brain [1, 25]. Messenger RNA and protein for NO-synthase is present throughout cerebral endothelium [10, 56, 65 for examples, see 19 for a review]. Although there are now a few examples of changes in expression of eNOS protein in disease states [19], relatively little is known about mechanisms that regulate promoter activity and expression of eNOS in cerebral endothelium.

Influence of Nitric Oxide on Vascular Tone

Nitric oxide is a potent vasodilator that produces relaxation of both large cerebral arteries and cerebral arterioles (both in vitro and in vivo [6, 11, 33, 78]. Several lines of evidence suggest that expression and activity of NOS in endothelium is sufficient to influence tone in cerebral blood vessels under basal conditions [19]. Biochemical assays have shown that basal levels of cyclic GMP [cGMP, which is produced by soluble guanylate cyclase (sGC) in response to nitric oxide, see below] are much greater in cerebral arteries with endothelium than in vessels without endothelium [19]. Inhibitors of NOS decrease basal levels of cGMP, produce endothelium-dependent contraction of cerebral blood vessels [12, 16, 17, 19, 60], and decrease cerebral blood flow in several species including humans [19, 74]. Reductions in cerebral blood flow in response to inhibition of NOS are absent in mice which are deficient in expression of the gene for eNOS [4, 40, 41] suggesting that endothelium is the primary source of NO that influences basal tone in vivo.

Lee was the first to demonstrate endothelium-dependent relaxation in cerebral blood vessels using acetylcholine [38]. It is now known that many receptor mediated agonists and shear stress are known to produces endothelium-dependent relaxation of cerebral blood vessels [15, 19]. A summary of endothelium-dependent agonists (of which acetylcholine is the most studied) that produce predominantly nitric oxide-mediated relaxation of cerebral microvessels is presented in Table 1. Although such data was first obtained in experimental animals [16, 17, 60], more recent studies have described the same mechanism in human cerebral vessels. For example, relaxation of human cerebral arterioles in response to acetylcholine is completely inhibited by N^G-nitro-L-arginine (L-NNA), an inhibitor of NOS [12]. In addition to these findings obtained on individual vascular segments (Table 1), several studies have shown that increases in cerebral blood flow in response to acetylcholine are mediated very predominantly by nitric oxide [28, 49, 77].

Although nitric oxide appears to be the major EDRF in the cerebral circulation, an EDHF may be functionally important in mediating endothelium-dependent responses to some stimuli. For example, Bryan et al. have suggested that relax-

Table 1. Endothelium-dependent agonists that produce predominantly nitric oxide mediated relaxation of cerebral microvessels

Agonist/stimulus	Species	Blood vessel	References
Acetylcholine	Rat	Pial arterioles	16, 34, 35, 45, 50, 55, 56
	Mouse	Pial arterioles	60, 63
	Rabbit	Pial arterioles	8, 13, 18
	Human	Parenchymal arterioles	12
	Rat	Parenchymal arterioles	50
	Juvenile pig	Pial arterioles	2
	Cat	Pial arterioles	3, 72
ADP	Rat	Pial arterioles	34, 42, 55
	Cat	Pial arterioles	3
ATP	Rat	Parenchymal arterioles	31
Substance P	Newborn pig	Pial arterioles	7, 75
	Mouse	Pial arterioles	61
	Rat	Pial arterioles	37
Intraluminal flow	Rat	Parenchymal arterioles	50

ation of cerebral vessels in responses to purines in vitro may be mediated by both nitric oxide and an EDHF [79]. In cerebral arterioles of the mouse in vivo, dilatation to acetylcholine is essentiallly abolished by L-NNA while a large component of the response to ADP is L-NNA-insensitive [Faraci, unpublished observations], consistent with the possibility that ADP may cause release of EDHF in the cerebral microcirculation.

Nitric Oxide-Mediated Signaling in Cerebral Blood Vessels

Nitric oxide can potentially produce relaxation of vascular muscle by sGC-dependent or sGC-independent mechanisms (Fig. 1). sGC has a high affinity for nitric oxide, and when active, converts guanosine-5'-triphoshate (GTP) to cGMP. Nitric oxide (and nitric oxide-donors) produce marked increases in cGMP and relaxation of cerebral blood vessels [6, 11, 33, 51, 78]. Recent studies using a selective inhibitor of sGC indicate that relaxation of both large cerebral arteries and cerebral microvessels in response to exogenously applied and endogenously produced nitric oxide is mediated very predominantly be sGC [21, 39, 44, 51, 57, 63, 64, 76]. Similar results were obtained in a very recent study using cerebral arteries from non-human primates [11].

   Potassium channels play a major role in regulation of cerebral vascular tone by mediating cerebral vasodilatation in response to diverse stimuli including receptor mediated agonists, second messengers and calcium sparks [20, 30, 48]. Potassium channels may contribute to mechanisms that produce relaxation of cerebral vessels in response to nitric oxide. Electrophysiological studies suggest that nitric oxide and cGMP increase activity of calcium-activated potassium channels and

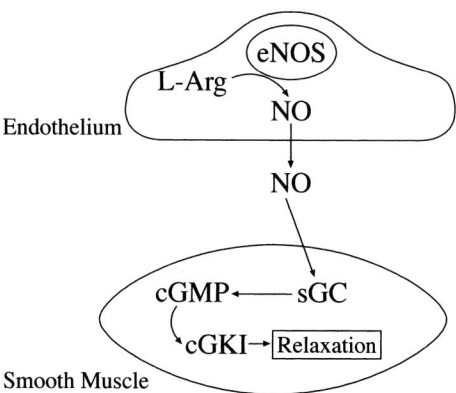

Fig. 1. Schematic representation of the major mechanism of endothelium-dependent relaxation of vascular muscle in cerebral arterioles. Nitric oxide (NO) is produced by the endothelial isoform of NO-synthase (eNOS) from the amino acid L-arginine (L-Arg). NO diffuses to vascular muscle where it activates soluble guanylate cyclase (sGC), causing increased production of cyclic GMP (cGMP) and activation of cGMP-dependent protein kinase I

produce hyperpolarization of cerebral vascular muscle [20]. In addition, membrane hyperpolarization and vasorelaxation in response to nitric oxide or cGMP can be attenuated by inhibitors of potassium channels (inhibitors of calcium-activated potassium channels in most studies) consistent with a role for potassium channels in nitric oxide-mediated responses [20, 54].

Interaction of Nitric Oxide and Superoxide

The bioactivity of nitric oxide depends, in part, on its interaction with the reactive oxygen species superoxide anion. Although there has been considerable effort to define the role of nitric oxide in regulation of cerebral vascular tone [19], the role of vascular superoxide in brain is poorly understood. Pharmacological agents that spontaneously generate superoxide (pyrogallol) or result in generation of superoxide by mechanisms such as auto-oxidation (tetrahydrobiopterin, ß-amyloid) impairs relaxation of cerebral blood vessels in response to endothelium-dependent stimuli [23, 58, 68]. In addition to preventing the activation of sGC by nitric oxide, the reaction of nitric oxide with superoxide results in the formation of peroxynitrite (Fig. 2), a potent oxidant which has the potential to produce cytotoxicity [5].

There are several potential sources of superoxide in blood vessels and all major components of the vessel wall have the potential to produce superoxide [24]. These sources include NAD(P)H oxidase, xanthine oxidase, cyclooxygenase and potentially nitric oxide synthases (Fig. 2). Local steady-state levels of superoxide are dependent on both the rate of production of superoxide as well as activity of endogenous superoxide dismutase(s) (SOD; Fig. 2). Nitric oxide reacts with superoxide at a rate three times faster than the dismutation of superoxide by SOD [5, 9]. Because of the efficiency of this reaction, the local concentration of SOD is likely to be an important determinant of activity (the biological half-life) of nitric oxide (Fig. 2).

There are three main isoforms of SOD (Mn-SOD, Cu/Zn-SOD, and extracellular (EC) SOD. Within blood vessels, the predominant isoforms of SOD are Cu/Zn-

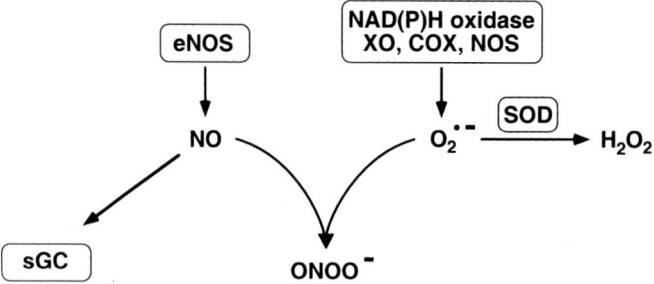

Fig. 2. Schematic representation of the interaction of nitric oxide (NO) and superoxide (O_2^-). NO is produced by eNOS. NO can then normally activate soluble guanylate cyclase (sGC) resulting in vasorelaxation. NO can also rapidly react with superoxide to form peroxynitrite (ONOO$^-$). Superoxide can be formed within blood vessels by several sources including NAD(P)H oxidase, cyclooxygease (COX), xanthine oxidase (XO) and perhaps NOS. Superoxide is dismuted by superoxide dismutase (SOD) to hydrogen peroxide (H_2O_2)

SOD and EC-SOD [52, 53, 66]. Although some evidence has suggested that Mn-SOD levels are higher in intracranial than in extracranial arteries [46], relatively little is known regarding the role of endogenous SOD in protecting nitric oxide mediated responses in the cerebral circulation. In recent studies using an inhibitor of CuZn SOD, we and others have provided evidence that endogenous SOD plays an important role in protecting endothelium-dependent responses in the basilar artery in vitro [71] and in the cerebral microcirculation in vivo [Didion & Faraci, unpublished observations].

Although expression and activity of SODs is a key determinant of local levels of superoxide, very little is known as to whether the functional importance of endogenous vascular SODs changes in disease states. A recent report suggested that activity of SOD in the basilar artery is markedly reduced during subarachnoid hemorrhage [67]. It was suggested that such reduction in the antioxidant capacity within the vessel wall may contribute to vasospasm following subarachnoid hemorrhage.

Pathophysiology Related to Superoxide and Nitric Oxide

Several lines of evidence support the concept that normal endothelial function is protective for the circulation including in the brain. In addition to producing vasodilatation, endothelium inhibits adherence of leukocytes and aggregation of platelets [19]. Several lines of evidence, including the use of mice which are deficient in expression of the gene for eNOS, suggest that nitric oxide produced by endothelium plays a protective role during and/or following cerebral ischemia [19, 27]. Endothelial dysfunction is known to occur in brain, under several pathophysiological conditions including acute and chronic hypertension, subarachnoid hemorrhage, ischemia, traumatic brain injury, and diabetes [19]. Outside of the brain, such endothelial dysfunction correlates with risk factors for vascular disease and is associated with clinical events [64]. A genetic analysis has demonstrated cosegregation of impaired endothelium-dependent relaxation with a stroke-prone phenotype [70].

As discussed above, superoxide (and potentially other reactive oxygen species) are known to inhibit nitric oxide mediated vascular responses. This concept was first demonstrated in studies performed by Kontos and Wei which provided evidence that superoxide inactivates nitric oxide (EDRF) in vivo [72]. Since that initial finding, other studies have suggested that inactivation of nitric oxide by superoxide contributes to impaired nitric oxide-mediated dilatation of cerebral blood vessels under several pathophysiological conditions. For example, impaired endothelium-dependent relaxation in animal models of traumatic brain injury, ischemia, diabetes, inflammation, and Alzheimer's disease can be improved with SOD alone or the combination of SOD and catalase [14, 26, 29, 43, 47]. Proinflammatory stimuli are also known to impair endothelial function and recent evidence obtained in genetically altered mice suggest that interleukin-10 (an antiinflammatory cytokine) limits increases in superoxide and endothelial dysfunction during inflammation [26]. Because ischemia, Alzheimer's disease, carotid artery disease, and diabetes all have an inflammatory component, these findings have potentially broad implications for regulation of local levels of superoxide and endothelial function. Thus, inactivation of nitric oxide by superoxide contributes to endothelial dysfunction in several disease states. The role of superoxide in vascular dysfunction may extend beyond its interaction with nitric oxide at the level of endothelium. For example, mice which overexpress CuZn-SOD are protected from vasospasm following experimental subarchnoid hemorrhage [32].

In summary, nitric oxide is the major EDRF in brain and mediates responses of cerebral microvessels to a variety of stimuli. The interaction of nitric oxide with superoxide is a key determinant of the biological half-life of nitric oxide. Nitric oxide mediated signalling in cerebral blood vessels can by impaired in several pathophysiological conditions that are associated with increased local levels of superoxide.

Acknowledgements. Studies described in this review were supported by NIH grants HL-38901, NS-24621 and HL-62984. The author thanks Dr. Christopher G. Sobey for critical evaluation of the manuscript.

References

1. Anouk-Martine T, TL Miller, SC Tai, Y Wang, X Bei, GB Robb, MJ Phillips and PA Marsden. In vivo expression profile of an endothelial nitric oxide synthase promoter-reporter transgene. Am J Physiol 278:H1352-H1361, 2000.
2. Armstead WM, SL Zuckerman, M Shibata, H Parfenova, and CW Leffler. Different pial arteriolar to acetylcholine in the newborn and juvenile pig. J Cerebral Blood Flow Metabol 14:1088–1095, 1994.
3. Asano Y, RC Koehler, JA Ulatowski, RJ Traystman, and E Bucci. Effect of cross-linked hemoglobin transfusion on endothelial-dependent dilation in cat pial arterioles. Am J Physiol 275:H1313-H1321, 1998.
4. Ayata C, J Ma, W Meng, P Huang, and MA Moskowitz. L-NA-sensitive rCBF augmentation during vibrissal stimulation in type III nitric oxide synthase mutant mice. J Cerebral Blood Flow Metabol 16:539–541, 1996.
5. Beckman JS, and WH Koppenol. Nitric oxide, superoxide, and peroxynitrite: the good, the bad, and the ugly. Am J Physiol 271:C1424-C1437, 1996.
6. Brian JE, DD Heistad, and FM Faraci. Effect of carbon monoxide on rabbit cerebral arteries. Stroke 25:639–644, 1994.
7. Busija DW and J Chen. Effects of trigeminal neurotransmitters on piglet pial arterioles. J Develop Physiol 18:67–72, 1992.
8. Colonna DM, W Meng, DD Deal, and DW Busija. Nitric oxide promotes arteriolar dilation during cortical spreading depression in rabbits. Stroke 25:2463–2470, 1994.
9. Darley-Usmar V, H Wiseman, and B Halliwell. Nitric oxide and oxygen radicals: a question of balance. FEBS Letters 369:131–135, 1995.
10. Demas GE, LJ Kriegsfeld, S Blackshaw, P Huang, SC Gammie, RJ Nelson, and SH Synder. Elimination of aggresive behavior in male mice lacking endothelial nitric oxide synthase. J Neurosci 19:RC30(1–5), 1999.
11. Didion SP, DD Heistad, and FM Faraci. Mechanisms tuct produce nitric oxide – Mediatec relaxation of cerebral arteries during atherosclerosis. Stroke 32:761–766, 2001.
12. Elhusseiny A, and E Hamel. Muscarinic – but not nicotinic – acetylcholine receptors mediate a nitric oxide-dependent dilation in brain cortical arterioles: A possible role for the M5 receptor subtype. J Cerebral Blood Flow Metabol 20:298–305, 2000.
13. Ellis, EF, SF Moore, and KA Willoughby. Anandamide and delta 9-THC dilation of cerebral arterioles is blocked by indomethacin. Am J Physiol 269:H1859-H1864.1995.

14. Ellison MD, DE Erb, HA Kontos, and JT Povlishock. Recovery of impaired endothelium-dependent relaxation after fluid-percussion brain injury in cats. Stroke 20:911–917, 1989.

15. Faraci FM. Regulation of the cerebral circulation by endothelium. Pharmacol Ther 56:1–22, 1992.

16. Faraci, FM. 1991. Role of endothelium-derived relaxing factor in cerebral circulation: large arteries vs. microcirculation. Am J Physiol 261:H1038-H1042.

17. Faraci FM. Role of nitric oxide in regulation of basilar artery tone in vivo. Am J Physiol 259:H1216-H1221, 1990.

18. Faraci FM, KR Breese, and DD Heistad. Nitric oxide contributes to dilatation of cerebral arterioles during seizures. Am J Physiol 265:H2209-H2212, 1993.

19. Faraci FM, DD Heistad. Regulation of the cerebral circulation: Role of endothelium and potassium channels. Physiological Reviews 78:53–97, 1998.

20. Faraci FM and CG Sobey. Role of potassium channels in regulation of cerebral vascular tone. J Cerebral Blood Flow Metab 18:1047–1063, 1998.

21. Faraci FM and CG Sobey. Role of soluble guanylate cyclase in dilator responses of the cerebral microcirculation. Brain Res 821:368–373, 1999.

22. Forstermann U, and H Kleinert. Nitric oxide synthase: expression and expressional control of the three isoforms. Naunyn-Schmied Archiv Pharmacol 352:351–364, 1995.

23. Girard P, R Sercombe, C Sercombe, G LeLem, J Seylaz, P Potier. A new synthetic flavonoid protects endothelium-derived relaxing factor-induced relaxation in rabbit arteries in vitro: evidence for superoxide scavenging. Biochem Pharmacol 49:1533–1539, 1995.

24. Griendling KK, D Sorescu D. M Ushio-Fukai. NAD(P)H oxidase: Role in cardiovascular biology and disease. Circ Res 86:494–501, 2000.

25. Guillot PV, J Guan, L Lui, JA Kuivenhoven, RD Rosenberg, WC Sessa WC, WC Aird. A vascular bed-specific pathway regulates cardiac expression of endothelial nitric oxide synthase. J Clin Invest 103:799–805, 1999.

26. Gunnett CA, DD Heistad, DJ Berg, and FM Faraci. Interleukin-10 (IL-10) deficiency increases superoxide and endothelial dysfunction following lipopolysaccharide: A protective role for IL-10 in inflammation. Am J Physiol (In press).

27. Huang Z, PL Huang, J Ma, W Meng, C Ayata, MC Fishman, and MA Moskowitz.Enlarged infarcts in endothelial nitric oxide synthase knockout mice are attenuated by nitro-L-arginine. J Cerebral Blood Flow Metab 16:981–987, 1996.

28. Iadecola C and F Zhang. Permissive and obligatory roles of NO in cerebrovascular responses to hypercapnia and acetylcholine. Am J Physiol 271:R990-R1001, 1996.

29. Iadecola C, F Zhang, K Niwa, C Eckman, SK Turner, E Fischer, S Younkin, DR Borchel, KK Hsiao, and GA Carlson. SOD1 rescues cerebral endothelial dysfunction in mice overexpressing amyloid precursor protein. Nature Neurosci 2:157–161, 1999.

30. Jaggar JH, VA Porter, WJ Lederer, and MT Nelson. Calcium sparks in smooth muscle. Am J Physiol 278:C235-C256.2000.

31. Janigro D, TS Nguyen, EL Gordon, and HR Winn. Physiological properties of ATP-activated cation channels in rat brain microvascular endothelial cells. Am J Physiol 270:H1423-H1434.1996.

32. Kamii H, I Kato, H Kinouchi, PH Chan, CJ Epstein, A Akabane, H Okamoto and Yoshimoto. Amelioration of vasospasm after subarachnoid hemorrhage in transgenic mice overexpressing CuZn-superoxide dismutase. Stroke 30:867–872, 1999.

33. Katusic ZS, JJ Marshall, HA Kontos, and PM Vanhoutte. Similar responsiveness of smooth muscle of the canine basilar artery to EDRF and nitric oxide. Am J Physiol 257:H1235-H1239, 1989.

34. Koenig HM, DA Pelligrino, and RF Albrecht. Halothane vasodilation and nitric oxide in rat pial vessels. J Neurosurg Anesthesiol 5:264–271, 1993.

35. Koenig HM, DA Pelligrino, Q Wang, and RF Albrecht. Role of nitric oxide and endothelium in rat pial vessel dilation response to isoflurane. Anesth Analg 79:886–891, 1994.

36. Kontos HA, and EP Wei. Endothelium-dependent responses after experimental brain injury. J Neurotrauma 9:349–354, 1992.

37. Lagaud GJL, PL Skarsgard, I Laher, and C Van Breemen. Heterogeneity of endothelium-dependent vasodilation in pressurized cerebral and small mesenteric resistance arteries of the rat. J Pharmacol Exp Ther 290:832–839, 1999.

38. Lee TJF. Direct evidence against acetylcholine as the dilator transmitter in the cat cerebral artery. Eur J Pharmacol 68:393–394, 1980

39. Lindauer U, D Megow, H Matsuda, and U Dirnagl. Nitric oxide: a modulator, but not a mediator, of neurovascular coupling in rat somatosensory cortex. Am J Physiol 277:H799-H811, 1999.

40. Ma J, C Ayata, PL Huang, MC Fishman, and MA Moskowitz. Regional cerebral blood flow response to vibrissal stimulation in mice lacking type I NOS gene expression. Am J Physiol 270:H1085-H1090, 1996.

41. Ma J, W Meng, C Ayata, PL Huang, MC Fishman, and MA Moskowitz. L-NNA-sensitive regional cerebral blood flow augmentation during hypercapnia in type III NOS mutant mice. Am J Physiol 271:H1717-H1719, 1996.

42. Mayhan WG. Endothelium-dependent responses of cerebral arterioles to adenosine 5'-diphosphate. J Vasc Res 29:353–358, 1992.

43. Mayhan WG. Superoxide dismutase partially restores impaired dilatation of the basilar artery during diabetes mellitus. Brain Research 760:204–209, 1997.

44. Mayhan WG. VEGF increases permeability of the blood-brain barrier via a nitric oxide synthase/cGMP-dependent pathway. Am J Physiol 276:C1148-C1153, 1999.

45. Mayhan WG, LK Simmons and GM Sharpe. Mechanism of impaired responses of cerebral arterioles during diabetes mellitus. Am J Physiol 260:H319-H326, 1991.

46. Napoli C, JL Witztum, F de Nigris, G Palumbo, FP D'Armiento, and W Palinski. Intracranial arteries of human fetuses are more resistant to hypercholesterolemia-induced fatty streak formation than extracranial arteries. Circulation 99:2003–2010, 1999.

47. Nelson CW, EP Wei, JT Povlishock, HA Kontos, and MA Moskowitz. Oxygen radicals in cerebral ischemia. Am J Physiol 263:H1356-H1362, 1992.

48. Nelson MT, and JM Quayle. Physiological roles and properties of potassium channels in arterial smooth muscle. Am J Physiol 268:C799-C822, 1995.

49. Ngai AC, JR Meno, and HR Winn. L-NNA suppresses cerebrovascular response and evoked potentials during somatosensory stimulation in rats. Am J Physiol 269:H1803-H1810, 1995.

50. Ngai AC, and HR Winn. Modulation of cerebral arteriolar diameter by intraluminal flow and pressure. Circ Res 77:832–840, 1995.

51. Onoue H, and ZS Katusic. The effect of 1H [1,2,4]oxadiazolo [4,3-a]quinoxalin-1-one (ODQ) and charybdotoxin on relaxations of isolated cerebral arteries to nitric oxide. Brain Res 785;107–113, 1998.

52. Oury TD, BJ Day, and JD Crapo. Extracellular superoxide dismutase: A regulator of nitric oxide bioavailability. Lab Invest 75:617–636, 1996.

53. Oury TD, BJ Day, and JD Crapo. Extracellular superoxide dismutase in vessels and airways of humans and baboons. Free Radical Biol Med 20:957–965, 1996.

54. Paterno R, FM Faraci, and DD Heistad. Role of Ca^{2+}-dependent K^+ channels in cerebral vasodilatation induced by increases in cyclic GMP and cyclic AMP in the rat. Stroke 27:1603–1608, 1996.

55. Pelligrino DA, Q Wang, HM Koenig, and R F Albrecht. Role of nitric oxide, adenosine, N-methyl-D-aspartate receptors, and neuronal activation in hypoxia-induced pial arteriolar dilation in rats. Brain Res 704:61–70, 1995.

56. Pelligrino, DA, S Ye, F Tan, RA Santizo, DL Feinstein and Q Wang. Nitric-oxide-dependent pial arteriolar dilation in the female rat: Effects of chronic estrogen depletion and repletion. Biochem Biophys Res Comm 269:165–171, 2000.

57. Petersson J, PM Zygmunt, P Jonsson, and ED Hogestatt. Characterization of endothelium-dependent relaxation in guinea pig basilar artery–effect of hypoxia and role of cytochrome P450 mono-oxygenase. J Vasc Res 35:285–294, 1998.

58. Price JM, ET Sutton, A Hellermann, T Thomas. ß-Amyloid induces cerebrovascular endothelial dysfunction in the rat brain. Neurol Res 19:534–538, 1997.

Production of Lactate and Reduction of pH:
The Role of Pre-ischemic Hyperglycemia and of Diabetes

Following complete cessation of CBF, the available stores of glycogen and glucose are rapidly metabolized to lactate. In the cerebral cortex of the normoglycemic rat, glycogen and glucose concentrations are about 3 and 2.5 $\mu mol \cdot g^{-1}$, respectively. When all glycogen and glucose have been used up, the lactate content increases from about 2 to about 13 $\mu mol \cdot g^{-1}$ (Ljunggren et al. 1974). However, the tissue glucose concentrations vary directly with the plasma glucose concentrations. This means that hypoglycemic animals show a reduced, and hyperglycemic ones an increased tissue lactate content during complete ischemia, with the amount of lactate formed corresponding to the pre-ischemic tissue glycogen and glucose concentrations (Ljunggren et al. 1974, Katsura et al. 1992). When a trickle of blood flow persists, additional substrate (glucose) is carried to the tissue; as a result, tissue lactate contents can rise to excessive values (Eklöf and Siesjö 1972).

It has been argued that the H^+ ions which are generated during metabolism are not formed in the lactate dehydrogenase reaction but during ATP hydrolysis, and the argument has led to the confusing statement that anaerobic production of H^+ is not the cause of the acidosis observed. As pointed out already by (Krebs et al. 1975, Alberti and Cuthbert 1982) lactate is formed from glucose according to the following two reactions:

$$\text{glucose} + 2\ HPO_4^{2-} + 2ADP^{3-} \rightarrow 2\ \text{lactate}^- + 2\ ATP^{4-} \tag{4}$$

$$\text{glucose} + 2\ H_2PO_4^- + 2ADP^{3-} \rightarrow 2\ \text{lactate}^- + 2ATP^{4-} + 2H^+ \tag{5}$$

We recognize that equation (5) but not equation (4) generates H^+. However, the ATP formed does not accumulate but is hydrolyzed according to the equations:

$$ATP^{4-} + 2H_2O \rightarrow ADP^{3-} + HPO_4^{2-} + H^+ \tag{6}$$

$$ATP^{4-} + 2H_2O \rightarrow ADP^{3-} + H_2PO_4^- \tag{7}$$

We note that equation (4) is coupled to equation (6), and equation (5) to equation (7). The net result is that whenever one mole of glucose is metabolized to two moles of lactate$^-$ at constant ATP concentration, two moles of H^+ are released (Hochachka and Mommsen 1983). Thus, production of lactate in ischemic tissue is synonymous with production of H^+. If, in addition, ATP and other nucleoside triphosphates are hydrolyzed, an additional amount of H^+ is released. This amount has been estimated to 3–5 $mM \cdot kg^{-1}$ (Katsura et al. 1992). The amount should be compared to that released by lactate formation in normoglycemic animals subjected to ischemia (10–12 $mM \cdot kg^{-1}$), or to that released in hyperglycemic animals (15–18 $mM \cdot kg^{-1}$).

It is thus understandable that when hyperglycemic animals are subjected to complete or incomplete ischemia, they show an enhanced decrease in intra- and extracellular pH (pH_i and pH_e, respectively) which persists during, and for some time after, the ischemia (Smith et al. 1986, Chopp et al. 1988). Animals rendered acutely hyperglycemic by glucose injection, or chronically by streptozotocin diabetes, show exaggerated brain damage after transient ischemia, and most of those subjected to acute hyperglycemia develop postischemic seizures (Myers and Yamaguchi 1977, Siemkowicz and Hansen 1978, Warner et al. 1987; for data on diabetic animals, see Li et al. 1998). It is tempting to conclude that the worsened outcome in these animals is due to the additional decrease in pH_i (or pH_e). In support of this contention are results showing that damage caused by transient ischemia is aggravated when acidosis is enhanced by superimposed, excessive hypercapnia in normoglycemic subjects (Katsura et al. 1994; for data on subjects with hypoglycemic coma, see Kristián et al. 1994); however, it remains unexplained why these animals did not develop postischemic seizures (Katsura et al. 1994). This issue, and that related to the fact that cells in culture show <u>decreased</u> damage when subjected to glutamate or to an anoxic transient under conditions of low pH (Tombaugh and Sapolsky 1993), are discussed in recent review articles (Kristián and Siesjö 1996, Siesjo et al. 1996, Li and Siesjö 1997). The in vitro argument does not detract from the general usefulness of the concept that excessive acidosis wrecks the machinery.

Function and Dysfunction of Mitochondria

The primary function of mitochondria is to generate energy in the form of ATP. This is accomplished by the stepwise oxidation of pyruvate and other substrates to CO_2 and water. In this process, electrons are passed down a series of respiratory carriers ("complexes") to be finally accepted by O_2. At three steps, H^+ is extruded across the inner mitochondrial membrane. The large electrochemical potential for H^+, thus created, is dissipated when H^+ flows back into the mitochondrial matrix via an ATPase, generating ATP (Mitchell 1966). This process thus depends on the provision of substrate (such as pyruvate) and of electron acceptor (O_2), on the proper functioning of the respiratory complexes (I – V, where V is the ATPase), and on a low unspecific permeability of the inner mitochondrial membrane to H^+.

In ischemia (or hypoxia) the primary problem is that the provision of electron acceptor (O_2) is dwindling. This is a transient problem, though, if oxygen is re-supplied by reperfusion. Nonetheless, reperfusion may not adequately restore mitochondrial functions. One reason for this could be that the ischemia-reperfusion transition has caused oxidative damage to the lipid backbone of the mito-chondrial membranes, or to the respiratory complexes. Although this is a traditional way of explaining postischemic mitochondrial dysfunction, it is now realized that the reason could be the assembly of a mitochondrial permeability transition (MPT) pore i.e. a Ca^{2+}-triggered and voltage-sensitive inner mitochondrial membrane channel which is indiscriminately permeable to solutes with a molecular mass <1500 Daltons (Zoratti and Szabó 1995, Bernardi et al. 1999). An MPT is assumed to be assembled under special conditions such as redox stress or mitochondrial calcium overload. This suggests that should such stress, or calcium overload, be present after an ischemic transient, an MPT pore could be assembled, leading to secondary mitochondrial dysfunction.

The role of an MPT in causing reperfusion damage in heart and liver tissue has been discussed by several authors (Halestrap et al. 1998, Lemasters et al. 1998). The importance of an MPT is underscored by results demonstrating a coupling between the accompanying depolarization and the mitochondrial release of an apoptosis-inducing factor (AIF) and of cytochrome c (cyt c). Both of these factors have the potential to induce cell death. The pathway has been best worked out for cyt c, which is known to activate caspase-9, which in turn activates caspase-3, a serine-threonine protease that has been called the executioner of cell death since it activates a series of enzymes, causing breakdown of DNA, fodrin, and poly (ADP-ribose) polymerase (PARP) (MacManus and Linnik 1997, Reed 1997, Green and Reed 1998, Susin et al. 1999).

The assembly of an MPT pore probably also contributes to reperfusion damage in the brain. Indirect evidence supporting this notion was obtained when it was found that the immunosuppressant cyclosporin A (CsA), when given in such a way that the low permeability to CsA across the BBB was bypassed, dramatically decreased the neuronal necrosis in the CA1 sector and other areas in the brain (Uchino et al. 1995, Uchino et al. 1998), and aborted postischemic seizures in hyperglycemic animals (Li et al. 1997). CsA proved effective when given 30 min after the start of reperfusion (Uchino et al. 1998), but not when given after 2 h (Friberg et al. 2000), suggesting that a CsA-sensitive MPT is not likely to operate many hours or days after the ischemia, i.e. at the time when the delayed damage becomes manifest.

The importance of this apoptotic program is underscored by the anti-ischemic effects of caspase-3 inhibitors (see below). However, there are several caveats in the data. First, release of ATP and of cyt c is believed to trigger not only programmed cell death ("apoptosis") but also a cascade of events leading to necrosis. The occurrence of these parallel pathways is shown in Fig. 3, which also suggests that apoptotic cells can be transformed into necrotic ones. We also recall that AIF can act on both nuclear and mitochondrial membranes, causing internal damage without the involvement of caspase activation (Susin et al. 1998, 1999).

Another caveat is that cyt c can be released in the absence of inner membrane depolarization, i.e. in the absence of an MPT (Andreyev and Fiskum 1999). Since cyt c resides in the space between the outer and inner mitochondrial membranes, once dislocated from its binding sites cyt c can cross a leaky outer membrane or one in which pores have been formed (Green and Reed 1998). Clearly, although mitochondrial dysfunction is a likely trigger of cell death, the detailed mechanisms have not been worked out yet. What seems likely is that mitochondrial dysfunction and membrane instability are important factors in the pathogenesis of cell death. It is also clear that the Bcl-2 family of proteins tend to stabilize (Bcl-2, Bcl-X_L) or destabilize (Bax, Bic, Bad) the membranes (see Fig. 3).

Immediate and Delayed Events in the Triggering of Ischemic Brain Damage

All of the events discussed, i.e. bioenergetic failure, release of glutamate, loss of ion homeostasis (with uncontrolled influx of calcium into cells) and acidosis, qualify as triggering events that can contribute to the final damage incurred. However, it must be explained how these triggering events can give rise to damage that is delayed by hours and days. In order to discuss the causes of this delay,

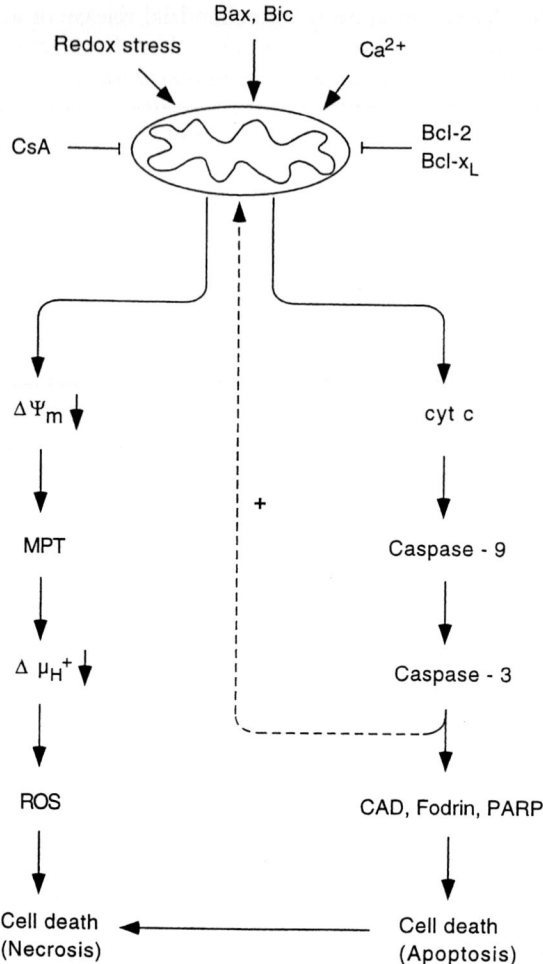

Fig. 3. This schematic diagram, modified from Green and Reed (1998), illustrates how mitochondria can trigger necrotic and apoptotic cell death. We envisage that the cell death trigger is a decrease in $\Delta\psi_m$, which is promoted by mitochondrial calcium accumulation or oxidative stress and counteracted by cyclosporin A (CsA) and the anti-apoptotic members of the Bcl-2 gene family. A sustained mitochondrial permeability transition (MPT) is apt to cause large amplitude mitochondrial swelling with outer membrane rupture, leading to massive release of mitochondrial proteins (and of glutathione). The immediate result is collapse of the $\Delta\mu_{H+}$, uncoupling of phosphorylation, a spurt of production of reactive oxygen species (ROS) and cessation of ATP production, while the ultimate result is cell necrosis. The right-lower part of the figure shows that apoptotic cell death, triggered by release of cytochrome c and other apoptotic factors, involves a series of events that involve Apaf-1 and activation of caspases, including caspase-3, the "executioner" of cell death

it seems justified to consider two major types of ischemia, viz. forebrain ischemia of brief duration, and focal ischemia of long duration. In the former, the transient period of ischemia is followed by a long maturation period during which cells resume some basic metabolic and electrical functions, and in which light microscopic signs of cell death are absent. In the latter, the ischemic insult is so severe (or prolonged) that the maturation period is brief; indeed the initial recovery of mitochondrial functions may be incomplete.

Forebrain Ischemia

Forebrain ischemia is usually dense, indicating that the bioenergetic failure and the loss of ion homeostasis are rapidly setting in. Presynaptic release of glutamate, activation of glutamate receptors, depolarization, and massive influx of calcium act as triggers of a host of reactions leading to cell death (for literature, see Siesjö 1991, Siesjö 1992). As Fig. 4 shows, such reactions encompass (a) lipolysis, secondary to calcium activation of PLA_2 and to transmitter activation of metabotropic glutamate receptors, with an ensuing production of IP_3 and IP_3-triggered release of Ca^{2+} from endoplasmic reticulum (REA) and other internal stores, (b) massive changes in the phosphorylation of proteins, reflecting the Ca^{2+} sensitivity of many kinases and phosphatases, (c) activation of enzymes, some of which are sensitive to calcium, others to the calcium-calmodulin complex: one such enzyme is constitutive NOS, and another one the serine-threonine phosphatase calcineurin, (d) Ca^{2+}-dependent DNA fragmentation, (e) dissolution of the cytoskeleton by Ca^{2+}-activated calpains, and by disassembly of microtubuli.

Many of the reactions elicited by a ischemic transient secondarily produce bioactive or toxic products. The production of some of these require reperfusion, i.e. the return of oxygen. For example, the AA accumulated will be converted to cyclo-oxygenase and lipoxygenase products which encompass chemotactic molecules and other compounds that trigger an inflammatory response. The cyclo-oxygenase enzyme is a known source of ROS, notable $\cdot O_2^-$. Additional sources of $\cdot O_2^-$ are the xanthine oxidase reaction, and the mitochondria themselves. There is thus an abundant source of $\cdot O_2^-$ (and H_2O_2) around. This is of pathogenetic importance since Ca^{2+}-calmodulin activation of NOS produces NO which reacts with $\cdot O_2^-$ to yield peroxynitrite according to the following reactions:

$$\cdot O_2^- + NO^\cdot \rightarrow ONOO^- + H^+ \rightarrow ONOOH \tag{7}$$

$$ONOOH \rightarrow \cdot OH + NO_2^\cdot \tag{8}$$

In general, reactions that give rise to ROS, whether they emanate from the cyclo-oxygenase reaction, the xanthine oxidase reaction, or from the mitochondria, require oxygen to produce the post-ischemic burst of free radical production (Carney and Floyd 1991, Piatandosi and Zhang 1996), thus representing typical reperfusion events.

It is possible, therefore, to identify a series of triggering events during ischemia, and in the immediate reperfusion period, which gives rise to brain damage. Such damage is likely due to involve breakdown of DNA, as well as of the

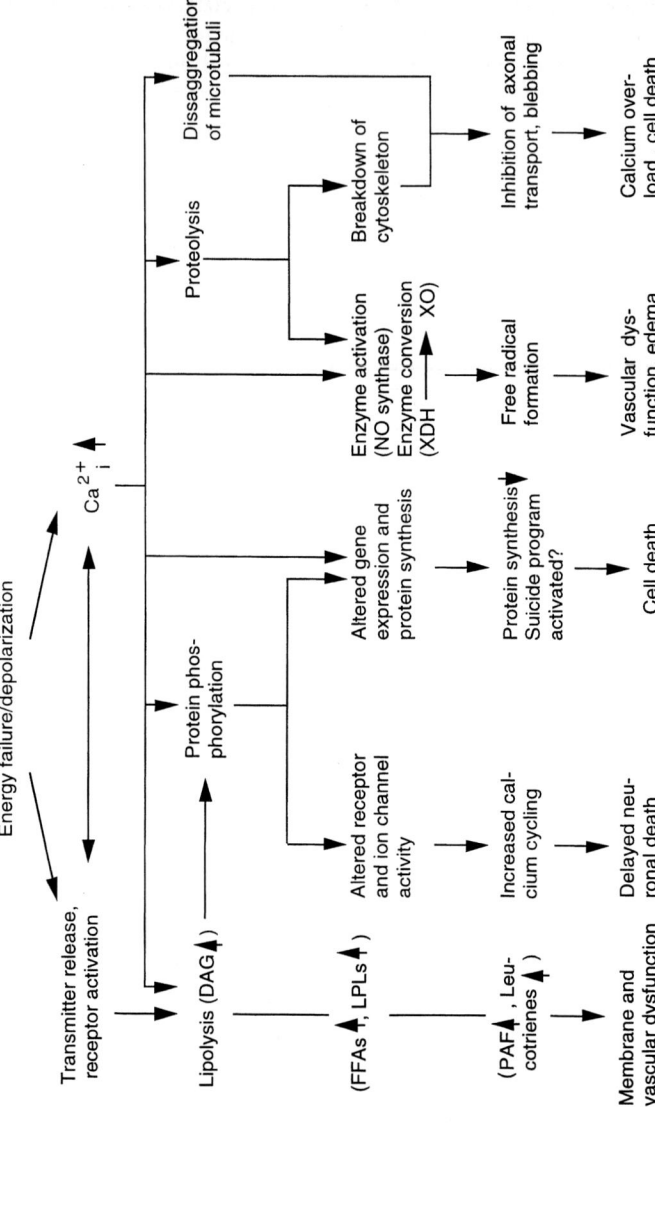

Fig. 4. Schematic diagram illustrating both the primary effects of depolarization and receptor activation and the secondary effects of an increased intracellular calcium concentration (Ca^{2+}_i). The major adverse effects of a massive rise in Ca^{2+}_i involve lipolysis, altered protein phosphorylation, proteolysis, and disassembly of microtubules. Lipolysis leads to production of diacylglycerides (DAG), lysophospholipids (LPL), free fatty acids (FFA), and platelet activating factor (PAF). An altered protein phosphorylation is thought to influence protein synthesis and to lead to changes in gene transcription, possibly with activation of a latent suicide program. A rise in Ca^{2+}_i also activates enzymes (e.g., cyclo-oxygenase, lipoxygenase, and nitric oxide synthetase), which lead to the production of free radicals; calcium-activated proteolysis could act similarly by converting xanthine dehydrogenase (XDH) to xanthine oxidase (XO). Modified from Siesjö, BK. Basic mechanisms of traumatic brain damage. Annals of Emergency Medicine 1993: 22: 959–969

cytoskeleton. If extensive, the DNA damage caused by Ca^{2+} and free radicals may be incompatible with cell survival, as would extensive breakdown of the cytoskeleton and interruption of axoplasmic transport.

Clearly, though, many of the reactions outlined could give rise to delayed damage. For example, one can envisage that accumulation of AA metabolites such as FFAs, lysophospholipids, prostanoids, and leukotrienes could cause membrane and vascular dysfunction, and that PAF leads to the expression of new genes, e.g. those coding for COX-2 (Bazan 1997, 1998). This would set the stage for a delayed inflammatory reaction. Similar effects would result if inducible NOS (iNOS) is expressed (Floyd 1999).

In this context, two additional mechanisms should be mentioned. One is the change in the subunit composition of the AMPA receptor rendering the channel gated by the AMPA receptor permeable to Ca^{2+} (Pelligrino-Giampietro et al. 1992). The other mechanisms are triggered by Ca^{2+}-induced activation of the phosphatase calcineurin. Calcineurin is a pro-apoptotic substance which may work by dephosphorylating Bad, a member of the Bcl-2 family which, when dephosphorylated, can heterodimerize with Bcl_2 or BCX_L, causing apoptosis (Wang et al. 1999). We recognize that such an effect would be blocked by either CsA or FK506. A change in the subunit composition of the AMPA-receptor-gated ion channel could represent a secondary source of calcium, which is responsible for delayed mitochondrial calcium overload (Deshpande et al. 1987). However, it does not seem likely that this triggers a classical MPT since CsA given 2 h after reperfusion does not ameliorate the ischemic damage (see above). It remains to be studied if an initial MPT triggers damage to mitochondrial membranes and complexes that matures with time. Another possibility is that the secondary mitochondrial dysfunction is caused by upregulation of proapoptotic members of the Bcl-2 family, or downregulation of anti-apoptotic members; alternatively, one may envisage that expression of proinflammatory enzymes (iNOS, COX-2) causes damage to still functioning mitochondria.

It remains unexplained why secondary edema and epileptic seizures develop after 18–24 h of recirculation following recovery after 10–15 min of forebrain ischemia in hyperglycemic animals. One can speculate that expression of trophic factors is suppressed (Uchino et al. 1994), or that mitochondrial failure with early release of cyt c is responsible (Li et al. 2000). If the latter would be the case, one can envisage that delayed mitochondrial failure represents depolarization from several adverse stimuli acting in the late recirculation period some of which may emanate from gene expression, and others from inflammatory responses.

Focal Ischemia

When ischemia is of relatively long duration (e.g. 2 h), reperfusion does not give rise to a complete recovery of the bioenergetic state; besides, a further deterioration is observed during the first 4–6 h (Folbergrová et al. 1995). The concept has been developed that recirculation after long periods of MCA occlusion is hindered by compromised reflow, particularly due to capillary plugging by polymorphonucleocytes (PMPNs), or by swelling of pericytes and pericapillary glial cells (del Zoppo et al. 1991, Garcia et al. 1994). However, measurements of blood flow or capillary patency during the first 6 h of reperfusion have failed to support this notion (Tsuchidate et al. 1997, Li et al. 1998) and other data suggest that reperfusion for 1 h is followed by partial recovery of mitochondrial respiratory functions, as studied *in vitro*, with secondary deterioration thereafter (Kuroda et al. 1996a, Kuroda et al. 1996b). The secondary deterioration of the bioenergetic state, as well as of mitochondrial respiratory functions, is ameliorated by the spin trap nitrone PBN, of the bioenergetic state, as well as when given 1 or 3 h after the start of reperfusion, following 2 h of MCA occlusion. It is thus of considerable interest that four drugs: PBN, NXY-059, FK506, and CsA act within a window of therapeutic opportunity of 1 – 3 h following the start of reperfusion, following 2 h of MCA occlusion, and that they all prevent the secondary deterioration of mitochondrial function after the first hour of reperfusion (Kuroda et al. 1999, Yoshimoto et al. 2000). Clearly, primary mitochondrial dysfunction and secondary aggravation of such dysfunction, are major pathogenetic factors in the maturation of focal ischemic brain damage.

Acknowledgements. Studies from the authors' laboratory were supported by an NIH grant (5RO1NS07838–31) as well as by a grant from Centaur Pharmaceuticals, Inc., Sunnyvale, CA and by the Queen Emma Foundation, Honolulu, Hawaii.

References

Alberti K, Cuthbert C (1982) The hydrogen ion in normal metabolism: a review. In: Metabolic acidosis., (R. Porter and G. Lawrensons, eds), Bath, The Pitman Press; pp 1–19.

Andreyev A, Fiskum G (1999) Calcium induced release of mitochondrial cytochrome c by different mechanisms selective for brain versus liver. Cell Death Differ 6:825–832.

Ankarcrona M, Dypbukt J, Boncoffo E, Zhivotovsky B, Orrenius S, Lipton S, Nicotera P (1995) Glutamate-induced neuronal death: A succession of necrosis or apoptosis depending on mitochondrial function. Neuron 15:961–973.

Auer R, Siesjö B (1988) Biological differences between ischemia, hypoglycemia and epilepsy. Ann Neurol 24:699–707.

Bazan N (1997) Lipid messengers and prostaglandin endoperoxide synthase-2 in neuronal cell death. Primer on Cerebrovascular Diseases 193–195.

Bazan N G (1998) The neuromessenger platelet-activating factor in plasticity and neurodegeneration. Prog Brain Res 118:281–291.

Bernardi P, Scorrano L, Colonna R, Petronilli V, Di Lisa F (1999) Mitochondria and cell death. Mechanistic aspects and methodological issues. Eur J. Biochem 264:687–701.

Blaustein M (1988) Calcium transport and buffering in neurons. Trends in Neuroscience 11: 438–443.

Carafoli E (1987) Intracellular calcium homeostasis. Ann Rev Biochem 56:395–433.

Carney J, Floyd R (1991) Protection against oxidative damage to CNS by a-phenyl-tert-butyl nitrone (PBN) and other spin trapping agents: A novel series of non-lipid free radical scavengers. J Mol Neurosci 3:47–57.

Chapman A, Westerberg E, Siesjö B (1981) The metabolism of purine and pyrimidine nucleotides in rat cortex during insulin-induced hypoglycemia and recovery. J Neurochem 36:179–189.

Chen J, Nagayama T, Jin K, Stetler RA, Zhu RL, Graham SH, Simon RP (1998) Induction of caspase-3-like protease may mediate delayed neuronal death in the hippocampus after transient cerebral ischemia. J Neurosci 18:4914–28.

Chopp M, Li Y (1996) Apoptosis in focal cerebral ischemia. Acta Neurochir [Suppl] 66:21–26.

Chopp M, Welch K, Tidwell C, and Helpern J (1988) Global cerebral ischemia and intracellular pH druing hyperglycemia and hypoglycemia in cats. Stroke 19:1383–1387.

Clapham D (1995) Calcium Signaling. Cell 80:259–268.

del Zoppo GJ, Schmid-Schönbein GW, Mori E, Copeland BR, Chang CM (1991) Polymorphonuclear leukocytes occlude capillaries following middle cerebral artery occlusion and reperfusion in baboons. Stroke 22:1276–1283.

Deshpande JK, Siesjö BK, Wieloch T (1987) Calcium accumulation and neuronal damage in the rat hippocampus following cerebral ischemia. J. Cereb. Blood Flow Metab 7:89–95.

Ekholm A, Katsura K, Siesjö BK (1992) Ion fluxes in ischemia: relationship to excitatory amino acids. In: Drug Research Related to Neuroactive Amino Acids., (A. Schousboe, N. H. Diemer and H. Kofods, eds), Copenhagen, Munksgaard, Copenhagen; pp 351–362.

Eklöf B, Siesjö BK (1972) The effect of bilateral carotid artery ligation upon acid-base parameters and substrates levels in the rat brain. Acta physiol scand 86:528–538.

Erecinska M, Silver I (1989) ATP and brain function. J Cereb Blood Flow Metab 9:2–19.

Floyd RA (1999) Antioxidants, oxidative stress, and degenerative neurological disorders. Proc Soc Exp Biol Med 222:236–245.

Folbergrová J, Zhao Q, Katsura K, Siesjö B (1995) N-tert-butyl-a-phenylnitrone improves recovery of brain energy state in the rats following transient focal ischemia. Proc Natl Acad Sci USA 92:5057–5061.

Friberg H, Elmér E, Wieloch T (2000) Effects of cyclosporin A and FK506 on brain damage when administered after transient forebrain ischemia in the rat. Manuscript

Fujie W, Kirino T, Tomukai N, Iwasawa T, Tamura A (1990) Progressive shrinkage of the thalamus following middle cerebral artery occlusion in rats. Stroke 21:1485–1488.

Garcia J, Liu K-F, Ho K-L (1995) Neuronal necrosis after middle cerebral artery occlusion in Wistar rats progresses at different time intervals in the caudoputamen and the cortex. Stroke 26:636–643.

Garcia J, Liu K-F, Yoshida Y, Chen S, Lian J (1994) Brain microvessels: factors altering their patency after the occlusion of a middle cerebral artery (wistar rat). Am J Pathol 145:728–740.

Green DR, Reed JC (1998) Mitochondria and apoptosis. Science 281:1309–1312.

Halestrap A, Kerr P, Javadov S, Woodfield K-Y (1998) Elucidating the molecular mechanism of the permeability transition pore and its role in reperfusion injury of the heart. Biochim Biophys Acta 1366:79–94.

Hansen AJ (1985) Effects of anoxia on ion distribution in the brain. Physiol Rev 65(1):101–148.

Hochachka P, Mommsen T (1983) Protons and Anaerobiosis. Science 219:1391–1397.

Ito U, Spatz M, Walker JT, Klatzo I (1975) Experimental cerebral ischemia in mongolian gerbils. I. Light microscopic observations. Acta Neuropathol (Berl) 32:209–223.

Jones T, Morawetz R, Crowell R, Marcoux F, Fitzgibbon S, DeGirolami U, Ojemann R (1981) Threshold of focal cerbral ischemia in awake monkeys. J Neurosurg 54:773–782.

Katsura K, Asplund B, Ekholm A, Siesjö BK (1992) Extra- and intracellular pH in the brain during ischemia, related to tissue lactate content in normo- and hypercapnic rats. Eur J Neurosci 4:166–176.

Katsura K, Folbergrová J, Gidö G, Siesjö B (1994a) Functional, metabolic, and circulatory changes associated with seizure activity in the postischemic brain. J Neurochem 62:1511–1515.

Katsura K, Kristian T, Smith M, Siesjö B (1994b) Acidosis induced by hypercapnia exaggerates ischemic brain damage. J Cerebr Blood Flow Metab 14:243–250.

Kerr J, Wyllie A, Currie A (1972) Apoptosis: a basic biological phenomenon with wide-ranging implications in tissue kinetics. Br J Cancer 26:239–257.

Kirino T (1982) Delayed neuronal death in the gerbil hippocampus following transient ischemia. Brain Res 239:57–69.

Kleihues P, Kobayashi K, Hossman K-A (1974) Purine nucleotide metabolism in the cat brain after one hour of complete ischemia. J Neurochem 23:417–425.

Krebs H, Woods H, Alberti K (1975) Hyperlactataemia and lactic acidosis. Essays Med Biochem 1:81–103.

Kristián T, Katsura K, Gidö G, Siesjö BK (1994) The influence of pH on cellular calcium influx during ischemia. Brain Res 641:295–302.

Kristián T, Siesjö B (1996) Calcium-related damage in ischemia. Life Sci 59:357–367.

Kuroda S, Katsura K, Hillered L, Bates TE, Siesjö B (1996b) Delayed treatment with a-phenyl-N-tert-butyl nitrone (PBN) attenuates secondary mitochondrial dysfunction after transient focal cerebral ischemia in the rat. Neurobiol Dis 3:149–157.

Kuroda S, Katsura K, Tsuchidate R, Siesjö B (1996a) Secondary bioenergetic failure after transient focal ischemia is due to mitochondrial injury. Acta Physiol Scand 156:149–150.

Leist M, Nicotera P (1997) The shape of cell death. Biochem. Biophys. Res Commun 236:1–9.

Lemasters J, Nieminen A-L, Qian T, Trost L, Elmore S, Nishimura Y, Crowe R, Cascio W, Bradham C, Brenner D, Herman B (1998) The mitochondrial permeability transition in cell death: a common mechanism in necrosis, apoptosis and autophagy. Biochim Biophys Acta 1366:177–196.

Li C, Li P-A, He Q-P, Ouyang Y-B, Siesjö BK (1998) Effects of diabetic hyperglycemia on brain damage following transient ischemia. Brain Res in press:

Li P-A, Shuaib A, Miyashita H, He Q, Siesjö B (2000) Hyperglycemia enhances extracellular glutamate accumulation in rats subjected to forebrain ischemia. Stroke 31:183–192.

Li P-A, Siesjö B (1997) Role of hyperglycaemia-related acidosis in ischaemic brain damage. Acta Physiol Scand 161:567–577.

Li P-A, Vogel J, Smith M, He Q P, Kuschinsky W, and Siesjo BK (1998) Capillary patency after transient middle cerebral artery occlusion of 2 h duration. Neurosci Lett 253:191–194.

Li P-A, Uchino H, Elmer E, Siesjö BK (1997) Amelioration by cyclosporin A of brain damage following 5 and 10 min of ischemia in rats subjected to preichemic hyperglycemia. Brain Res 753:133–140.

Ljunggren B, Schutz H, Siesjö BK (1974) Changes in energy state and acid-base parameters of the rat brain during complete compression ischemia. Brain Res 73:277–289.

MacManus J, Linnik M (1997) Gene expression induced by cerebral ischemia: an apoptotic perspective. J Cereb Blood Flow Metab 17:815–832.

Myers R, Yamaguchi, S (1977) Nervous system effects of cardiac arrest in monkeys. Arch Neurol 34:65–74.

Nedergaard M, Hansen AJ (1993) Characterization of cortical depolarizations evoked in focal cerebral ischemia. J Cereb Blood Flow Metab 13:568–574.

Pelligrino-Giampietro D, Zukin R, Bennett M, Cho S, Pulsinelli W (1992) Switch in glutamate receptor subunit gene expression in CA1 subfield of hippocampus following global ischemia in rats. Proc Natl Acad Sci USA 89:10499–10503.

Piatandosi CA, Zhang J (1996) Mitochondrial generation of reactive oxygen species after brain ischemia in the rat. Stroke 27:327–332.

Pulsinelli WA, Brierley JB, Plum F (1982a) Temporal profile of neuronal damage in a model of transient forebrain ischemia. Ann Neurol 11:491–498.

Reed J (1997) Cytochrome c: Can't live with it-can't live without it. Cell 91:559–562.

Saji M, Reis D (1987) Delayed transneuronal death of substantia nigra neurons prevented by g-aminobutyric acid agonist. Science 235:66–69.

Samdani AF, Dawson TM, Dawson VL (1997) Nitric oxide synthase in models of focal ischemia. Stroke 28:1283–1288.

Siemkowicz E, Hansen A (1978) Clinical restitution following cerebral ischemia in hypo-, normo-, and hyperglycemic rats. Acta Neurol Scand 58:1–8.

Siesjö B (1991) The role of calcium in cell death. In: Neurodoegenerative disorders: Mechanisms and prospects for therapy., (D. Price, A. Aguayo and H. Thoenens, eds), Chichester, John Wiley & Sons Ltd; pp 35–59.

Siesjo B, Katsura K, Kristian T (1996) Molecular mechanisms of acidosis-mediated damage. Acta Neurochir 66:8–14.

Siesjö BK (1984) Cell damage in the brain: A speculative synthesis. Acta Phys Scand 69:313.

Siesjö BK (1988) Mechanisms of ischemic brain damage. Crit Care Med 16:954–963.

Siesjö BK (1992a) Basic mechanisms of traumatic brain damage. Annals of Emergency Medicine 22:959–969.

Siesjö BK (1992b) Calcium-related damage in the brain. In: Calcium antagonists and neurological disorders., (J. G. de Yebeness, eds), pp ?

Smith M, Auer R, Siesjö B (1984) The density and distribution of ischemic brain injury in the rat following 2–10 min of forebrain ischemia. Acta Neuropathol (Berl) 64:319–332.

Smith M, von Hanwehr R, Siesjö B (1986) Changes in extra- and intracellular pH in the brain during and following ischemia in hyperglycemic and in moderately hypoglycemic rats. J Cereb Blood Flow Metab 6:574–583.

Susin S, Zamzami N, Kroemer G (1998) Mitochondria as regulators of apoptosis: doubt no more. Biochim Biophys Acta 1366:151–165.

Susin SA, Lorenzo HK, Zamzami N, Marzo I, Snow BE, Brothers GM, Mangion J, Jacotot E, Costantini P, Loeffler M, Larochette N, Goodlett DR, Aebersold R, Siderovski DP, Penninger JM, Kroemer G (1999) Molecular characterization of mitochondrial apoptosis-inducing factor [see comments]. Nature 397:441–446.

Tamura A, Kirino T, Sano K, Takagi K, Oka H (1990) Atrophy of the ipsilateral substantia nigra following middle cerebral artery occlusion in the rat. Brain Res 510:154–157.

Tombaugh GC, Sapolsky RM (1993) Evolving concepts about the role of acidosis in ischemic neuropathology. J Neurochem 61:793–803.

Tominaga T, Kure S, Narisawa K, Yoshimoto T (1993) Endonuclease activation following focal ischemic injury in the rat brain. Brain Res 608:21–26.

Tsuchidate R, Qing-Ping H, Smith M, Siesjo BK (1997) Regional cerebral blood flow during and after 2 hours of middle cerebral artery occlusion in the rat. J Cereb Blood Flow Metab 17:1066–1073.

Uchino H, Elmér E, Uchino K, Li P-A, He Q-P, Smith M-L, Siesjö B (1998) Amelioration by cyclosporin A of brain damage in transient forebrain ischemia in the rat. Brain Res 812:216–226.

Uchino H, Elmér E, Uchino K, Lindvall O, Siesjö B (1995) Cyclosporin A dramatically ameliorates CA1 hippocampal damage following transient forebrain ischemia in the rat. Acta Physiol Scand 155:469–471.

Uchino H, Lundgren J, Smith M, Siesjo B (1994) Preischemic hyperglycemia leads to delayed postischemic hyperthermia.

Wang TH, Wang HS (1999) Apoptosis: (2) characteristics of apoptosis. J Formos Med Assoc 98:531–542.

Warner DS, Smith M-L, Siesjö BK (1987) Ischemia in normo- and hyperglycemic rats: effects on brain water and electrolytes. Stroke 18:464–471.

Wyllie A, Kerr J, Currie A (1981) Cell death: The significance of apoptosis. Internat Rev Cytology 68:251–307.

Yoshimoto T, Kristian T, Hu B, Ouyang Y-B, Siesjo B (2000) Cyclosporin A and NXY-059 ameliorates secondary deterioration of mitochondrial function following transient focal ischemia. submitted

Zoratti M, Szabó I (1995) The mitochondrial permeability transition. Biochim Biophys Acta 1241:139–176.

Ischemic Mechanisms in Traumatic Brain Injury

P.M. Kochanek, K.S. Hendrich, K.D. Statler, R.S.B. Clark,
L.W. Jenkins, D.S. Williams, C. Ho, and D.W. Marion

Introduction

Despite considerable evidence supporting the occurrence of ischemic damage after traumatic brain injury in both experimental animal models and in the clinical condition, the precise role of ischemia in the evolution of secondary damage after traumatic brain injury has remained difficult to define. Similarly, studies of the effects of the application of therapies targeting secondary ischemic damage in traumatic brain injury are limited. In this chapter, the classical and contemporary studies supporting a role for ischemic mechanisms in experimental and clinical traumatic brain injury will be reviewed. In addition, based on our own research interest, early posttraumatic ischemia will serve as a point of focus. Again, in light of our own current work in experimental models of traumatic brain injury, the potential value of the application of perfusion magnetic resonance imaging using the continuous arterial spin labeling (CASL) method will be highlighted.

The Role of Ischemia After Severe Traumatic Brain Injury: Clinical Studies

A possible role of cerebral ischemia in human head injury was suggested as early as 1897 by Phelps [1], and in 1939 by Helfand [2] in their descriptions of the contribution of secondary insults (shock) and cerebral infarction, respectively. Subsequently, Graham and Adams [3] published one of the earliest detailed descriptions of the putative role of ischemia in patients with severe traumatic brain injury as reflected by histopathological evidence of ischemic damage. In that classic work, fifty-three cases of fatal human head injury were reviewed after excluding cases where ischemic damage resulted from herniation. In their series, ischemic damage was observed in thirty-two of the fifty-three cases, including hippocampal lesions in twenty-three of the victims. However, much of the focus by pioneers in the field on ischemic damage in both clinical and experimental traumatic brain injury centered around the role of secondary insults– either shock or hypoxemia in the field or emergency department, or secondary insults in the neurointensive care unit as a result of refractory intracranial hypertension [4–6]. Obrist et al. [7, 8] published some of the first work quantifying the time course of changes in cerebral blood flow after severe traumatic brain injury in humans. Despite the fact that delayed hyperemia (blood flow in excess of cerebral metabolic rate for oxygen, $CMRO_2$) and its contribution to cerebral swelling was the focus of the investigation, cerebral blood flow, measured with the ^{133}Xe method, was frequently observed to be reduced during the initial twelve hours after injury. Similarly, the arterial-jugular venous oxygen content difference was noted to be greatest early after injury, consistent with the possibility of early ischemia.

A shift from a focus on delayed hyperemia to concern with early posttraumatic hypoperfusion and/or ischemia was given considerable impetus by the work of Muizelaar et al. [9] in the investigation of the effect of prophylactic hyperventilation on the management of 113 adults with severe traumatic brain injury. At 3 and 6 months after injury the number of patients with a favorable outcome (good or moderately disabled) was significantly lower in the hyperventilated patients, although evidence of exacerbation of cerebral ischemia was not demonstrated in the hyperventilated group. Concurrently, Marion et al. [10] demonstrated early cerebral blood flow reduction after severe traumatic injury by using the xenon-computerized tomography method in 32 severely head-injured adults. In that study, forty-three percent of the flow determinations were made within seven days after injury. During the first day, patients with an initial Glasgow Coma Scale (GCS) score of 3 or 4 and no surgical mass had significantly lower flows than did those patients with a higher GCS score or mass lesions. Similarly, patients without surgical mass lesions who died tended to have a lower global cerebral blood flow than did those with better outcomes. Bouma et al. [11] subsequently confirmed this finding applying the xenon-computerized tomography method in adults on admission to the hospital. Overall, global or regional cerebral ischemia (defined as a cerebral blood flow less than 18 ml/100 g/min) was seen in over thirty percent of patients. More recently Adelson et al. [12] demonstrated similarly early hypoperfusion after severe traumatic brain injury in infants and children. Specifically, global cerebral blood flow less than 20 ml/100 g/min was associated with poor outcome.

The acute reduction in cerebral blood flow after injury certainly is consistent with the considerable vulnerability of the injured brain to secondary insults. Chesnut et al. [13] demonstrated a powerful association of hypotension (systolic blood pressure less than 90 mmHg) with poor outcome in a study of 717 cases of severe traumatic brain injury in the Traumatic Coma Data Bank. Notably, hypotension was seen in almost thirty-five percent of cases and was associated with a 150 percent increase in mortality rate. Early posttraumatic increases in cerebral glucose utilization supporting astrocyte uptake of glutamate and other excitotoxic neurotransmitters released in injured brain regions is also proposed to contribute to the enhanced vulnerability of the traumatically injured brain to blood flow reductions [14–16]. Bergsneider et al. [16] recently demonstrated increased cerebral glucose utilization in a series of humans with severe traumatic brain injury. Under such conditions, even moderate flow reductions may produce relative ischemia in hypermetabolic brain regions unable to regulate cerebral blood flow in the face of increased needs for substrate delivery. Further study of this putative mechanism of secondary damage in human head injury is needed.

The Role of Ischemia After Severe Traumatic Brain Injury: Laboratory Studies

In the late 1970s, Nilsson and Nordstrom [17] described flow reductions after impact in a rat model of cerebral concussion. Subsequently, Lewelt et al. [18] used a cat model of fluid percussion and demonstrated that traumatic brain injury attenuates the vasodilatory response to hypoxemia. This work, and the investigation by Ishige et al. [4, 19] and Jenkins et al. [20] of the exacerbation of neuronal damage with the application of secondary hypoxemic or ischemic insults in the rat model of fluid percussion represent some of the earliest animal studies of the dramatic deleterious consequences of secondary insults after experimental traumatic brain injury. Laboratory studies have shown that the brain is more vulnerable to secondary insults after traumatic brain injury as the result of changes in both susceptibility of the vasculature and neurons. Vascular susceptibility involves vascular dysfunction that increases the likelihood of cerebral ischemia, such as the reduced ability of the cerebral vasculature after traumatic brain injury to autoregulate (dilate) in response to decreased blood pressure or oxygen content [18, 21], while increased sensitivity of neurons involves a decreased ability of selective brain regions to withstand hypoxia/ischemia after traumatic brain injury compared to the normal brain [20, 22]. The mechanisms mediating enhanced vulnerability are largely unknown but some mechanisms, such as impaired vascular responses to hypotension and receptor-mediated injury through muscarinic and NMDA receptors, have been identified [18, 20–22].

Yamakami and McIntosh [23] provided one of the first comprehensive descriptions of the time course of cerebral blood flow after experimental traumatic brain injury. Moderate fluid-percussion injury produced an acute and profound reduction in cerebral blood flow, as quantified using the radiolabeled microsphere technique. Oligemia persisted for at least two hours in the injured region that went on to develop cystic necrosis at four weeks postinjury. In the controlled cortical impact model of traumatic brain injury in rats, Bryan et al. [24], and Kochanek et al. [25] reported marked flow reductions in the injured cortex to ischemic levels. In both of these reports, cerebral blood flow was quantified using the ^{14}C-iodoantipyrine method. Focal ischemia at the contusion site was accompanied by global flow reductions of a more modest degree, that was generally proportional to the proximity of the location to the impact site.

Application of the CASL Method to Experimental Traumatic Brain Injury in Rats

A major limitation to the traditional methods applied to the investigation of posttraumatic cerebral blood flow in experimental models has been the inability to generate serial non-invasive maps of perfusion. This is particularly important in traumatic brain injury in light of the heterogeneity of damage, such as within and surrounding a focal cerebral contusion. In 1992, Detre et al. [26] introduced the non-invasive technique of CASL for the magnetic resonance imaging (MRI) quantification of perfusion. This technique uses arterial water as

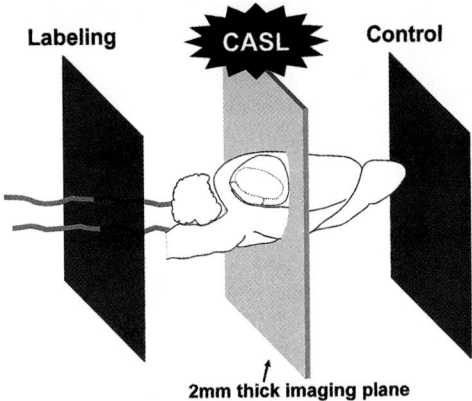

Fig. 1. Cartoon illustrating the quantification of cerebral blood flow (CBF) using the non-invasive continuous arterial spin-labeling (CASL) magnetic resonance imaging technique. After defining the appropriate position of the rat for perfusion acquisition, a steady low-power radiofrequency (RF) field is applied in the presence of a magnetic field gradient to label endogenous arterial water proton spins. When a single RF coil is used for both arterial spin-labeling (labeling) and for detection (imaging plane), the labeling pulse also saturates macromolecules in the imaging plane, resulting in reduction in tissue water signal intensity in that plane. Therefore, an additional experiment without arterial spin labeling (control) is performed by centering the RF irradiation symmetrically opposite to the detection plane. In our studies, a 2-mm thick imaging plane is used near the contusion center. Percent-change maps are generated from the magnetization intensity in the control image (M_C) and the labeled image (M_L). CBF is then calculated from the equation, CBF $= \lambda \cdot (T_{1obs} - 2\alpha)^{-1} \cdot (M_C - M_L) \cdot M_C^{-1}$, where λ is the brain-blood partition coefficient of water, α represents the arterial spin-labeling efficiency, and T_{1obs} is the experimentally observed spin-lattice relaxation time of tissue water

an endogenous tracer by magnetically labeling the water proton spins at the level of the carotid arteries (Fig. 1). A quantitative map of cerebral blood flow is then generated from magnetization changes measured in the brain images (Fig. 2; reprinted from the work of Hendrich et al., with permission). Our group has utilized this method in a number of studies to investigate the cerebrovascular response to experimental traumatic brain injury, in addition to studying various aspects of normal cerebrovascular physiology [27–34].

In our initial application of this method to the controlled cortical impact model of traumatic brain injury, we studied the reactivity of the cerebral circulation to changes in $PaCO_2$ at 24 hours after injury. This method facilitated the generation of the first maps of CO_2 reactivity of the cerebral circulation of the rat in any brain injury model. In the cortex, CO_2 reactivity was reduced from baseline values of about 3.1 percent (per mmHg change in CO_2) to 1.4 percent in a contusion-enriched region of interest [27]. In a subsequent study [28], we reported the extent of hypoperfusion early after injury and defined the important contribution of increases in the *in vivo* spin-lattice relaxation time (T_{1obs}) early after injury within and around the contusion site to the quantification of perfusion in our trauma model. Indeed, if a homogenous normal value for T_{1obs} is used rather than either a pixel-by-pixel or region of interest-specific value in our model, cerebral

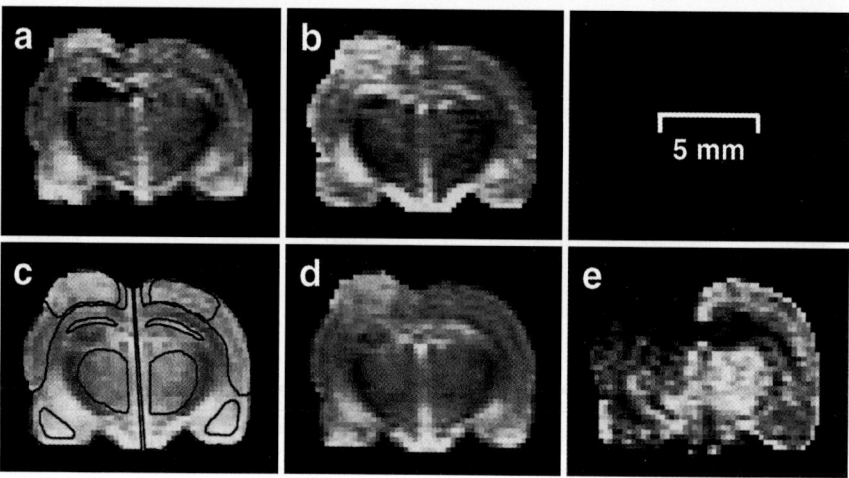

Fig. 2a–e. Images from a study at 2–3.5 hours after controlled cortical impact in rat. **a** Hemorrhage appears hypointense in the T_2-weighted image. **b** Tissue in the contused region, which is presumably edematous, appears hyperintense on the T_{1obs} map. **c** Outlines of the anatomic regions of interest defined are overlaid on the control image from the perfusion experiment, where mean regional pixel values represent M_c in the equation defined in Fig. 1. **d** The labeled image contains pixel values for M_L in the same equation. **e** Control and labeled images were used to generate the perfusion percent-change map, where areas of perfusion deficit are easily detected as low intensity. Reprinted from the work of Hendrich et al. (28) with permission

blood flow in injured hypoperfused regions can be overestimated by as much as 87 percent. Currently, we use a region-of-interest adjusted perfusion calculation to optimize flow determinations with this method.

More recently, we have used the CASL method in a variety of ways including: 1) coupled assessment of cerebral blood flow and blood-brain barrier permeability after controlled cortical impact [29], 2) assessment of perfusion in follow-up as long as one year after injury [30], 3) assessment of early and delayed perfusion after experimental traumatic brain injury in immature (post-natal day 17) rats [31], 4) investigation of the effect of a variety of anesthetics (isoflurane, pentobarbital, or fentanyl) on perfusion in the normal rat brain [32], and 5) assessment of novel anti-excitotoxic and flow promoting strategies in the normal and injured rat brain [33, 34].

Relationship of CBF to Metabolic Demands and Neuronal Death After Experimental Traumatic Brain Injury

Clinical studies have demonstrated that $CMRO_2$ is reduced early after severe traumatic brain injury and this reduction persists– at least for the duration of coma [7, 8]. However, a number of studies in experimental models of traumatic brain injury carried out in the laboratory of Hovda et al. [14, 35–38] have demonstrated that early during the period of posttraumatic hypoperfusion, considerable increases in metabolic rate for glucose (CMRglu) are observed. These increases have been termed "hyperglycolysis," and are proposed to develop, at least in part, as a result of local excitotoxicity. Yoshino et al. [35] used the lateral fluid percussion injury in rats and reported 30–50% and 80–90% increases in CMRglu in ipsilateral cortex and hippocampus, respectively, immediately after injury. This effect was still seen at 30 min after injury. However, by 6 hours after injury, ipsilateral cortex and hippocampus went into a state of metabolic depression that persisted for at least 5 days. Subsequently, by chemically lesioning CA3, Yoshino et al. [36] demonstrated that hippocampal CA3 projections to CA1 are critical to this response, implicating glutamatergic input into CA1 as mediating this metabolic response. Kawamata et al. [37] similarly supported a role of all subtypes of glutamate receptors in mediating this response in cortex by demonstrating that the hyperglycolytic response could be inhibited via the *in situ* local infusion (via microdialysis) of a variety of glutamate-receptor antagonists. Glucose utilization secondary to increases in local neuronal activation and as consequence of glutamate uptake by astrocytes is posed to be involved [14, 15]. This acute hyperglycolytic response, coupled with the previously described loss of blood pressure autoregulation of cerebral blood flow, is likely to play a key role in producing the enhanced vulnerability of the traumatically injured brain to secondary hypotensive or hypoxemic insults (Fig. 3). The potential role of this process in the evolution of secondary damage, even in the absence of a secondary extracerebral insult is discussed below.

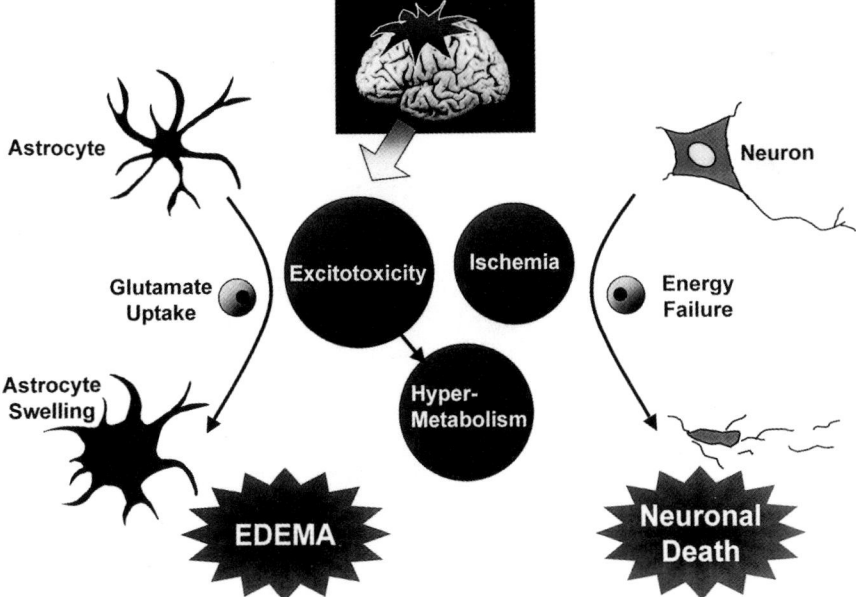

Fig. 3. Cartoon depicting pathological cascade and consequences of combination of early excitotoxicity and hypoperfusion after severe traumatic brain injury

Therapies Targeting Either Early Posttraumatic Hypoperfusion or the Combination of Early Posttraumatic Hypoperfusion and Hypermetabolism After Experimental Traumatic Brain Injury

A question that remains unanswered in traumatic brain injury is whether strategies promoting cerebral blood flow early after injury could improve outcome. This is a current area of active laboratory and clinical investigation (Fig. 4). Minchenko [39] reported fluid-percussion injury-induced release of the potent vasoconstrictor peptide endothelin-1 (ET-1). In addition, ET-1 antagonism partially restored impaired hypotensive pial artery dilation and improved cerebral blood flow. DeWitt et al. [40] demonstrated that early hypoperfusion after experimental fluid percussion injury could be attenuated by treatment with L-arginine– presumably by supplying substrate for endothelial nitric oxide synthase (eNOS). Cherian et al. [41] studied the effect of L-arginine on both early posttraumatic cerebral blood flow and ultimate lesion volume in a rat model of controlled cortical impact injury. In vehicle treated rats, flow decreased to <25% of baseline at the impact site and stayed at that level for 3 hours. Infusion of L-arginine increased blood flow back to near-baseline levels, without a concomitant increase in intracranial pressure. In addition, treatment with L-arginine reduced the contusion volume. These in addition to other strategies deserve investigation

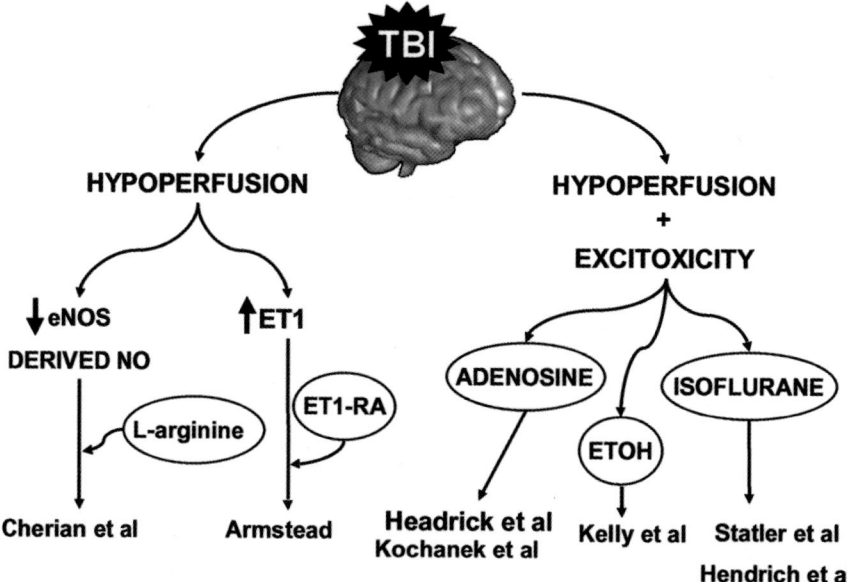

Fig. 4. *(Left)* Two putative mechanisms involved in the development of early posttraumatic hypoperfusion that are currently being investigated in experimental and/or clinical traumatic brain injury. *(Right)* Three putative strategies (augmentation of adenosine, administration of ethanol, and optimization of anesthesia and/or sedation) currently being tested to target the combination of early excitotoxicity and hypoperfusion after severe traumatic brain injury. See references for the specific citations identified at the bottom of the figure; *TBI* = traumatic brain injury

to determine if early posttrauma blood flow promotion may have merit for translation to the clinic. Notably, L-arginine is currently being tested in a clinical trial in adults with severe traumatic brain injury [Personal communication, C.S. Robertson].

We and others are investigating an alternative strategy to isolated flow promotion after severe traumatic brain injury, namely simultaneous enhancement of cerebral blood flow and attenuation of excitotoxicity (Fig. 4). Adenosine is an endogenous neuroprotectant produced in response to both ischemia and excitotoxicity [42]. Breakdown of adenosine triphosphate (ATP) leads to formation of adenosine, a purine nucleoside that decreases neuronal metabolism and increases cerebral blood flow, among other mechanisms. Adenosine binding to A1 receptors decreases metabolism by increasing K^+ and Cl^- and decreasing Ca^{++} conductances in the neuronal membrane [43, 44]. A1 receptors are located on neurons in brain regions that are susceptible to ischemia and traumatic brain injury (i.e., hippocampus) and are spatially associated with NMDA receptors [45]. Thus, released adenosine minimizes excitotoxicity. Binding of adenosine to A2 receptors (on cerebrovascular smooth muscle) causes vasodilation, although binding to A2a receptors on neurons may be detrimental.

Brain interstitial levels of adenosine are increased early after experimental traumatic brain injury in rats [46–48]. Using cortical or hippocampal microdialysis, interstitial adenosine was found to increase immediately after injury to levels 50- to 100-fold greater than baseline [47, 48]. In clinical studies, we recently observed marked increases in brain interstitial levels of adenosine and purine degradation products in adults with severe traumatic brain injury during episodes of jugular venous desaturation (documented secondary insults), supporting a role of adenosine as a "retaliatory" defense metabolite [49]. We previously reported considerable increases in cerebrospinal fluid adenosine concentration in adults with severe head injury [50]. Neuroprotection is afforded by a variety of strategies augmenting endogenous levels of adenosine. Headrick et al. [51], in a rat model of moderate fluid percussion injury, reported that administration of the non-selective adenosine analog 2-chloroadenosine improved energy failure and functional outcome after fluid percussion injury in rats. Similarly, we recently reported that local injection of low doses of 2-chloroadenosine (0.3 nanomoles) reduces early posttraumatic edema after controlled cortical impact in rats [33]. 2-chloroadenosine activates both A1 and A2a receptors [52, 53], suggesting the possibility that both anti-excitotoxic and flow promoting effects are operating. However, our recent studies of parenchymal injection in normal rats suggests that higher doses of 2-chloroadenosine (~6 and ~12 nanomoles) are needed to produce increases in regional and hemispheric cerebral blood flow, respectively [34]. A variety of strategies are available to augment local adenosine concentration or activate adenosine receptors in injured brain and these deserve additional investigation in experimental traumatic brain injury.

Another clue suggesting the possible benefit of simultaneously attenuating early posttraumatic hypoperfusion and excitotoxicity was demonstrated by the recent work of Kelly et al. [54] who demonstrated a beneficial effect of systemic administration of ethanol in the controlled cortical impact model in rats. Ethanol was shown to reduce contusion volume after injury [55], and subsequently (administered at a dose of 1 g/kg, 30 min before injury) was shown to simultaneously reduce posttraumatic increases in CMRglu and attenuate the early flow reduction. Related to this approach, Statler et al. [56] in our group recently demonstrated a marked reduction in hippocampal CA1 neuronal death and improved motor and cognitive functional outcomes in rats anesthetized with isoflurane versus fentanyl after controlled cortical impact injury. Hendrich et al. [32] recently demonstrated, using identical anesthetic regimens, that cerebral blood flow was about 3-fold higher on isoflurane than fentanyl. In addition, isoflurane is associated with considerably greater anti-excitotoxic properties than fentanyl [57, 58]. Recent work by Statler et al. [59] suggests that CMRglu in the CA1 hippocampus is greater in rats anesthetized with fentanyl versus isoflurane after controlled cortical impact. We are currently comparing the effect of early posttrauma sedation/anesthesia with seven different anesthetics in our controlled cortical impact model in rats [60]. Remarkably, despite routine use of sedatives and analgesics in patients with severe traumatic brain injury, this area has received limited investigation in either laboratory models or the clinic.

Finally, one of the clinical impediments to the application of such an approach is the risk of herniation. It will be important in experimental models to address this possibility in carefully designed studies, preferentially in models in which there is an intact cranium.

Acknowledgements. Supported in part by NIH grants NS 38087, NS 30318, and RR-10962, the US Army DAMD 17–97–1–7009, the Laerdal Foundation, and the Whitaker Foundation. We thank Marci Provins for preparation of this manuscript and Bradley Stezoski for preparation of Figs. 1, 3, and 4. We thank Drs. Peter Safar, Edwin Jackson, C. Edward Dixon, and David Warner for helpful suggestions.

References

1. Phelps C. Principles of Treatment, in Traumatic Injuries of the Brain and Its Membranes, M Critchley, et al., Editors. 1897, D. Appleton and Company: New York. p. 207.
2. Helfand M. Cerebral lesions due to vasomotor disturbances following brain trauma. J Nerv Ment Dis. 1939;90:157.
3. Graham DI, Adams JH. Ischaemic Brain Damage in Fatal Head Injuries, in Brain Hypoxia, JB Brierley, BS Meldrum, Editors. 1971, William Heinemann Medical Books Ltd., London. pp. 34–40.
4. Ishige N, Pitts LH, Berry I, et al. The effect of hypoxia on traumatic head injury in rats: Alterations in neurologic function, brain edema, and cerebral blood flow. J Cereb Blood Flow Metab. 1987;7:759–767.
5. Marshall LF, Graham DI, Durity F, et al. Experimental cerebral oligemia and ischemia produced by intracranial hypertension. Part 2: Brain morphology. J Neurosurg. 1975;43:318–322.
6. Rosner MJ, Becker DP. Origin and evolution of plateau waves. Experimental observations and a theoretical model. J Neurosurg. 1984;60:312–324.
7. Obrist WD, Gennarelli TA, Segawa H, Dolinskas CA, Langfitt TW. Relation of cerebral blood flow to neurological status and outcome in head-injured patients. J Neurosurg. 1979;51:292–300.
8. Obrist WD, Langfitt TW, Jaggi JL, Cruz J, Gennarelli TA. Cerebral blood flow and metabolism in comatose patients with acute head injury. Relationship to intracranial hypertension. J Neurosurg. 1984;61:241–253.

9. Muizelaar JP, Marmarou A, Ward JD, et al. Adverse effects of prolonged hyperventilation in patients with severe head injury: A randomized clinical trial. J Neurosurg. 1991;75:731–739.

10. Marion DW, Darby J, Yonas H. Acute regional cerebral blood flow changes caused by severe head injuries. J Neurosurgery. 1991;74:407–414.

11. Bouma GJ, Muizelaar JP, Stringer WA, et al. Ultra-early evaluation of regional cerebral blood flow in severely head-injured patients using xenon-enhanced computerized tomography. J Neurosurg. 1992;77:360–368.

12. Adelson PD, Clyde B, Kochanek PM, et al. Cerebrovascular response in infants and young children following severe traumatic brain injury: A preliminary report. Pediatr Neurosurg. 1997;26:200–207.

13. Chesnut RM, Marshall LF, Klauber MR, et al. The role of secondary brain injury in determining outcome from severe head injury. J Trauma. 1993;34:216–222.

14. Hovda DA, Lee SM, Smith ML, et al. The neurochemical and metabolic cascade following brain injury: Moving from animal models to man. J Neurotrauma. 1995;12:903–906.

15. Pellerin L, Magistretti PJ. Glutamate uptake into astrocytes stimulates aerobic glycolysis: A mechanism coupling neuronal activity to glucose utilization. Proc Natl Acad Sci USA. 1994;91:10625–10629.

16. Bergsneider M, Hovda DA, Shalmon E, et al. Cerebral hyperglycolysis following severe traumatic brain injury in humans: a positron emission tomography study. J Neurosurg. 1997;86:241–251.

17. Nilsson B, Nordstrom CH. Experimental head injury in the rat. Part 3: Cerebral blood flow and oxygen consumption after concussive impact acceleration. J Neurosurg. 1977;47: 262–273.

18. Lewelt W, Jenkins LW, Miller JD. Effects of experimental fluid-percussion injury of the brain on cerebrovascular reactivity of hypoxia and to hypercapnia. J Neurosurg. 1982;56:332–338.

19. Ishige N, Pitts LH, Berry I, Nishimura MC, James TL. The effects of hypovolemic hypotension on high-energy phosphate metabolism of traumatized brain in rats. J Neurosurg. 1988;68:129–136.

20. Jenkins LW, Lyeth BG, Lewelt W, et al. Combined pretrauma scopolamine and phencyclidine attenuate posttraumatic increased sensitivity to delayed secondary ischemia. J Neurotrauma. 1988;5:275–287.

21. Lewelt W, Jenkins LW, Miller JD. Autoregulation of cerebral blood flow after experimental fluid percussion injury of the brain. J Neurosurg. 1980;53:500–511

22. DeWitt DS, Jenkins LW, Prough DS. Enhanced vulnerability to secondary ischemic insults after experimental traumatic brain injury. New Horizons. 1995;3:376–383.

23. Yamakami I, McIntosh TK. Alterations in regional cerebral blood flow following brain injury in the rat. J Cereb Blood Flow Metab. 1991;11:655–660.

24. Bryan RM, Cherian L, Robertson C. Regional cerebral blood flow after controlled cortical impact injury in rats. Anesth Analg. 1995;80:687–695.

25. Kochanek PM, Marion DW, Zhang W, et al. Severe controlled cortical impact in rats: Assessment of cerebral edema, blood flow, and contusion volume. J Neurotrauma. 1995;12:1015–1025.

26. Detre JA, Leigh JS, Williams DS, Koretsky AP. Perfusion imaging. Magn Reson Med. 1992; 23:37–45.

27. Forbes ML, Hendrich KS, Kochanek PM, et al. Assessment of cerebral blood flow and CO2 reactivity after controlled cortical impact by perfusion magnetic resonance imaging using arterial spin labeling in rats. J Cereb Blood Flow Metab. 1997;17:865–874.

28. Hendrich KS, Kochanek PM, Williams DS, et al. Early perfusion after controlled cortical impact in rats: Quantification by arterial spin-labeled MRI and the influence of spin-lattice relaxation time heterogeneity. Magn Reson Med. 1999;42:673–681.

29. Hendrich KS, Schiding JK, Kochanek PM, et al. Sequential MRI assessment of cerebral blood flow and blood-brain barrier permeability early after traumatic brain injury in rats. J Cereb Blood Flow Metab. 1997;17:S76.

30. Kochanek PM, Hendrich KS, Dixon CE, et al. Perfusion magnetic resonance imaging at one year after controlled cortical impact in rats. J Neurotrauma. 1997;14:783.

31. Adelson PD, Hendrich K, Robichaud P, et al. Magnetic resonance imaging (MRI) assessment of traumatic brain injury (TBI) in immature rats: A preliminary report. J Neurotrauma. 1998;15:853.

32. Hendrich KS, Kochanek PM, Melick JA, et al. Cerebral perfusion during anesthesia with fentanyl, isoflurane, or pentobarbital in normal rats studied by arterial spin-labeled MRI. Magn Reson Med (in press) 2001.

33. Robertson CL, Hendrich KS, Kochanek PM, et al. Assessment of 2-chloroadenosine treatment after experimental traumatic brain injury in the rat using arterial spin-labeled MRI. Proc Intl Soc Magn Reson Med. 1999;7:896.

34. Kochanek PM, Hendrich KS, Robertson CL, et al. Assessment of the effect of 2-chloroadenosine on cerebral blood flow in normal rats using arterial spin labeled MRI. Magn Reson Med. 2000;45:924–929.

35. Yoshino A, Hovda DA, Kawamata T, Katayama Y, Becker DP. Dynamic changes in local cerebral glucose utilization following cerebral concussion in rats: Evidence of a hyper- and subsequent hypometabolic state. Brain Res. 1991;561:106–119.

36. Yoshino A, Hovda DA, Katayama Y, Kawamata T, Becker DP. Hipocampal CA3 lesion prevents postconcussive metabolic dysfunction in CA1. J Cereb Blood Flow Metab. 1992;12:996–1006.

37. Kawamata T, Katayama Y, Hovda DA, Yoshino A, Becker DP. Administration of excitatory amino acid antagonists via microdialysis attenuates the increase in glucose utilization seen following concussive brain injury. J Cereb Blood Flow Metab. 1992;12:12–24.

38. Sutton RL, Hovda DA, Adelson PD, Benzel EC, Becker DP. Metabolic changes following cortical contusion: relationships to edema and morphological changes. Acta Neurochir Suppl (Wien). 1994;60:446–448.

39. Minchenko AG, Armstead VE, Opentanova IL, Lefer AM. Endothelin-1, endothelin receptors and ecNOS gene transcription in vital organs during traumatic shock in rats. Endothelium. 1999;6:303–314.

40. DeWitt DS, Smith TG, Deyo DJ, et al. L-arginine and superoxide dismutase prevent or reverse cerebral hypoperfusion after fluid-percussion traumatic brain injury. J Neurotrauma. 1997;14:223–233.

41. Cherian L, Chacko G, Goodman JC, Robertson CS. Cerebral hemodynamic effects of phenylephrine and L-arginine after cortical impact injury. Crit Care Med. 1999;27(11):2512–2517.

42. Matsumoto K, Graf R, Rosner G, Shimada N, Heiss WD. Flow thresholds for extracellular purine catabolite elevation in cat focal ischemia. Brain Res. 1992;579:309–314.

43. Siggins GR, Schubert P. Adenosine depression of hippocampal neurons in vitro: an intracellular study of dose dependent actions on synaptic and membrane potentials. Neurosci Lett. 1981;23:55–60.

44. Segal M. Intracellular analysis of a postsynaptic action of adenosine in the rat hippocampus. Eur J Pharmacol. 1982;79:193–199.

45. Bowery NG, Wong EHF, Hudson AL. Quantitative autoradiography of (3H) MK-801 binding sites in mammalian brain. Br J Pharmacol. 1988;93:948–954.

46. Nilsson P, Hillered L, Ponten U, Ungerstedt U. Changes in cortical extracellular levels of energy-related metabolites and amino acids following concussive brain injury in rats. J Cereb Blood Flow Metab. 1990;10:631–637.

47. Bell MJ, Kochanek PM, Carcillo JA, et al. Interstitial adenosine, inosine, and hypoxanthine, are increased after experimental traumatic brain injury in the rat. J Neurotrauma. 1998;15:163–170.

48. Robertson CL, Kochanek PM, Jackson EA, et al. Inhibition of adenosine deaminase after severe traumatic brain injury in rats. J Neurotrauma. 1998;15:893.

49. Bell M, Robertson C, Kochanek P, et al. Interstitial brain adenosine during jugular venous desaturations after human traumatic brain injury (TBI): Evidence of energy failure. Crit Care Med Suppl. 1998;26:A31.

50. Clark RSB, Carcillo JA, Kochanek PM, et al. Cerebrospinal fluid adenosine concentration and uncoupling of cerebral blood flow and oxidative metabolism after severe head injury in humans. Neurosurgery. 1997;41:1284–1293.

51. Headrick JP, Bendall MR, Faden AI, Vink R. Dissociation of adenosine levels from bioenergetic state in experimental brain trauma: Potential role in secondary injury. J Cereb Blood Flow Metab. 1994;14:853–861.
52. Daly JW, Bruns RF, Snyder SH. Adenosine receptors in the central nervous system: relationship to the central actions of methylxanthines. Life Sci. 1981;28:2083–2097.
53. Bruns RF, Lu GH, Puglsey TA. Characterization of the A2 adenosine receptor labeled by [3H]NECA in rat striatal membranes. Mol Pharmacol. 1986;29:331–346.
54. Kelly DF, Kozlowski DA, Haddad E, et al. Ethanol reduces metabolic uncoupling following experimental head injury. J Neurotrauma. 2000;17:261–272.
55. Kelly DF, Lee SM, Pinanong PA, Hovda DA. Paradoxical effects of acute ethanolism in experimental brain injury. J Neurosurg. 1997;86:876–882.
56. Statler KD, Kochanek PM, Dixon CE, et al. Fentanyl versus isoflurane anesthesia: Effect on outcome after traumatic brain injury in rats. J Neurotrauma. 1999;16:965.
57. Bickler PE, Buck LT, Hansen BM. Effects of isoflurane and hypothermia on glutamate receptor-mediated calcium influx in brain slices. Anesthesiology. 1994;81:1461–1469.
58. Dildy-Mayfield JE, Eger EI, Harris RA. Anesthetics produce subunit-selective actions on glutamate receptors. J Pharmacol Exp Ther. 1996;276:1058–1065.
59. Statler KD, Kochanek PM, Dixon CE, et al. Isoflurane improves long-term neurologic outcome vs fentanyl after traumatic brain injury in rats. J. Neurotrauma 2000;17:1179–1189.
60. Alexander H, Statler KD, Kochanek PM, et al. Effects of seven anesthetics on outcome in experimental traumatic brain injury. J Neurotrauma 2000;17:792

Coupling and Compartmentation of Cerebral Blood Flow and Metabolism

A. Gjedde

Introduction

Is there a link between brain function and brain energy metabolism? If there is a link, is it important to the understanding of brain function and its organization? To answer these general questions, we must understand at least four relationships which reasonable considerations suggest underlie the link between brain function and brain energy metabolism. These relationships link:

- The function of the brain to the work carried out in the brain (the function-work couple),
- the work of the brain to the cells which carry out the work (cellular compartmentation),
- the cells which carry out the work to the relative and absolute magnitudes of oxidative and non-oxidative energy metabolism of brain (work-metabolism couple), and
- the energy metabolism of the brain to its blood supply (metabolism-flow couple).

The sodium theory defined the work of the excited brain as largely electrochemical, i.e., subserving the transport of ions against their concentration gradients to maintain these gradients. According to the sodium theory, depolarized neurons accumulate extra sodium and lose potassium and thus stimulate the hydrolysis of adenosine triphosphate (ATP) and generation of adenosine diphosphate (ADP) by membrane-bound adenosine triphosphatase (ATPase). The sodium theory assigned this work to neurons and it explained how the generation of ADP in turn would stimulate the oxidative phosphorylation of ADP to ATP. It also suggested that the change of ions, ATP, ADP, or brain metabolites would alter the resistance of the brain vasculature and hence increase blood flow in proportion to the need for oxidative phosphorylation.

A recent alternative theory places the work of the excited brain under the control of a neurochemical process called neurotransmitter cycling (Shulman and Rothman 1998). This process subserves the import and amination of the excitatory amino acid glutamate by astrocytes. According to the theory, the import stimulates the rate of aerobic glycolysis in astrocytes and leads to generation of lactate, which cannot be oxidized in situ but must be exported to neurons, where it undergoes oxidation to carbon dioxide. This theory revives an ancient, now abandoned, claim that astrocytic foot-processes play a nutritive role in brain: The theory claim that the circulation supplies glucose only to astrocytes, which in turn supply lactate to neurons. It is a condition of this claim that the glycolytic and oxidative components of brain metabolism are strictly compartmentalized, aerobic glycolysis taking place only in astrocytes in proportion to the magnitude of glutamatergic neurotransmission, and the combustion of lactate taking place only in neurons in proportion to the rate of glycolysis in astrocytes (Magistretti et al. 1999). The theory is based on a selective interpretation of the evidence to be discussed below, and it is open to rejection by alternative interpretations.

The Brain's Work

Entropy

Energy is the measure of an ability to do work. The calculation of the work of information processing in the brain is based on the concept of entropy, according to which information creates order in a system. The order can be increased only by work which requires a supply of energy and consequent loss of entropy. The identification of information with a loss of entropy is based on the number of ways in which the state of the system can be reached, i.e., on the probability of the state occurring randomly. The lower this probability is, the higher the information content and the lower the entropy are.

The Brain As Intelligent Machine

If electrochemical work is required to support the processing of the information on which the brain as an intelligent system bases its decisions (Szilard 1929), then the work of brain functions should be calculable from the combustion of fuels measured during functional activity of the brain. According to one calculation, a single binary decision, i.e., a unity *bit*, requires a minimum energy supply of 3.10^{-24} kJ (Morowitz 1978). The hydrolysis of ATP yields free energy of about 3.10^{-5} kJ μmol^{-1}. The brain tissue hydrolyzes about 10 μmol^{-1} ATP g^{-1} min^{-1} (see below). Assuming an upper limit of thermodynamic efficiency of 50%, brain tissue would have the capacity to perform binary decisions at the maximum rate of 10^{11} megabytes g^{-1} s^{-1}, or about 10^{18} floating point operations (flops) s^{-1} for one whole-brain. Considering that the largest computer devised by man now has a capacity of about 2 teraflops s^{-1}, half-a-million of these would be required to match the decision-making work and energy flow of a single human brain.

Cognitive Versus Cellular Work

Not all of the brain's work subserves the processing of information; as much as 50% of the average work supports general cellular functions. The proportions of cellular and cognitive work in the brain were estimated in numerous studies, ranging from electrical stimulation of brain slices to measurements of anesthesia

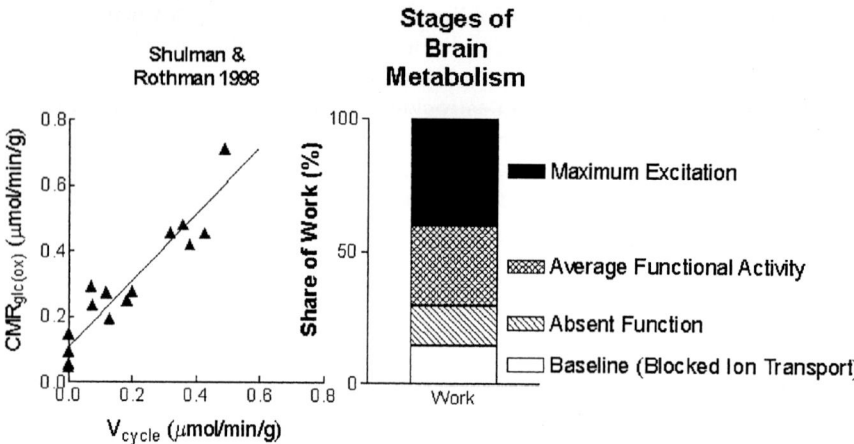

Fig. 1. Stages of brain metabolism in comparison with rate of glutamate cycling and corresponding rate of brain oxidative metabolism measured by Shulman and Rothman (1998)

in animals, and coma and stupor in humans (see Gjedde 1996b). These findings were recently supplemented with magnetic resonance studies of rats at various stages of activity (Shulman and Rothman 1998). A summary of the stages of brain activation gleaned from these studies is presented in Fig. 1. The figure shows that the basic cellular work of brain tissue may represent as little as 10% of the maximally achievable metabolic rate.

Energy Cost of Depolarization

The sodium theory holds that the functioning of the brain itself is non-energy-requiring but the maintenance of the steady-state related to the functioning requires work because the functions depend on the de- and repolarization of neurons. Depolarization is the loss of membrane potential by increased permeability of the neuronal membranes to sodium ions, and repolarization is the subsequent reestablishment of the membrane potential by increased permeability of the membranes to potassium ions. The permeabilities allow the sodium ions to leak into neurons and potassium ions to leak out. The extracellular and intracellular concentrations of sodium and potassium ions established by the leakage stimulate the phosphorylation-type (P-type) Na^+-K^+-ATPase to exchange three intracellular sodium ions for two extracellular potassium ions (Skou 1960), a discovery for which the Aarhus University professor Jens C. Skou received the 1997 Nobel Prize in chemistry.

The ATPase activity simultaneously converts ATP to ADP which much be rephosphorylated. The membrane permeabilities of sodium and potassium form a continuum, each pair associated with a specific magnitude of ion leakage and hence with a specific turnover of ATP, as shown in Fig. 2. The relationship between the membrane potential and the ATP turnover was calculated by Gjedde (1993) on the basis on the Goldman-Hodgkin-Katz constant field equation, the steady-state

Fig. 2. Relationship between sodium and potassium ion permeabilities, membrane potential, and corresponding requirement for oxidative glucose metabolism calculated by Gjedde (1993), on condition a of constant chloride ion permeability of 0.549 ml g^{-1} min^{-1} (see Table 1)

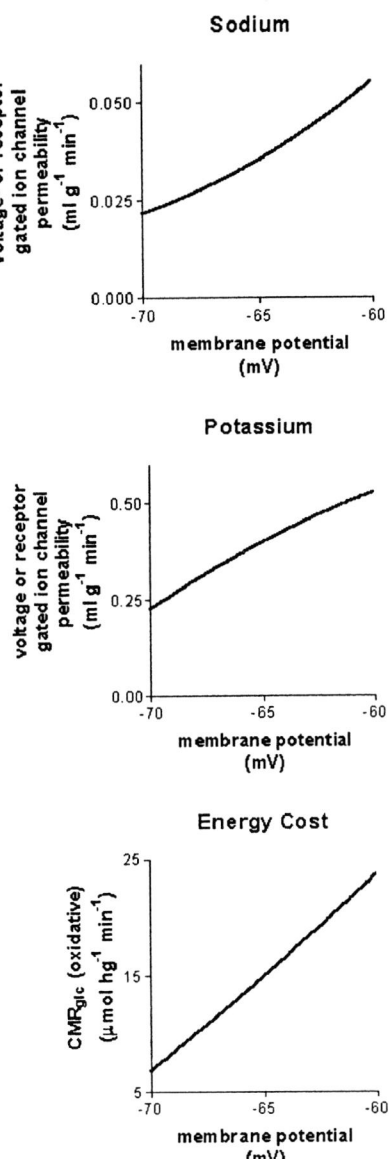

3:2 ratio between the fluxes of sodium and potassium, and a constant chloride permeability.

Figure 2 predicts that the ATP requirements change with the degree of membrane polarization, when the chloride permeability is kept constant. While there is no doubt that the ion fluxes and resulting field potentials change with the functioning of the brain, as evidenced by evoked potential recordings, electroencephalography and magnetoencephalography, the real question is whether the

Table 1. Ion movements across nerve cell membranes

Variable	Unit	Ion Sodium		Potassium		Chloride	
Transmembrane Leakage	μmol g^{-1} min^{-1}	15	36	10	24	5	12
PS product at –65 mV	ml g^{-1} min^{-1}	0.038		0.404		0.549	
PS product at –55 mV	ml g^{-1} min^{-1}	0.044	0.082	0.285	0.617	0.246	0.549

From Gjedde (1993), assuming 50% of ATP turnover dedicated to ion transport, calculated from the concentrations measured by McCormick (1990). To estimate the chloride permeability, it was necessary to use a simplified form of the Goldman-Hodgkin-Katz constant field equation.

steady-state ATP requirements actually change as a function of the potential changes. The analysis underlying Fig. 2 also shows that it is possible to depolarize the membranes without a change of the ion fluxes when the permeabilities of all three ions are allowed to change in a coordinated manner, that of sodium increasing and those of potassium and chloride decreasing. Table 1 lists two membrane potentials with the same fluxes of the sodium, potassium, and chloride ions. In other words, with certain changes of the membrane permeability, neurons may undergo de- and repolarization without actually having to change their ATP turnover and hence without a need to change the rate of oxidative phosphorylation of ADP.

The claim that it possible to maintain different levels of membrane polarization with no change of ATP requirement is of interest to the discussion of where and how the changes of membrane permeability are effected and when neurotransmitter action leads to increased metabolism. There is agreement that the ion fluxes associated with the rapidly changing action potential changes of axonal membranes (AC potentials) are small compared to the fluxes associated with the more slowly changing potentials of pre- and post-synaptic, dendritic and somatic membranes (DC potentials).

Energy Cost of Neurotransmitter Cycling

AC and DC potential changes are effected in different ways, the AC potentials by means of voltage-gated ion channels, the DC potentials by means of receptor-gated ion channels linked to neurotransmitter receptors. The DC potentials are excitatory or inhibitory. The predominant excitatory neurotransmitter in cerebral cortex is glutamate. This excitatory amino acid is stored presynaptically in vesicles and released to the synaptic cleft upon adequate stimulation. From the synaptic cleft, it is reimported into neurons and astrocytes in symport with sodium ions, three sodium ions for each glutamate molecule. The import leads to intracellular accumulation of sodium ions which must be extruded at the expense of ATP, one ATP molecule per glutamate molecule imported. If imported into astrocytes, glutamate must undergo amination to glutamine. Otherwise, the neurotransmitter could not be returned to neurons, as cell membranes are largely impermeable to glutamate but permeable to glutamine. The amination by the glutamine synthase reaction with ammonium ions occurs at the expense of yet another ATP molecule. In addition, there are the costs of vesicular storage and release, perhaps of a similar magnitude as the reuptake and amination of the transmitter.

The study of Shulman and Rothman (1998) indicates that the oxidative cost of the glutamate reuptake and amination is 5% of the total oxidative metabolism of the rat brain. As the need for amination only applies to uptake of glutamate into non-neuronal cells, it is a reasonable estimate that 5–10% of the total energy cost associated with excitation subserves the cost of excitatory neurotransmitter cycling, while the remainder 90–95% subserves the cost of depolarization.

Metabolic Compartmentation

Large and Small Compartments

The two major cell populations of the brain tissue are the neurons and the astrocytes, the latter extending their processes from the perivascular space to the space immediately adjacent to the synaptic cleft. The exact role of the astrocytes in the metabolism and function of the brain has remained a mystery, inviting much speculation about the significance of the peculiar connection between the brain's microvessels and the synapses, its functional elements. One such speculation postulated that astrocytes feed neuron terminals by extracting a steady stream of nutrients directly from the microvessels through the foot processes and delivering these nutrients to immediate vicinity of the terminals (Andriezen 1893). After lingering unconvincingly for decades, this postulate was finally and definitively rejected when Brightman and Reese (1969) proved that the foot processes form no part of the blood-brain barrier, even to the largest macromolecules, and thus could not possibly extract nutrients directly from the capillaries (Brightman et al. 1970).

Newman and Paulson (1987) speculated that astrocytes could carry out the reverse function of siphoning potassium ions from the extrasynaptic to the perivascular space. They reasoned that the inside route through the foot processes would permit the potassium to arrive at the perivascular space with a much lower time constant (66 ms) than if it were left to diffuse through the much more voluminous extracellular space (2.5 s).

Traditionally, the concept of compartmentation refers to the exchange between glutamate and glutamine in large and small compartments of brain tissue (Cremer 1976, Cremer et al. 1979), now generally believed to represent neurons and glial cells, respectively. The compartmentation ensures that glutamate is converted to glutamine in astrocytes. The intriguing question is whether the concept of separation of reactions can be extended to a host of other processes, including some involved in the linking of brain function and metabolism.

In addition to the specific enzymes and transporters involved in the glutamate-glutamine compartmentation, a number of other enzyme and transporter subtypes are differentially expressed in neurons and astrocytes. The most important to the present discussion include the glucose transporters (GLUT-3 vs. the 45 kDa GLUT-1, Drewes 1999), monocarboxylic acid transporters (MCT-1 vs. MCT-2, Gerhart et al. 1997, 1998), excitatory amino acid transporters (EAAT2 vs. EAAT3 in humans, Vandenberg 1998), and lactate dehydrogenases and their associated mRNA (LD_1 vs. LD_5, Tholey et al. 1981, Bittar et al. 1996, Laughton et al. 2000).

Compartmentation of Metabolism

Recent measurements summarized in Fig. 3, indicate that about 30% of the total glucose consumption occurs in glial cells, of which one-sixth (5% of the tissue total) is converted to lactate, while neurons are the sites of 70% of the glucose consumption, of which only one-fourteenth (also 5% of the total) is converted to lactate (Silver and Erecinska 1997, Sokoloff 1999). The capacity of oxidative metabolism is now believed to reflect the habitual level of energy turnover of the cells, averaged over longer periods of time, and is thought to be unchangeable except by sustained stimulation (Hevner et al. 1995).

Oxidative phosphorylation proceeds from pyruvate in near-equilibrium with lactate. If neurons are responsible for 72% (65/90) of this process, the issue of metabolic compartmentation is therefore a question of the origin of the pyruvate which is oxidized in neuronal mitochondria: Which are the relative contributions of neuronal and glial glycolysis to neuronal oxidative phosphorylation? Given the magnitudes of the oxidative and non-oxidative metabolic rates in the two populations of cells, the estimate of the glial origin of the pyruvate oxidized in neurons is 3% (2/65). This percentage may rise during excitation of nervous tissue, of course, depending on the degree of differential activation of the two populations of cells.

Oxidative metabolism is 19 times more efficient than non-oxidative metabolism. For this reason, it is an intriguing coincidence that the fraction of oxidative brain metabolism in the service of neurotransmitter cycling in glia (4.6%) is not unlike the fraction of efficiency ascribed to non-oxidative metabolism (5.3%). Thus, if the fueling of neurotransmitter cycling in glia were entirely non-oxidative and neuronal metabolism entirely oxidative, glycolysis and subsequent oxidative phosphorylation could occur only in response to neurotransmitter cycling.

This coincidence has led to the claim that all glucose supplied to the brain undergoes glycolysis to lactate in astrocytes which in turn supply all their lactate to neurons which themselves take up no glucose (Magistretti et al. 1999). The metabolism of neurons would be entirely oxidative, because all glycolysis would take place in astrocytes, which would have to feed the neurons with all the pyruvate they need.

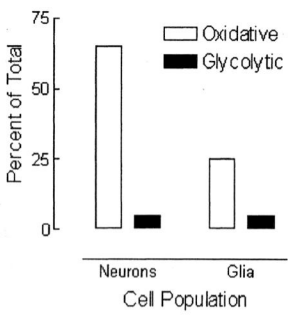

Fig. 3. Proportions of oxidative and glycolytic metabolism in neuronal and glial tissue compartments measured by Silver and Erecinska (1994)

This is an extension of the early claim that astrocytic end-feet serve to siphon glucose from the circulation. The claim was ultimately abandoned when the blood-brain barrier was shown not to include the end-feet. However, there is little direct evidence in favor of the basic oxidativeness of metabolism being substantially different in neurons and glia, nor of a substantial net transfer of lactate to neurons in vivo. In theory, a difference could be imposed by excitation during which the firing frequency may require commensurate time-constants of removal of neurotransmitter which may outstrip the habitually established capacity of the oxidative phosphorylation in glial cells.

Lactate Dehydrogenase

The equilibrium lactate-pyruvate ratio depends on the affinities of the prevailing isozymes of LDH (LD_1-LD_5) towards its two substrates, as influenced by the NAD^+-NADH ratio and the pH, because the K_m of LDH for pyruvate varies with the subtype, the aerobic heart form LD_1 (H_4) having the lowest K^{lact}_m/K^{pyr}_m ratio and the anaerobic muscle and liver form LD_5 (M_4) having the highest K^{lact}_m/K^{pyr}_m ratio (Kaplan and Everse 1972).

The brain has both the H_4 (LD_1), which causes pyruvate to rise quickly for a given increase of glycolysis, and the M_4 (LD_5), which causes pyruvate to rise more slowly (Tholey et al. 1981, Bittar et al. 1996, Laughton et al. 2000). Thus, the higher the ratio between LDH's affinities (i.e., the lower the ratio between the Michaelis constants) for lactate and pyruvate, the more rapid the approach to a new steady-state, with a time constant of $[1 + (K^{lact}_m/K^{pyr}_m/[\Sigma T_{max}/K_t]$ (see equation 3). LDH is also present in mitochondria, apparently with the same distribution of subtypes as in the cytosol, although additional subtypes also have been identified (Brandt et al. 1987).

Transporters

Excitatory Amino Acid Transporters

Astrocytes remove glutamate from excitatory synaptic clefts, where the astrocytic processes engulf the synapses, in humans by means of the glutamate transporters EAAT-1–5 (Vandenberg 1998). Glutamate transporters reside also on neurons but recent gene knock-out studies suggest that the glial EAAT-3 is indispensable for normal brain function, unlike the neuronal EAAT-2 (Tanaka et al. 1997). Knockout or blockade of this transporter inhibits the increase of the rate of glucose phosphorylation in the tissue which accompanies simple somatosensory stimulation of the rat whisker barrels in vivo (Cholet et al. 2001), although it is not known in which tissue compartment or population of cells the inhibition occurs.

Monocarboxylic Acid Transporters

The near-equilibrium between pyruvate and lactate and the abundance of monocarboxylate transporters ensures rapid and reversible exchange between the cellular and extracellular pools of pyruvate and lactate. Pyruvate and lactate cross the membranes of brain tissue by means of facilitative proton-dependent transport catalyzed by the MCT family of membrane spanning proteins (Oldendorf 1973, Halestrap 1975, Poole and Halestrap 1993, Halestrap and Price 1999). In brain tissue, the important transporters appear to be MCT-1 and MCT-2. The MCT-1 protein spans the membranes of the capillary endothelium. Gerhart et al. (1997, 1998) claim that MCT-1 also resides on neurons, while the MCT-2 protein belongs to astrocytes, apparently particularly their foot processes, in disagreement with Broer et al. (1997) who originally assigned MCT-1 to astrocytes and MCT-2 to neurons. As proton symport, the transport is influenced by the pH of the cells. The MCT-2 is of higher affinity than the MCT-1, indicating that it is saturated by pyruvate and lactate at much lower concentrations than the MCT-1. For this reason, the MCT-2 may be more efficient at transporting pyruvate than MCT-1.

Glucose Transporters

Glucose is the source of pyruvate and enters brain tissue, neurons and astrocytes by means of facilitative insulin and sodium insensitive transport by several members of the GLUT family of membrane spanning proteins (Gjedde 1992). In brain, the important members are GLUT-1 and GLUT-3 (Drewes 1999). The 55 kDa GLUT-1 resides in the membranes of the capillary endothelium, while the slightly modified 45 kDa GLUT-1 resides in the membranes of astrocytes and choroid plexus. The GLUT-3 protein resides in the membranes of neurons. The exchange of glucose among the tissue compartments of the brain is essentially equilibrative (Diemer et al. 1985), ensuring that the glucose concentration everywhere in brain tissue is the same substantial fraction of the plasma glucose (Gjedde and Diemer 1983, Silver and Erecinska 1994). The significance of the difference between the subtypes of glucose transporters in neurons and glia is not known.

Oxidative and Non-Oxidative Metabolism

Average Cerebral Metabolic Rate in Awake Humans

Kety (1949) and Lassen (1959) first measured the magnitudes of resting brain energy metabolism and blood flow in human brain. More recently determined resting or average steady-state values of energy metabolism and blood flow of the human brain are listed in Table 2, together with the steady-state turnover rates of ATP and lactate, calculated from the stoichiometric relationships,

$$J_{ATP} = 2 J_{glc} + 6 J_{O_2} \tag{1}$$

and

$$J_{lact} = 2 J_{glc} - \frac{1}{3} J_{O_2} \tag{2}$$

where J_{ATP} is the ATP production, J_{glc} the glucose consumption, and J_{lact} the lactate production. Blood flow and metabolic rates were all measured by positron emission tomography (PET), blood flow by i.v. bolus injection of $[^{15}O]$water according to the method of Ohta et al. (1996), oxygen consumption by single-breath inhalation of $[^{15}O]O_2$ according to the method of Ohta et al.(1992), and glucose consumption by i.v. bolus injection of [^{18}F]fluorodeoxyglucose according to the method of Kuwabara et al.(1990).

In the baseline, total glucose consumption of cerebral cortex is about 30 µmol hg^{-1} min^{-1}. The 10% non-oxidative metabolism leads to a lactate production of 5 µmol hg^{-1} min^{-1}, of which 50% is generated in neurons and 50% in glia according to the oxidative efficiency of the two populations of cells. The lactate flux is about 25% of the T_{max} of the blood-brain barrier MCT-1, consistent with a tissue lactate concentration of 1.5 mM.

Cerebral Metabolic Rate During Brain Activation

Glycolyis

Recent measurements of oxygen consumption during simple primary somatosensory stimulation of human cerebral cortex, summarized in Table 2, generally show little or no change of oxygen consumption of the human brain (Fox and Raichle 1986, Fox et al. 1988, Seitz and Roland 1992, Ohta et al. 1999, Fujita et al 1999).

With the single-inhalation method of measuring oxygen consumption, changes of blood flow and oxygen consumption were compared during 30 minutes of vibrotactile stimulation of one hand's fingers. In primary sensory cortex, the blood flow change was 18% both at the onset of stimulation and still 11% after 20 minutes of stimulation, but the oxygen consumption failed to increase for as long as 30 min (Fujita et al. 1999). Yet, increases of as much as 50% of the rate of glucose phosphorylation were measured during the primary somatosensory stimulations listed in Table 2. Because many of these studies were complicated by the long circulation of tracer fluorodeoxyglucose required to determine glucose consumption accurately (Sokoloff et al. 1977). Kuwabara et al. (1992) and Ribeiro et al. (1993) shortened the method from 45 to 20 minutes, with the same result (Murase et al 1998).

When not coupled to oxidative phosphorylation, even tiny increases of energy demand must of course be accompanied by substantial increases of the glucose supply (Ginsberg et al. 1988). When maximally stimulated, the rate of pyruvate generation can rise to 3–4 µmol hg^{-1} min^{-1} (Robin et al. 1984, Gjedde 1984) which is several fold the calculated maximum velocity of pyruvate oxidation, and close to the calculated T_{max} of the mMCT symporter in mitochondria.

In the absence of an increase of oxidative phosphorylation, a 50% increase of the glucose phosphorylation rate causes the lactate generation to rise to as much as 35 µmol hg^{-1} min^{-1} and the fraction of non-oxidative metabolism to rise from the 10% baseline to as much as 50%, although the total ATP flux rises by a mere 5%. When the rate of generation of lactate exceeds the T_{max} of the blood-brain barrier MCT-1, lactate concentration continues to rise, and the concentration of pyruvate rises with it, until the transport into mitochondria by the mMCT and the rate of the reaction catalyzed by the pyruvate dehydrogenase complex match the rate of generation.

The reason for the failure of the oxygen consumption to increase is not known, but it has long been surmised that oxidative phosphorylation cannot match the 7-fold increase of pyruvate production seen under the most extreme circumstances of glycolytic stimulation of the mammalian brain (van den Berg and Bruntink

Table 2. Neuronal activation of brain metabolism

Stimulus	Duration [min]	Supply			Products	
		ΔF [%]	ΔJ_{glc}	ΔJ_{O_2}	ΔJ_{ATP} [µmol g^{-1} min^{-1}]	ΔJ_{lact}
Simple primary						
Somatosensory	1a	28	[17]	9*	0.96*	0.05
	1b	31	[18]	13*	1.35*	0.03
	1c	18	[8]	−3	0.04	0.04
	20c	11	[8]	−1	0.04	0.04
	20d	18	8	[0]	0.04	0.04
	45e	27	17	[0]	0.10	0.10
Visual (Photic)	30f	43	27	0	0.15	0.15
	45 g	49	51	5*	0.76*	0.26
Complex secondary and motor						
Visual (checkerboard)	5[h] (8 Hz)	25	[28]	28	2.83	0.008
	10[h] (8 Hz)	26	[29]	29	2.93	0.009
	4[i] (1 Hz)	32	[10]	10	1.07	0.004
	4[i] (4 Hz)	38	[16]	16	1.71	0.006
	4[i] (8 Hz)	42	[6]	6	0.64	0.002
Thalamic stimulation	8[j]	88	[47]	47	5.02	0.019
Internal visualization	1[k]	31	[37]	37	3.95	0.015
Tactile learning	1[l]	23	–	–	3.95	0.015
Hand grip	8[m]	30	[40]	40	4.27	0.016

From [a]Fox and Raichle (1986), [b]Seitz and Roland (1992), [c]Fujita et al. (1999), [d]Kuwabara et al. (1992), [e]Ginsberg et al. (1998), [f]Ribeiro et al. (1993), [g]Fox et al. (1998), [h]Marrett and Gjedde (1997), [i]Vafaee and Gjedde (2000), [j]Katayama (1986), [k]Roland et al. (1987), [l]Roland et al. (1989), [m]Raichle (1976), values in brackets are estimates; *J_{O_2} increase not significant.

1983). The time constant for the LDH reaction is of the order of milliseconds, depending on the LDH subtype, while the time constant of the pyruvate sym-porter is of the order of seconds. From the presence of the LDH subtypes LD_1 and LD_5, it is predicted that the increases of pyruvate and lactate would occur with a time constant that is lower for LD_1 than for LD_5.

Given the experimentally observed increases of lactate, it is possible to determine the steady-state lactate-pyruvate concentration ratio by regression of the following equation to the data,

$$\Delta C_{lact}(t) = 2\left[\frac{K_m^{lact}}{K_m^{pyr}}\right]\frac{\Delta J_{glc}}{\left[\sum \frac{T_{max}}{K_t}\right]}\left(1 - e^{-t\left[\sum \frac{T_{max}}{K_t}\right]/\left[1 + \left[\frac{K_m^{lact}}{K_m^{pyr}}\right]\right]}\right)$$

(3)

where ΔJ_{glc} represents the increase of glycolysis, $\sum T_{max}/K_t$ the sum of the clearances of pyruvate into the mitochondrial matrix and across all membranes,

Fig. 4. Estimation of rate constant of lactate increase calculated from measurements reported by Shram et al. (1998). Rate constant is consistent with glycolytic ("white") LDH subtype

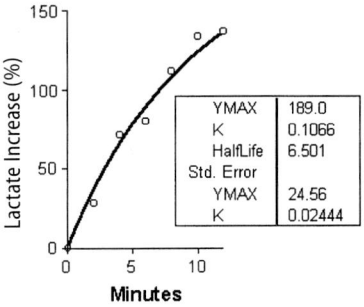

including the endothelium (assuming C_{pyr} always to be small relative to K_t), and K^{lact}_{m}/K^{pyr}_{m} the equilibrium lactate-pyruvate ratio. The equilibrium $\Sigma T_{max}/K_t$ ratio can be calculated from the ratio between the average net rate of glucose consumption and the steady-state pyruvate concentration such that $\Sigma T_{max}/K_t = 2$ J_{glc}/C_{pyr}. With a steady-state pyruvate concentration of 0.1 µmol g^{-1}, the average $\Sigma T_{max}/K_t$ ratio is 6 min^{-1}. Shram et al. (1998) used lactate-sensitive electrodes to measure the increase of lactate shown in Fig. 4 as it occurred after application of the glutamate receptor agonist N-methyl-D-aspartate to brain tissue in vivo. The change is consistent with a steady-state lactate-pyruvate ratio of 55, consistent with the LDH subtype LD$_5$.

Oxidative Phosphorylation

Contrary to the results of no change of oxygen consumption upon simple primary somatosensory stimulation, both motor stimulation and more complex stimulation of visual cortex with a reversing checkerboard pattern for 5 or 10 minutes caused significant increases of oxygen consumption (Raichle 1976, Marrett and Gjedde 1997, Vafaee et al 1998, 1999, Vafaee and Gjedde 2000). The reported values of J_{O_2} and the calculated ATP flux are listed in Table 2.

The reason for the slow initial rise of oxygen consumption may be the slow rise of the pyruvate concentration in the presence of a substantial lactate sink when the bulk of the acceleration of glycolysis occurs in astrocytes. If pyruvate transport were indeed rate-limiting in state 3 activation (Shearman and Halestrap 1984), the consumption of oxygen would depend on the cytosolic pyruvate concentration and hence on the rate of glycolysis as described by the equation,

$$\Delta J_{O_2}(t) = 5.6\Delta J_{glc}(1 - e^{-kt}) \tag{4}$$

where k is the rate constant of the pyruvate and lactate accumulations shown in equation (3) above. The predicted time-course of the increase of oxygen consumption is shown in Fig. 5, according to which the half-time of change is two minutes for a lactate-pyruvate ratio of 15 (LD$_1$, $k=0.375$) but as much as 15 minutes for a ratio of 100 (LD$_5$, $k=0.06$).

Table 2 identifies two kinds of oxidative responses, both relative to baseline, the primary somatosensory response in which the rise of oxygen consumption averages only 10% of the rise of blood flow, and the motor and secondary somatosensory response in which the rise of oxygen consumption averages 75% of the rise of blood

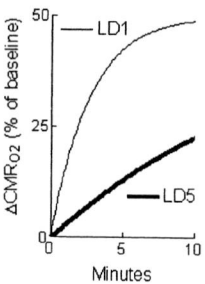

Fig. 5. Estimation of rate of increase of oxidative metabolism for two different rate constants dictated by different subtypes of lactate dehydrogenase, according to equation (4). LD_1 subtype was modeled with rate constant $k=0.375^{-1}$, LD_5 subtype with rate constant $k=0.050$ min^{-1}

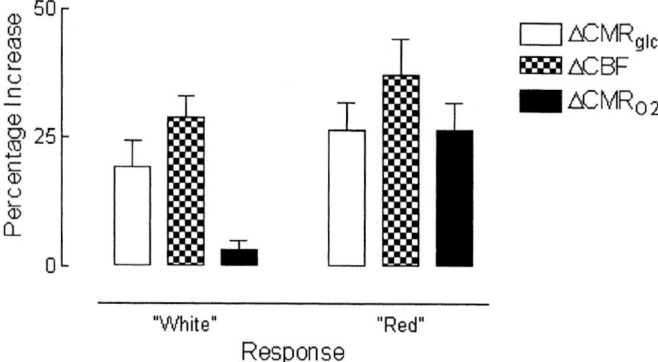

Fig. 6. Relative increases of glycolysis, blood flow, and oxidative metabolism, estimated for the two categories of stimulation (simple primary somatosensory, "white"; and complex secondary somatosensory or motor, "red") listed in Table 2

flow. The average primary somatosensory response is a 3% increase of CMR_{O_2} for a 29% increase of CBF, while the average motor and secondary somatosensory response is a 27% increase of CMR_{O_2} for a 39% increase of CBF (see Fig. 6).

From the oxidativeness of the complex secondary somatosensory and motor responses, it is to be expected that the rise of oxygen consumption after an acute stimulation of glycolysis would reflect a rise of pyruvate concentration indicative of LD_1, the subtype of LDH claimed to be characteristic of tissues with a comparatively high ratio of oxidative to glycolytic metabolism. Marrett and Gjedde (1997) determined the time-course of increase of oxygen consumption shown in Fig. 7: Upon complex checkerboard stimulation of the visual system, the oxygen consumption rose at a rate of 0.44 min^{-1}, which is consistent with a steady-state lactate-pyruvate ratio of 13, and hence with the presence of LD_1 in the cells so stimulated.

Blood Flow Regulation

It is puzzling that oxygen consumption sometimes does not rise at all upon stimulation of brain tissue (primary somatosensory stimulation, e.g., vibrotactile stimula-

Fig. 7. Estimation of rate constant of increase of oxidative metabolism calculated from measurements reported by Marrett and Gjedde (1997). Rate constant is consistent with "aerobic" ("red") LDH subtype LD_1 ($k=0.445$ min^{-1})

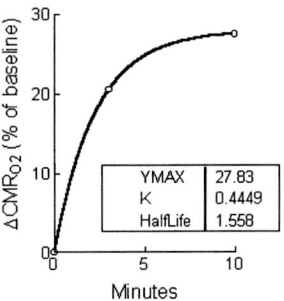

YMAX	27.83
K	0.4449
HalfLife	1.558

tion), despite an increase of blood flow, suggesting either that additional factors prevent neurons from using the available oxygen, or that the blood flow rises to satisfy other needs than a demand for oxygen. It may be important that blood flow supplies substances other than oxygen, including glucose and amino acids, and removes substances such as water, lactate, pyruvate, hydrogen ions, and carbon dioxide.

Blood Flow in Service of Glucose Delivery

The responses of blood flow to stimulation of brain tissue show that on the average the flow change is independent of the oxidativeness of the metabolic response but they also show that the blood flow response generally exceeds the response of oxidative metabolism. Thus, there seems to be little direct relation between the rise of blood flow and the demand for oxygen. In contrast, the relationship between the rise of blood flow and the rise of glucose consumption appears to be almost linear as shown in Fig. 6.

The findings suggest that a signal from glycolysis elicits the blood flow increase, also when no additional oxygen is used. The absent use of additional oxygen may be physiological (absent post-synaptic depolarization in cases of inhibition, absent calcium ion accumulation in mitochondria), as in the cases of primary somatosensory stimulation, or pathological, as in cases of ischemia or hypoxemia. This suggestion raises the questions of the agent which mediates the increase of blood flow in the absence of an increased need for oxygen, and of the situations in which the demand for glucose is increased but the demand for oxygen is not. There is evidence that this agent may be potassium ions in situations in which the extracellular depolarization is not induced by a glutamate release. In these situations, the need for glutamate transport into glial cells may be greatly elevated.

Potassium

Neuronal excitation raises the extracellular potassium and glutamate ion concentrations. Both are imported by glia but in different ways. Potassium enters astrocytes by several non-energy-requiring routes, as well as in response to glutamate import. The glutamate symport with sodium activates the P-type ATP-ase which exchanges the intracellular sodium ions with extracellular potassium ions. Only the process linked to glutamate transport represents an energy-requiring net transfer of potassium ions from neurons to astrocytes via the extracellular space (Takahashi et al. 1997, Longuemare et al. 1999).

Glutamate is released when excitatory neurons fire but the degree of resulting post-synaptic depolarization and activation depends on the sum of excitatory and inhibitory impulses converging on the post-synaptic neurons. In the conditions of post-synaptic inhibition, post-synaptic loss of potassium can be prevented when opposite changes of sodium, and potassium and chloride, ion permeabilities clamp the ion fluxes to some resting average value, as exemplified in Table 1. The primary energy-demanding process in this situation would be the removal of the glutamate released from the excitatory pre-synaptic terminals, which leads to accumulation of potassium in astrocytes. Because of the high membrane permeability to potassium ions, this potassium escapes passively to the extracellular space surrounding astrocytes, including the perivascular space surrounding capillaries.

Newman and Paulson (1987) speculated that potassium released passively to the perivascular space may cause relaxation of smooth muscle and dilatation of resistance vessels and hence increased blood flow. They reasoned that the time constant of delivery of potassium to the perivascular space is much smaller when the potassium is siphoned to the vessels inside the foot processes (66 ms) than when the potassium is left to diffuse through the extracellular space (2.5 s). The lower time constant may assure an immediate increase of blood flow to match the increase of glycolysis induced by the removal of glutamate.

The role of potassium ions in mediating functionally induced increases of blood flow in the brain was tested by Caesar et al. (1999), who found that the relative contributions of extracellularly applied potassium ions and adenosine to the blood flow regulation in cerebellum varied among the cell populations, potassium (and nitric oxide) having the greatest effect in parallel fiber connections, and adenosine (and nitric oxide) having the greatest effect in climbing fiber connections.

Lactate

Minimal post-synaptic depolarization would have two important consequences: Post-synaptic mitochondrial dehydrogenases would not be activated by calcium, but astrocytes nevertheless would be stimulated to remove glutamate rapidly, hence possibly exceeding their oxidative capacity and generating lactate to be metabolized neither in neurons nor in astrocytes. Lactate generation could reflect the situation in which glutamate is released but excitation is subliminal and post-synaptic depolarization is prevented by parallel inhibitory input. Mathiesen et al. (1998) showed that stimulation of cerebellar neurons in some cases led to increased blood flow despite partly GABAergic inhibition of post-synaptic spiking activity, presumably by prevention of post-synaptic depolarization.

Thus, in inhibited or otherwise uncommonly excited states it is possible that rapid removal of glutamate (Kojima et al. 1999), achievable only by glycolysis, may generate pyruvate in excess of the average oxidative capacity of glial cells. Thus, although recent measurements of the relative contributions of oxidative phosphorylation to the energy turnover in neurons and astrocytes suggest that only 30% of the total resting average energy conversion of brain tissue takes place in astrocytes, the astrocytes may contribute significantly more to the increase of non-oxidative metabolism when excitation of post-synaptic neurons is prevented by parallel inhibition. Skeletal muscle studies confirm that a correlation exists between the increase of blood flow and the increase of lactate (Connett et al. 1985), and Laptook et al. (1988) showed that lactate may contribute to the regulation of cerebral blood flow. The increased blood flow would contribute to the removal of the lactate from brain tissue, but the generated lactate would not be oxidized in neurons unless their oxidative metabolism were similarly stimulated.

Blood Flow in Service of Oxygen Delivery

Diffusion-Limited Oxygen Transport

The mechanism underlying the regulation of oxygen delivery is important to the issues of physiologic and pathologic re- or uncoupling of flow and metabolism during changes of brain activity (Gjedde 1996a, 1996b). A recent hypothesis claims that blood flow must rise to supply more oxygen during excitation of brain tissue to maintain a constant mitochondrial oxygen tension in brain tissue. At a constant mitochondrial oxygen tension, oxygen consumption depends solely on the mean capillary oxygen tension for a given capillary density. Sudden changes of brain function are subserved by changes of blood flow which adjust the mean capillary oxygen tension upwardly. Oxygen extraction fraction declines with higher blood flow rates, thus establishing a higher average capillary partial pressure of oxygen and a higher oxygen saturation of hemoglobin.

Cytochrome c oxidase cannot remain saturated if the mitochondrial P_{O_2} declines relative to the average capillary P_{O_2} when an imbalance exists between the delivery of oxygen and the cytochrome oxidase activity. The imbalance can be expressed as a simple Michaelis-Menten relationship between the mitochondrial oxygen tension and the kinetic properties of the cytochrome oxidase,

$$J_{O_2} = V_{max}^{cytox} \sigma_e \sigma_{O_2} \tag{5}$$

where J_{O_2} is the net oxygen consumption, V_{max}^{cytox} is the maximum cytochrome c oxidase reaction rate, and σ_e and σ_{O_2} are the cytochrome c oxidase saturation fractions for electrons and oxygen, respectively. The oxygen tension in mitochondria $P_{O_2}^{mit}$ is the tension consistent with the observed oxygen consumption rate relative to the half-saturation tension (P_{50}^{cytox}),

$$P_{O_2}^{mit} = \frac{P_{50}^{cytox} J_{O_2}}{\left(\sigma V_{max}^{cytox}\right) - J_{O_2}} \tag{6}$$

from which it follows that the average capillary oxygen tension ($P_{O_2}^{cap}$) driving the delivery is given by

$$P_{O_2}^{cap} = J_{O_2} \left[\frac{1}{L} + \frac{P_{50}^{cytox}}{\left(\sigma_e V_{max}^{cytox}\right) - J_{O_2}} \right] \tag{7}$$

where L is the oxygen diffusion capacity. The equation is illustrated in Fig. 8, which shows the resulting mitochondrial oxygen tension and rate of oxygen consump-

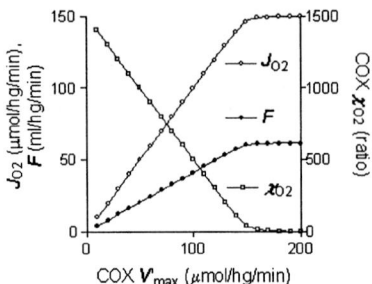

Fig. 8. Oxygen diffusion capacity ceiling of oxidative metabolism in brain, calculated from equations (7) and (11). Abscissa is cytochrome oxidase ("cox") activity ($V'_{max} = \sigma_e V_{max}$), ordinates are (left) oxygen consumption and blood flow at constant ratio, and (right) mitochondrial oxygen tension relative to cytochrome oxidase ("cox") half-saturation tension ($J_{O_2}^{max} = P_{O_2}^{cap}$ 150 = μmol hg-1 min-1, $J_{O_2}^{max} + J_{50}^{cytox} = P_{O_2}^{cap} + P_{50}^{hb}$ 150.1 = μmol hg-1 min-1)

tion for a range of cytochrome oxidase activities ($\sigma_e V^{cytox}_{max}$), given a constant capillary oxygen tension, established by a constant oxygen extraction fraction, and hence a constant ratio between oxygen consumption and blood flow (linear flow-metabolism coupling). Figure 8 shows that the rate of oxygen consumption fails to rise above a certain threshold despite further increases of the cytochrome oxidase activity. The threshold is dictated by the mitochondrial oxygen tension and is reached when the tension declines below the level associated with sufficient oxygen saturation of the cytochrome oxidase. Only increases of the oxygen diffusion capacity (recruitment) or the mean capillary oxygen tension (increased blood flow) allow the rate of oxygen consumption to rise above this threshold.

Oxygenation of Hemoglobin in Brain

The kinetic analysis of cytochrome oxidase activity shown in Fig. 8 revealed that increases of blood flow above the increase of oxygen consumption may deliver additional oxygen during excitation, when a decline of the mitochondrial oxygen tension threatens to reduce the oxygen saturation of cytochrome oxidase. At this threshold, oxygen consumption depends solely on the mean capillary oxygen tension for a given capillary density, and sudden changes of brain function must be subserved by changes of blood flow which adjust the mean capillary oxygen tension in the required direction.

We previously presented a simple one-dimensional model of oxygen diffusion to brain tissue (Gjedde 1996b, Vafaee and Gjedde 2000) to answer the question whether blood flow must rise to deliver more oxygen during functional activation. The model is based on the claim that the average capillary oxygen saturation of hemoglobin is a function of the net extraction of oxygen, assuming a reasonably even distribution of the oxygen delivery along the length of all capillaries,

$$\overline{S}_{O_2} = 1 - \frac{E_{O_2}}{2} \tag{8}$$

where $\overline{S}_{O_2}$ is the average capillary oxygen saturation of hemoglobin and E_{O_2} is the unidirectional oxygen extraction fraction, equal to the net oxygen extraction fraction when the tissue oxygen tension is negligible. The average capillary oxygen tension and average capillary hemoglobin saturation with oxygen are also related by the equation for the oxygen dissociation curve,

$$\bar{S}_{O_2} = \cfrac{1}{1 + \left[\cfrac{P^{hb}_{50}}{P^{cap}_{O_2}} \right]^h} \tag{9}$$

where P^{hb}_{50} is the hemoglobin half-saturation oxygen tension. The resulting equation establishes the inverse correlation between the net extraction fraction and the average capillary oxygen tension,

$$\bar{P}^{cap}_{O} = \sqrt[h]{\frac{2}{E_{O_2}} - 1} \tag{10}$$

where h is the Hill coefficient and E_{O_2} is the ratio J_{O_2}/FC_{O_2}, where F is the blood flow, and C_{O_2} is the arterial oxygen concentration. When the maximum delivery capacity is reached, the delivery is a function of the average capillary oxygen tension according to the relationship,

$$J^{max}_{O_2} = L\bar{P}^{cap}_{O_2} \tag{11}$$

where $J^{max}_{O_2}$ is the maximum oxygen delivery capacity and L is the average tissue oxygen diffusion capacity between the capillary lumen and the mitochondria. The relationship between the maximum oxygen delivery capacity and the blood flow estimated by means of this equation is shown in Fig. 9.

The degree of hemoglobin saturation is measurable by magnetic resonance imaging as the blood-oxygenation-level-dependent (BOLD) contrast due to the presence of deoxyhemoglobin. The measurements confirm that brain activity generally leads to increases of venous hemoglobin oxygenation, as evidenced by the decline of signal losses due to the paramagnetic deoxyhemoglobin (Ogawa et al. 1990, Kwong et al. 1992).

Fig. 9. Model of maximum oxygen delivery capacity ($J^{max}_{O_2}$) in non-linear relation to blood flow, as presented by Gjedde (1996b) and Vafaee and Gjedde (2000). The maximum oxygen delivery capacities were calculated from equations (10) and (11)

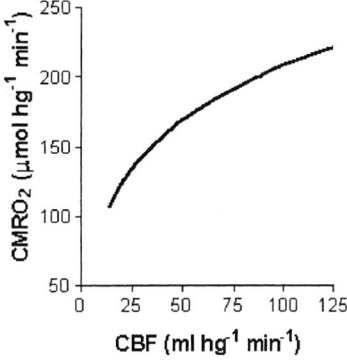

Nitric Oxide

Blood flow regulation is important to the maintenance of a constant oxygen tension in mitochondria, and neuronal activation can mediate blood flow changes by means of the endothelium-derived relaxation factor (EDRF) nitric oxide (NO). Many blood flow stimulators act by means of NO, including carbon dioxide and hydrogen ions which are products of oxidative metabolism (Iadecola 1992, Iadecola et al. 1994, Fabricius and Lauritzen 1994, Villringer and Dirnagl 1995). NO causes vasodilatation of brain resistance vessels, in addition to other effects. It is synthesized in neurons (and endothelial cells) in proportion to the cytosolic concentration of unbound calcium and is generated in reactions catalyzed by cell-specific NO synthases (NOS), either endothelial (eNOS) or neuronal (nNOS), of which nNOS is by far the most abundant.

It is not clear to which extent only nNOS activation is involved in functionally induced increases of cerebral blood flow. It is known that blocking of the vascular receptors suspected of being involved in the synthesis of nitric oxide by eNOS abolishes functionally induced blood flow increases, and focal changes of cortical blood flow induced by sensory stimulation can be eliminated by blocking endothelial acetylcholine receptors (Ogawa et al. 1994), including those involved in mediating synthesis of NO. Yet the underlying cellular activation (whether glial or neuronal) is unimpeded, as indicated by increased glycolysis (Ogawa et al. 1994), suggesting either that nNOS activation is not involved in the increase of glycolysis, or that eNOS activation is not required for the neuronal activation. Other evidence suggests that the cerebral vasodilatation associated with simple somatosensory stimulation in rodents is mediated by nNOS activity (Ayata et al. 1996, Ma et al. 1996, Cholet et al. 1997).

Conclusions

There are few facts in evidence of a rigid association in vivo between *changes* of oxygen consumption, glucose combustion, and blood flow in the human brain. The claim that blood flow must somehow equally satisfy the demands for oxygen and glucose during excitation is therefore without foundation. It is important to note that Roy and Sherrington (1890) measured neither glucose nor oxygen consumption. They observed pial *vasodilatation* after administration of post-mortem brain extracts to living animals. They surmised that a metabolite had caused the dilatation and that that metabolite might be lactate.

The theoretical analysis suggests that the cerebral energy demand reflects the steady-state level of post-synaptic membrane depolarization. Substantial increases of net energy turnover are required neither for neuronal inhibition caused by increased chloride conductance, nor for increased action potential frequency per se. Increased energy turnover is not required to sustain hyperpolarization caused by decreased conductance of sodium or increased conductance of potassium. Increased energy supply is only required to maintain dendritic and/or somatic membrane depolarization in the state of increased sodium and potassium conductances.

Substantial lactate generation may occur when glutamate release is not followed by post-synaptic depolarization. In these case, there may be a demand for glutamate removal of a magnitude exceeding the sum of the average glial and neuronal oxidative capacities. This lactate can be removed only by the circulation. The suggestion is consistent with the observation that simple primary somatosensory stimulation elicits a rapid 'white' metabolic response which may be of glial origin, while the bulk of the motor or complex secondary somatosensory excitation leads to a 'red' metabolic response which is primarily of neuronal origin.

References

Andriezen WL (1893)The neuroglia elements in the human brain. Brit Med J ii: 227–230

Ayata C, Ma J, Meng W, Huang P, Moskowitz MA (1996) L-NA-sensitive rCBF augmentation during vibrissal stimulation in type III nitric oxide synthase mutant mice. J Cereb Blood Flow Metab 16: 539–541

van den Berg CJ, Bruntink R (1983) Glucose oxidation in the brain during seizures: Experiments with labeled glucose and deoxyglucose. In: Hertz L, Kvamme E, McGeer EG, Schousboe A (eds) Glutamine, Glutamate and GABA in the Central Nervous System, Alan R Liss, New York, pp. 619–624.

Bittar PG, Charnay Y, Pellerin L, Bouras C, Magistretti PJ (1996) Selective distribution of lactate dehydrogenase isoenzymes in neurons and astrocytes of human brain. J Cereb Blood Flow Metab 16: 1079–1089.

Brandt RB, Laux JE, Spainhour SE, Kline ES (1987) Lactate dehydrogenase in rat mitochondria. Arch Biochem Biophys 259: 412–422.

Brightman MW; Reese TS (1969) Junctions between intimately apposed cell membranes in the vertebrate brain. J Cell Biol 40: 648–677.

Brightman MW; Klatzo I; Olsson Y; Reese TS (1970) The blood-brain barrier to proteins under normal and pathological conditions. J Neurol Sci 110: 215–239.

Broer S; Rahman B; Pellegri G; Pellerin L; Martin JL; Verleysdonk S; Hamprecht B; Magistretti PJ (1997) Comparison of lactate transport in astroglial cells and monocarboxylate transporter 1 (MCT 1) expressing Xenopus laevis oocytes. Expression of two different monocarboxylate transporters in astroglial cells and neurons. J Biol Chem 272: 30096–30102.

Caesar K, Akgoren N, Mathiesen C, Lauritzen M (1999) Modification of activity-dependent increases in cerebellar blood flow by extracellular potassium in anaesthetized rats. J Physiol (Lond) 520: 281–292.

Cholet N, Seylaz J, Lacombe P, Bonvento G (1997) Local uncoupling of the cerebrovascular and metabolic responses to somatosensory stimulation after neuronal nitric oxide synthase inhibition. J Cereb Blood Flow Metab 17: 1191–1201.

Cholet N, Pellerin L, Welker E, Lacombe P, Seylaz J, Magistretti P, Bonvento G (2001) Local injection of antisense oligonucleotides targeted to the glial glutamate transporter GLAST decreases the metabolic response to somatosensory activation. J Cereb Blood Flow Metab 21:404–412

Connett RJ, Gayeski TE, Honig CR (1985) Energy sources in fully aerobic rest-work transitions: A new role for glycolysis. Am J Physiol 248: H922-H929.

Cremer JE (1976) The influence of liver-bypass on transport and compartmentation in vivo. Adv Exp Med Biol 69: 95–102.

Cremer JE, Cunningham VJ, Pardridge WM, Braun LD, Oldendorf WH (1979) Kinetics of blood-brain barrier transport of pyruvate, lactate and glucose in suckling, weanling and adult rats. J Neurochem 33: 439–446.

Diemer NH, Benveniste H, Gjedde A (1985) In vivo cell membrane permeability to deoxyglucose in rat brain. Acta Neurol Scand 72: 87.

Drewes L (1999) Transport of brain fuels, glucose and lactate. In: Paulson OB, Knudsen GM, Moos T (eds.) Brain Barrier Systems, Alfred Benzon Symposium 45, Munksgaard, Copenhagen, pp. 285–295.

Fabricius M, Lauritzen M (1994) Examination of the role of nitric oxide for the hypercapnic rise of cerebral blood flow in rats. Am J Physiol 266: H1457–1464.

Fox PT, Raichle ME (1986) Focal physiological uncoupling of cerebral blood flow and oxidative metabollism during somatosensory stimulation in human subjects. Proc Natl Acad Sci USA 83: 1140–1144.

Fox PT, Raichle ME, Mintun MA, Dence CE (1988) Nonoxidative glucose consumption during focal physiological activity. Science 241: 462–464.

Fujita H, Kuwabara H, Reutens DC, Gjedde A (1999) Oxygen consumption of cerebral cortex fails to increase during continued vibrotactile stimulation. J Cereb Blood Flow Metab 19: 266–271.

Gerhart DZ, Enerson BE, Zhdankina OY, Leino RL, Drewes LR (1997) Expression of monocarboxylate transporter MCT1 by brain endothelium and glia in adult and suckling rats. Am J Physiol 273: E207–213.

Gerhart DZ, Enerson BE, Zhdankina OY, Leino RL, Drewes LR (1998) Expression of the monocarboxylate transporter MCT2 by rat brain glia. Glia 22: 272–281.

Ginsberg MD, Chang JY, Kelley RE, Yoshii F, Barker WW, Ingento G, Boothe TE (1988) Increases in both cerebral glucose utilization and blood flow during execution of a somatosensory task. Ann Neurol 23: 152–160.

Gjedde A (1984) On the measurement of glucose in brain. Neurochem Res 9: 1667–1671.

Gjedde A, Diemer NH (1983) Autoradiographic determination of regional brain glucose content. J Cereb Blood Flow Metab 3: 303–310.

Gjedde A, Ohta S, Kuwabara H, Meyer E (1991) Is oxygen diffusion limiting for blood-brain transfer of oxygen? In Lassen NA, Ingvar DH, Raichle ME, Friberg L (eds.) Brain Work and Mental Activity, Alfred Benzon Symposium 31, Munksgaard, Copenhagen, pp. 177–184.

Gjedde A (1992) Blood-brain glucose transfer. In: Physiology and Pharmacology of the Blood-Brain Barrier, Chapter 6a: Handbook of Experimental Pharmacology, MWB Bradbury, ed. Springer-Verlag, Berlin Heidelberg 1992, pp. 65–115.

Gjedde A (1993) The energy cost of neuronal depolarization. In Gulyas B, Ottoson D, Roland PE (eds.) Functional Organization of the Human Visual Cortex, Pergamon Press, Oxford, pp. 291–306.

Gjedde A (1996a) PET criteria of cerebral tissue viability in ischemia. Acta Neurol Scand 93: 3–5.

Gjedde A (1996b) The relation between brain function and cerebral blood flow and metabolism. Chapter 2, Cerebrovascular Disease (ed Batjer HH). Lippincott-Raven, Philadelphia, pp. 23–40.

Halestrap AP (1975) The mitochondrial pyruvate carrier. Biochem J 148: 85–96.

Halestrap AP (1978) Stimulation of pyruvate transport in metabolizing mitochondria through changes in the transmembrane pH gradient induced by glucagon treatment of rat. Biochem J 172: 389–398.

Halestrap AP, Armston AE (1984) A re-evaluation of the role of mitochondrial pyruvate transport in the hormonal control of rat liver mitochondrial pyruvate metabolism. Biochemical Journal 223: 677–85.

Halestrap AP, Price NT (1999) The proton-linked monocarboxylate transporter (MCT) family: structure, function and regulation. Biochem J 343: 281–299.

Hevner RF; Liu S; Wong-Riley MT (1995) A metabolic map of cytochrome oxidase in the rat brain: histochemical, densitometric and biochemical studies. Neuroscience 65: 313–342

Iadecola C (1992) Does nitric oxide mediate the increases in cerebral blood flow elicited by hypercapnia? Proc Natl Acad Sci U S A. 89: 3913–3916.

Iadecola C, Pelligrino DA, Moskowitz MA, Lassen NA (1994) Nitric oxide synthase inhibition and cerebrovascular regulation. J Cereb Blood Flow Metab 14: 175–192.

Kaplan NO, Everse J (1972) Regulatory characteristics of lactate dehydrogenases. Adv Enzyme Regul 10: 323–336.

Kety SS (1949) The physiology of the human cerebral circulation. Anesthesiology 10: 610–614.

Kojima S, Nakamura T, Nidaira T, Nakamura K, Ooashi N, Ito E, Watase K, Tanaka K, Wada K, Kudo Y, Miyakawa H (1999) Optical detection of synaptically induced glutamate transport in hippocampal slices. J Neurosci 19: 2580–2588:

Kuwabara H, Evans AC, Gjedde A (1990) Michaelis-Menten constraints improved cerebral glucose metabolism and regional lumped constant measurements with [^{18}F]fluoro-deoxyglucose. J Cereb Blood Flow Metab 10: 180–189.

Kuwabara H, Ohta S, Brust P, Meyer E, Gjedde A (1992) Density of perfused capillaries in living human brain during functional activation. Progr Brain Res 91: 209–215.

Kwong KK; Belliveau JW; Chesler DA; Goldberg IE; Weisskoff RM; Poncelet BP; Kennedy DN; Hoppel BE; Cohen MS; Turner R; et al (1992) Dynamic magnetic resonance imaging of human brain activity during primary sensory stimulation. Proc-Natl-Acad-Sci-U-S-A 89: 5675–5679.

Laptook AR, Peterson J, Porter AM (1988) Effects of lactic acid infusions and pH on cerebral blood flow and metabolism. J Cereb Blood Flow Metab 8: 193–200.

Lassen NA (1959) Cerebral blood flow and oxygen consumption in man. Physiol Rev 39: 183–238.

Laughton JD, Charnay Y, Belloir B, Pellerin L, Magistretti PJ, Bouras C (2000) Differential messenger RNA distribution of lactate dehydrogenase LDH-1 and LDH-5 isoforms in the rat brain. Neuroscience 96: 619–625.

Longuemare MC, Rose CR, Farrell K, Ransom BR, Waxman SG, Swanson RA (1999) K(+)-induced reversal of astrocyte glutamate uptake is limited by compensatory changes in intracellular Na+. Neuroscience 93: 285–292.

Ma J, Ayata C, Huang PL, Fishman MC, Moskowitz MA (1996) Regional cerebral blood flow response to vibrissal stimulation in mice lacking type I NOS gene expression. Am J Physiol 270: H1085–1090.

Magistretti PJ, Pellerin L, Rothman DL, Shulman RG (1999) Energy on demand. Science 283: 496–497.

Marrett S, Gjedde A (1997) Changes of blood flow and oxygen consumption in visual cortex of living humans. Adv Exp Med Biol 413: 205–208.

Mathiesen C, Caesar K, Akgoren N, Lauritzen M (1998) Modification of activity-dependent increases of cerebral blood flow by excitatory synaptic activity and spikes in rat cerebellar cortex. J Physiol (Lond) 512: 555–566.

McCormick DA (1990) Membrane properties and neurotransmitter actions. In Shepherd G (ed.) The Synaptic Organization of the Brain, 3rd Ed., Oxford University Press, New York, pp. 32–66.

Morowitz HJ (1978) Foundations of Bioenergetics. Academic Press, New York.

Murase K, Kuwabara H, Yasuhara Y, Evans AC, Gjedde A (1996) Mapping of change in cerebral glucose utilization using fluorine-18 fluorodeoxyglucose double injection and the constrained weighted-integration method. IEEE Transact Med Imag 15: 824–835.

Ogawa M, Magata Y, Ouchi Y, Fukuyama H, Yamauchi H, Kimura J, Yonekura Y, Konishi J (1994) Scopolamine abolishes cerebral blood flow response to somatosensory stimulation in anesthetized cats: PET study. Brain Res 650: 249–252.

Ogawa S, Lee TM, Nayak AS, et al. (1990a) Oxygenation-sensitive contrast in magnetic resonance imaging of rodent brain at high magnetic fields. Magn Reson Med 14: 68–78.

Ogawa S; Lee TM; Kay AR; Tank DW (1990b) Brain magnetic resonance imaging with contrast dependent on blood oxygenation. Proc Natl Acad Sci USA 87: 9868–72.

Ogawa S; Menon RS; Tank DW; Kim SG; Merkle H; Ellermann JM; Ugurbil K (1993) Functional brain mapping by blood oxygenation level-dependent contrast magnetic resonance imaging. A comparison of signal characteristics with a biophysical model. Biophys-J 64: 803–12.

Ohta S, Meyer E, Thompson CJ and Gjedde A (1992) Oxygen consumption of the living human brain measured after a single inhalation of positron emitting oxygen. J Cereb Blood Flow Metab 12: 179–192.

Ohta S, Meyer E, Fujita H, Reutens DC, Evans A, Gjedde A (1996) Cerebral [O-15]water clearance in humans determined by PET. I. Theory and normal values. J Cereb Blood Flow Metab 16: 765–780.

Ohta S, Reutens DC, Gjedde A (1999) Brief vibrotactile stimulation does not increase cortical oxygen consumption when measured by single inhalation of positron emitting oxygen. J Cereb Blood Flow Metab 19:} 260–265.

Oldendorf WH (1973) Carrier-mediated blood-brain barrier transport of short-chain monocarboxylic organic acids. Am J Physiol 224: 1450–1453.

Pardridge WM (1981) Transport of nutrients and hormones through the blood-brain barrier. Diabetologia 20: 246–254.

Paulson OB, Newman EA (1987) Does the release of potassium from astrocyte endfeet regulate cerebral blood flow? Science 237: 896–898.

Pette D (1985) Metabolic heterogeneity of muscle fibres. J Exp Biol 115: 179–189.

Poole RC, Halestrap AP (1993) Transport of lactate and other monocarboxylates across mammalian plasma membranes. Am J Physiol 264: C761–82.

Ribeiro L, Kuwabara H, Meyer E, Fujita H, Marrett S, Evans A, Gjedde A (1993) Cerebral blood flow and metabolism during nonspecific bilateral visual stimulation in normal subjets. In Uemura K, Lassen NA, Jones T, Kanno I (eds.) Quantification of Brain Function. Tracer Kinetics and Image Analysis in Brain PET, Elsevier, Amsterdam, pp. 217–224.

Robin ED, Murphy BJ, Theodore J (1984) Coordinate regulation of glycolysis by hypoxia in mammalian cells. J Cell Physiol 118: 287–290.

Roy CS, Sherrington CS (1890) On the regulation of the blood supply of the brain. J Physiol (Lond) 11: 85–108.

Seitz RJ, Roland PE (1992) Vibratory stimulation increases and decreases the regional cerebral blood flow and oxidative metabolism: A positron emission tomography (PET) study. Acta Neurol Scand 86: 60–67.

Shalit MN, Beller AJ, Feinsod M, Drapkin AJ, Cotev S (1970) The blood flow and oxygen consumption of the dying brain. Neurology 20: 740–748.

Shalit MN, Beller AJ, Feinsod M (1972) Clinical equivalents of cerebral oxygen consumption in coma. Neurology 22: 155–160.

Shearman MS, Halestrap AP (1894) The concentration of the mitochondrial pyruvate carrier in rat liver and heart mitochondria determined with alpha-cyano-beta-(1-phenylindol-3-yl)acrylate. Biochemical Journal 223: 673–676.

Shram NF, Netchiporouk LI, Martelet C, Jaffrezic-Renault N, Bonnet C, Cespuglio R (1998) In vivo voltammetric detection of rat brain lactate with carbon fiber microelectrodes coated with lactate oxidase. Anal Chem. 1998 Jul 1; 70(13):2618–22.

Shulman RG, Rothman DL (1998) Interpreting functional imaging studies in terms of neurotransmitter cycling. Proc Natl Acad Sci U S A. 95: 11993–11998.

Silver IA, Erecinska M (1994) Extracellular glucose concentration in mammalian brain: Continous monitoring of changes during increased neuronal activity and upon limitation in oxygen supply in normo-, hypo-, and hyperglycemic animals. J Neurosci 14: 5068–5076.

Silver IA, Erecinska M (1997) Energetic demands of the Na+/K+ ATPase in mammalian astrocytes. Glia 21: 35–45.

Skou JC (1960) Further investigations on a Mg^{++}-Na^+-activated adenosine-triphospha-tase, possibly related to the active, linked transport of Na^+ and K^+ across the nerve membrane. Biochim Biophys Acta 42: 6–23.

Sokoloff L, Reivich M, Kennedy C, DesRosiers MH, Patlak CS, Pettigrew KD, Sakurada O, Shinohara M (1977) The [^{14}C]deoxyglucose method for the measurement of local cerebral glucose utilization: Theory, procedure, and normal values in the conscious and anesthetized albine rat. J Neurochem 28: 897–916.

Sokoloff L (1999) Energetics of functional activation in neural tissues. Neurochem Res 24: 321–329.

Szilard L (1929) Uber die Entropie Verminderung in einem thermodynamischen System bei Eingriffen intelligenter Wesen. Zeitsch Physik 53: 840–856.

Takahashi S, Shibata M, Fukuuchi Y (1997) Effects of increased extracellular potassium on influx of sodium ions in cultured rat astroglia and neurons. Brain Res (Dev Brain Res) 104: 111–117.

Tanaka K, Watase K, Manabe T, Yamada K, Watanabe M, Takahashi K, Iwama H, Nishikawa T, Ichihara N, Kikuchi T, Okuyama S, Kawashima N, Hori S, Takimoto M, Wada K (1997) Epilepsy and exacerbation of brain injury in mice lacking the glutamate transporter GLT-1. Science 276: 1699–1702.

Tholey G, Roth-Schechter BF, Mandel P (1981) Activity and isoenzyme pattern of lactate dehydrogenase in neurons and astroblasts cultured from brains of chick embryos. J Neurochem 36: 77–81.

Vafaee M, Meyer E, Marrett S, Evans AC, Gjedde A (1998) Increased oxygen consumption in human visual cortex: Respond to visual stimulation. Acta Neurol Scand 98: 85–89.

Vafaee MS, Meyer E, Marrett S, Paus T, Evans AC, Gjedde A (1999) Frequency-dependent changes in cerebral metabolic rate of oxygen during activation of human visual cortex. J Cereb Blood Flow Metab 19:} 272–277.

Vafaee MS, Gjedde A (2000) Model of blood-brain transfer of oxygen explains non-linear flow-metabolism coupling during stimulation of visual cortex. J Cereb Blood Flow Metab 20:747–754.

Vandenberg (1998) Molecular pharmacology and physiology of glutamate transporters in the central nervous system. Vandenberg RJ Clin Exp Pharmacol Physiol 25: 393–400.

Villringer A, Dirnagl U (1995) Coupling of brain activity and cerebral blood flow: basis of functional neuroimaging. Cerebrovascular Brain Metabolism Reviews 7: 240–276.

The Genetic Control of Ischemic Neuronal Cell Death

S.H. Graham and R.W. Hickey

Apoptosis, Necrosis and Programmed Cell Death

Apoptosis is the final event in programmed cell death, the mechanism by which neurons die during development. Whether neurons die by apoptosis or necrosis after cerebral ischemia remains controversial. Strictly speaking, apoptosis includes certain key morphologic features: condensation and cleavage of nuclear chromatin, and the formation of budding cytoplasmic appendages known as apoptotic bodies. In addition, intracellular membranes and the plasma membrane remain intact until very late in apoptotic cell death, and there is little inflammation.

Programmed cell death requires an orderly expression and activation of gene products. These gene products include the initiators of the programmed cell death cascade, key-controlling genes, and genes that execute programmed cell death. Programmed cell death has been best characterized in the neurons of the roundworm *C. elegans* [1]. Three *C. elegans* death (*ced*) genes, *ced-3*, *ced-4*, and *ced-9*, regulate the key steps that irreversibly commit the cell to programmed cell death. *Ced-3* and *ced-4* activate programmed cell death whereas *ced-9* inhibits programmed cell death. A number of other genes execute programmed cell death, and when these genes are mutated, the dying neuron shows changes in morphology, phagocytosis, or DNA cleavage, but still dies even in the absence of activity of these genes [2].

The mammalian homologues of the *ced* genes have now been identified (Fig. 1) and include bcl-2 family genes, caspases and Apaf-1. Bcl-2 and its many family members are homologous to *ced-9* [3]. The bcl-2 genes can both inhibit and promote programmed cell death via their actions on mitochondrial permeability and release of cytochrome *c* into the cytoplasm [4]. Caspases are the mammalian homologue of ced-3 [5], and Apaf-1 is the mammalian equivalent of *ced-4* [6]. When cytochrome *c* is released into the cytoplasm, it complexes with Apaf-1 and procaspase-9. As a result, procaspase-9 is cleaved and activated caspase-9 is formed. Caspase-9 in turn cleaves procaspase-3 [7], and the result is activated caspase-3, a key executioner of programmed cell death. Activation of caspase-3 results in cleavage of a number of cytoskeletal proteins important in maintaining cellular morphology [8]. In developing neurons, cleavage in these proteins results in the morphologic changes known as apoptosis. In addition, caspases activate calcium activated DNAase (CAD), which, at boundaries between histones, cleaves DNA into fragments of discrete 400 base-multiples [9]. This produces the DNA damage that is characteristic of programmed cell death.

Fig. 1. Simplified schematic diagram illustrating the key changes in gene expression, location and activity that control programmed cell death in mammalian cells

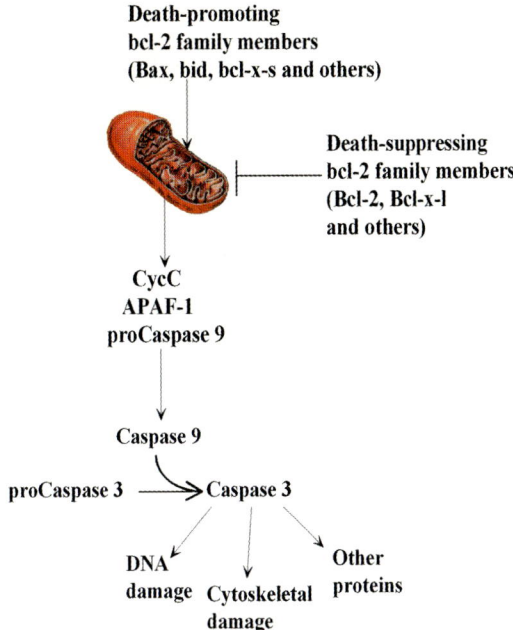

Death-promoting bcl-2 family members (Bax, bid, bcl-x-s and others)

Death-suppressing bcl-2 family members (Bcl-2, Bcl-x-l and others)

CycC
APAF-1
proCaspase 9

Caspase 9

proCaspase 3 ——→ Caspase 3

DNA damage   Cytoskeletal damage   Other proteins

Apoptosis in Cerebral Ischemia

Although some of the morphologic features of apoptosis may be found in some ischemic neurons, it is becoming increasingly clear that neurons dying by ischemia do not have all of the morphologic features of apoptosis. Nuclear condensation and cleavage have been reported in temporary focal ischemia models, but coagulative necrosis remains the pathological hallmark of brain ischemia. Colbourne et al. have carefully characterized morphologic changes that occur in neurons after global ischemia [10]. Although some of their findings suggest nuclear condensation and cleavage at the light microscopic level, they could not find evidence of morphologic changes consistent with apoptosis in over 400 neurons examined at the ultrastructural level. Instead, they found condensation and degeneration of the mitochondria, a morphologic change that is quite distinct from what is found in developing neurons that die by apoptosis. These and other results suggest that the classic morphologic changes of apoptosis often do not occur in cerebral ischemia.

Does the absence of the morphologic changes of apoptosis mean that programmed cell death is not occurring after ischemia? The presence of morphologic changes characteristic of apoptosis strongly support programmed cell death, but these changes may not occur in all cases of programmed cell death. For example, disruption of downstream *ced*/death genes in *C. elegans* does not prevent cell death, but the morphologic changes that characterize cell death, DNA fragmentation, or engulfment by neighboring cells may be altered [2]. Likewise, expression and activity of downstream genes is necessary for apoptosis to occur in mammalian cells. Cao et al. found that CAD, a caspase-dependent nuclease that cleaves DNA between histones as in apoptosis, may be inhibited by dominant negative inhibitors [11]. When CAD is inhibited in this fashion, PC12 cells still die but without their usual apoptotic nuclear morphology. Thus, these results suggest that programmed cell death can still occur without the classic morphologic changes of apoptosis.

There are several reasons why all of the death effector genes may not be expressed or active in ischemic neurons. Differentiation of adult post-mitotic cells results in differential expression of many genes. Furthermore, translation of many genes is blocked during ischemia [12]. Therefore, all of the downstream death effector genes that are expressed during programmed cell death during development may not be expressed in the ischemic neuron. Thus, programmed cell death could occur without the classic morphologic change known as apoptosis.

Evidence That Programmed Cell Death Occurs After Cerebral Ischemia

After cerebral ischemia, alteration has been observed in expression and activity of genes that control programmed cell death in mammals, including the bcl-2 family genes and caspases. This provides stronger evidence that programmed cell death occurs after cerebral ischemia. The most convincing evidence in support of this hypothesis is that alteration in expression of bcl-2 family genes and caspases determines whether ischemic neurons live or die after ischemia.

Bcl-2 Family Genes

Bcl-2 is the mammalian homologue of *ced-9* that inhibits programmed cell death. It is a mitochondrial membrane protein that stabilizes the mitochondrial membrane and prevents depolarization and opening of the mitochondrial permeability transition pore [13]. The bcl-2 family may play an important role in regulating neuronal susceptibility to ischemia (reviewed in Graham et al., 2000) [14]. Bcl-2 expression is found in neurons in the penumbral region in focal ischemia models that are ischemic yet survive [15]. Likewise, bcl-2 is expressed in CA-3 and in the dentate gyrus, neurons that are ischemic yet survive in model of global ischemia [16, 16]. Bcl-x-long is another death-suppressing bcl-2 family member [18] that is expressed and plays a protective role in CA-3 and the dentate gyrus in global ischemia [16]. Thus, the expression of bcl-2 family genes after ischemia suggests that they could play a role in promoting neuronal survival.

Other bcl-2 family members promote rather than suppress programmed cell death. One death-promoting member of the bcl-2 family is Bax [19]. Overexpression of Bax increases mitochondrial permeability and promotes egress of cytochrome *c* from the cytoplasm, which triggers activation of caspase-9 and the intrinsic cascade leading to programmed cell death [20]. In keeping with its death-promoting role, Bax expression is increased in selectively vulnerable CA1 neurons after ischemia [21, 22]. Furthermore, Bax is translocated from the cyto-plasm to the mitochondria [23]. Bcl-x-s, the proapoptotic slice variant of bcl-x, has been detected in the core regions after temporary focal ischemia [24].

Thus, expression of bcl-2 family genes is found to be altered in a pattern con-sistent with their proposed role in regulating cell death. This finding supports, but does not prove, the hypothesis that these genes are important in determining neu-ronal survival. A more direct test of the hypothesis is to alter expression of these genes by use of transgenic animal models, viral vectors, or antisense oligonu-cleotides. In the case of bcl-2, all three of these methods have been used. A trans-genic mouse that overexpresses human bcl-2 had significantly smaller infarction volumes after permanent focal ischemia compared to wild-type controls [25]. Several studies have shown that expression of bcl-2 by replication-deficient her-pes simplex viral vectors protects neurons against ischemic injury [26–28].

These studies show that expression of bcl-2 prior to the ischemic insult can protect neurons against ischemia. However, they do not address whether the bcl-2 that is endogenously expressed after ischemia has a protective role. To address this issue, Chen et al. used bcl-2 antisense oligonucleotides to block translation of bcl-2 protein induced by ischemia [29]. Antisense oligonucleotides are single strands of DNA that are complimentary to the bcl-2 messenger RNA and bind to the bcl-2 messenger RNA forming a double-stranded complex which blocks translation. Chen et al. used antisense oligonucleotide controls consisting of an oligonucleotide with its sequence scrambled, or the sense strand or vehicle con-trols perfused into the rat brain after ischemia. The antisense oligonucleotide, but not the controls, decreased the expression of bcl-2 found on Western blot from brain samples removed 24 hours after 30 minutes of ischemia. Treatment with the antisense oligonucleotides, but not the controls, increased infarction volume after 60 minutes of ischemia. These data demonstrate that endogenous expression of bcl-2 protects the brain against ischemic injury.

Caspases

A substantial number of studies have been published documenting an increase in caspase mRNA, caspase protein, and caspase activity in models of traumatic brain injury, spinal cord ischemia, focal brain ischemia, global brain ischemia and neu-rodegenerative conditions (reviewed by Eldadah and Faden) [30]. Importantly, administration of caspase inhibitors decreases the extent of brain injury following transient focal ischemia [31–34] and global ischemia in rodents [35, 36]. Similarly, transgenic mice overexpressing a dominant-negative caspase-1 have less brain injury following both transient [37, 38] and permanent focal ischemia [39, 40]. Furthermore, virally-mediated overexpression of the anti-apoptotic gene for the X chromosome-linked inhibitor of apoptosis protein (XIAP) attenuates loss of CA1 neurons and impairment of spatial learning after transient forebrain ischemia in rats [41].

In our lab, we have found that caspase-3 mRNA and protein are induced at 8–72 hours after 15 minutes of transient global ischemia in the rat. Brain cell extracts from ischemic brain demonstrate increased caspase-3-like activity and increased cleavage of the caspase-3 substrate PARP. In the hippocampus, caspase-3 mRNA and protein are predominantly increased in the selectively vulnerable CA1 sector. Furthermore, double-label experiments demonstrate that the majority of CA1 neurons overexpressing caspase-3 also stain positively for DNA fragmentation. Finally, intraventricular infusion of the caspase inhibitor Z-DEVD-FMK decreases caspase-3 activity in the hippocampus and attenuates CA1 neuronal loss up to 7 days after ischemia [35]. Taken together, our experiments and those published by other laboratories suggest that caspases are key mediators of programmed cell death following ischemic brain injury and are potential therapeutic targets.

The Spectrum of Necrosis and Programmed Cell Death

Despite the lack of apoptosis in ischemic models, there is now considerable evidence that changes in gene expression and activity characteristic of programmed cell death occur in these models. The extent to which cell death occurs via programmed cell death or necrotic mechanisms depends upon the severity and duration of the ischemic insult. This principle is well demonstrated in vitro, where brief exposures to low concentrations of excitotoxins can induce apoptosis, but exposures to higher concentrations or longer durations induce death with necrotic characteristics [42, 43]. Furthermore, brief sublethal durations of ischemia induce expression of genes that have protective effects. These include antiapoptotic genes such as bcl-2 [44] as well as heat shock proteins (reviewed by Massa et al.) [45].

The duration and severity of the ischemic insult may also determine the extent to which neurons die by programmed cell death mechanisms after ischemia in vivo (reviewed by Nicotera) [46]. In models of focal ischemia, neurons located in the severely stressed ischemic core demonstrate predominantly *necrotic* features of cell death, whereas neurons in the less stressed border regions (penumbra) demonstrate more *apoptotic* features [47–49]. Figure 2 portrays the relationship between duration of injury and the morphologic features of cell death. Brief durations of ischemia produce sublethal injury and are associated with expression of survival factors including antiapoptotic genes such as bcl-2 and heat shock proteins. With longer durations of ischemia, cell death occurs initially via programmed cell death, but as the duration of ischemia increases, necrosis predominates in the core region where ischemia is most severe. Further increasing duration of injury results in expansion of the ischemic core into the penumbra and thus increased necrosis and decreased apoptosis. Programmed cell death is limited to the cortical mantle, the so-called penumbral area where ischemia is less severe. Thus, there is a loss of protection from caspase inhibitors (and in caspase-deficient knockout mice) with increasing severity of ischemic injury [34, 38]. One potential mechanism for the switch from apoptosis to necrosis is the increased energy deprivation accompanying an increase in the duration/severity of ischemia. ATP is necessary for Apaf-1/cytochrome c cleavage of pro-caspase-9 [7]. Indeed, energy depletion in vitro can cause a shift from apoptotic cell death to necrotic cell death [50, 51].

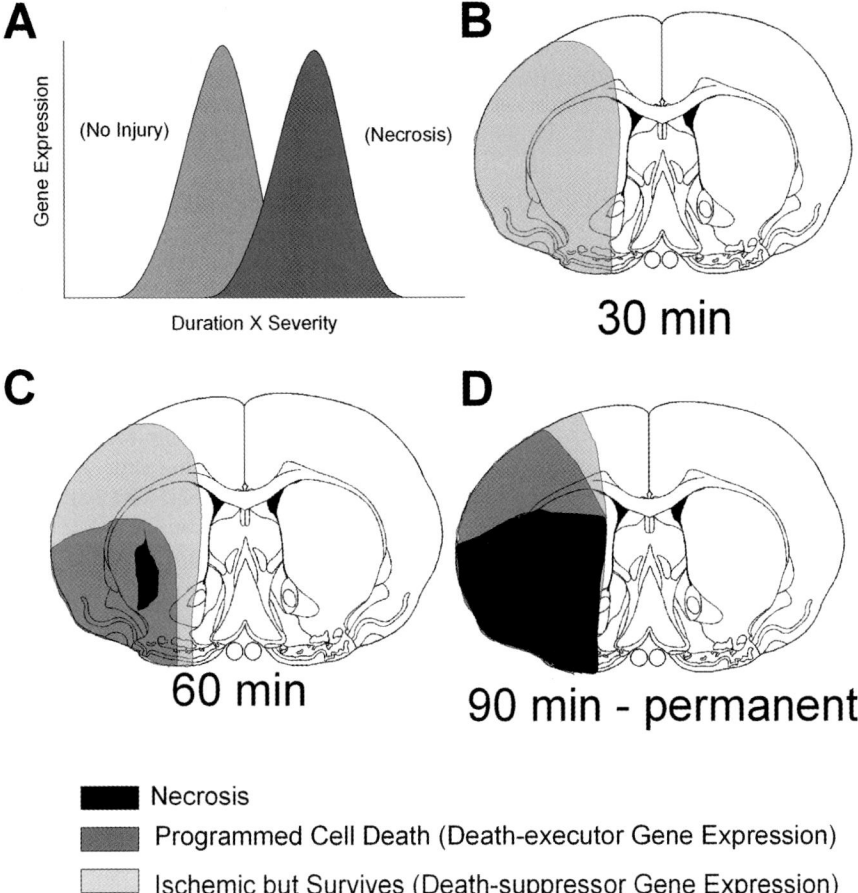

Fig. 2A–D. Idealized schematic drawings illustrating the spectrum of gene expression events produced by varying durations and severities of ischemia. **A** Very brief durations or very mild severities of ischemia produce no injury and no gene expression changes. More severe or prolonged ischemia can produce sublethal injury. This degree of injury is associated with expression of genes that act to increase neuronal survival including genes such as bcl-2 that inhibit programmed cell death and heat shock proteins *(light gray)*. More prolonged or severe ischemia may induce expression of genes that promote programmed cell death *(dark gray)*. If ischemia is severe or prolonged, ATP is not available and protein expression is blocked, so necrosis occurs *(black)*. Idealized schematic drawings of coronal sections of rat brain after 30 min **B** 60 min. **C** and 90 min to permanent middle cerebral artery occlusion **D** With 30 min ischemia, there is sublethal ischemia and induction of expression of genes that suppress programmed cell death and heat shock proteins. With 60 min of middle cerebral artery occlusion, there is lethal ischemia. In the center of the core region there is necrosis, but there is a surrounding zone of programmed cell death. When ischemia is prolonged to 90 min or longer, the necrotic area expanded and programmed cell death occurs only in the cortical mantle

Future Questions

Animal models of ischemia provide considerable evidence that programmed cell death may occur under conditions where ischemia is incomplete or transient. Expression and activity of the genes that regulate programmed cell death are altered in a manner consistent with the known effects of these genes upon cell death. Furthermore, alteration in expression of some of the key genes that control cell death after ischemia alters the fate of the ischemic neurons. However, a number of important questions remain.

Unlike in nematode cells, in mammalian cells there is a multitude of redundant pathways by which programmed cell death may be executed. Which of these pathways is responsible for programmed cell death depends upon the cell type and the exact death stimuli. Although caspase-3 was assumed to be the final common pathway by which programmed cell death is executed, it is now clear that caspase-3 activation via cytochrome c release is just one way by which the mitochondrion initiates programmed cell death. Caspase-independent mechanisms such as apoptosis-inducing factor (AIF) can also cause cell death [52]. The extent to which these and other mechanisms are active in ischemic neurons is not known.

Finally, although studies show that programmed cell death contributes to post-ischemic cell death in rodent models, little data is available regarding programmed cell death in humans. Future studies that examine whether the gene expression changes and DNA cleavage characteristic of programmed death are present in human tissue may determine whether programmed cell death is relevant to human stroke.

Acknowledgements. This work was supported by the NIH NINDS R01 NS37459, P01 NS35965 and P50 NS30318 (SHG) and the Department of Veteran Affairs Medical Service Merit Review Program and the V.A. / D.O.D. Traumatic Brain Injury Initiative (SHG). The authors thank Carol Culver for editorial assistance.

References

1. Ellis HM, Horvitz HR. Genetic control of programmed cell death in the nematode C. elegans. Cell 1986;44(6):817–29.
2. Ellis RE, Jacobson DM, Horvitz HR. Genes required for the engulfment of cell corpses during programmed cell death in Caenorhabditis elegans. Genetics 1991;129(1):79–94.
3. Hengartner MO, Horvitz HR. C. elegans cell survival gene ced-9 encodes a functional homolog of the mammalian proto-oncogene bcl-2. Cell 1994;76(4):665–76.
4. Reed JC. Bcl-2 family proteins. Oncogene 1998;17(25):3225–36.
5. Yuan J, Shaham S, Ledoux S, Ellis HM, Horvitz HR. The C. elegans cell death gene ced-3 encodes a protein similar to mammalian interleukin-1 beta-converting enzyme. Cell 1993;75(4):641–52.
6. Zou H, Henzel WJ, Liu X, Lutschg A, Wang X. Apaf-1, a human protein homologous to C. elegans CED-4, participates in cytochrome c-dependent activation of caspase-3. Cell 1997; 90(3):405–13.
7. Li P, Nijhawan D, Budihardjo I, Srinivasula SM, Ahmad M, Alnemri ES, et al. Cytochrome c and dATP-dependent formation of Apaf-1/caspase-9 complex initiates an apoptotic protease cascade. Cell 1997;91(4):479–89.

8. Thornberry NA, Lazebnik Y. Caspases: enemies within. Science 1998;281(5381):1312–6.

9. Enari M, Sakahira H, Yokoyama H, Okawa K, Iwamatsu A, Nagata S. A caspase-activated DNase that degrades DNA during apoptosis, and its inhibitor ICAD. Nature 1998;391(6662):43–50.

10. Colbourne F, Sutherland GR, Auer RN. Electron microscopic evidence against apoptosis as the mechanism of neuronal death in global ischemia. J Neurosci 1999;19(11):4200–10.

11. Chen D, Stetler RA, Cao G, Pei W, O'Horo C, Yin XM, et al. Characterization of the rat DNA fragmentation factor 35/Inhibitor of caspase-activated DNase (Short form). The endogenous inhibitor of caspase-dependent DNA fragmentation in neuronal apoptosis. J Biol Chem 2000;275(49):38508–17.

12. Hossmann KA. Disturbances of cerebral protein synthesis and ischemic cell death. Prog Brain Res 1993;96:161–77.

13. Hockenbery D, Nunez G, Milliman C, Schreiber RD, Korsmeyer SJ. Bcl-2 is an inner mitochondrial membrane protein that blocks programmed cell death. Nature 1990;348(6299):334–6.

14. Graham SH, Chen J, Clark RS. Bcl-2 family gene products in cerebral ischemia and traumatic brain injury. J Neurotrauma 2000;17(10):831–41.

15. Chen J, Graham SH, Chan PH, Lan J, Zhou RL, Simon RP. bcl-2 is expressed in neurons that survive focal ischemia in the rat. Neuroreport 1995;6(2):394–98.

16. Chen J, Graham SH, Nakayama M, Zhu RL, Jin KL, Stetler RA, et al. Apoptosis repressor genes bcl-2 and bcl-x-long are expressed in the rat brain following global ischemia. J. Cerebr. Blood Flow Metabol. 1997;17:1–10.

17. Shimazaki K, Ishida A, Kawai N. Increase in bcl-2 oncoprotein and the tolerance to ischemia-induced neuronal death in the gerbil hippocampus. Neuroscience Research 1994;20(1):95–99.

18. Boise LH, Gonzalez-Garcia M, Postema CE, Ding L, Lindsten T, Turka LA, et al. bcl-x, a bcl-2-related gene that functions as a dominant regulator of apoptotic cell death. Cell 1993;74(4):597–608.

19. Oltvai ZN, Milliman CL, Korsmeyer SJ. Bcl-2 heterodimerizes in vivo with a conserved homolog, Bax, that accelerates programmed cell death. Cell 1993;74(4):609–19.

20. Jurgensmeier JM, Xie Z, Deveraux Q, Ellerby L, Bredesen D, Reed JC. Bax directly induces release of cytochrome c from isolated mitochondria. Proc Natl Acad Sci U S A 1998;95(9):4997–5002.

21. Krajewski S, Mai JK, Krajewska M, Sikorska M, Mossakowski MJ, Reed JC. Upregulation of Bax protein levels in neurons following cerebral ischemia. Journal Of Neuroscience 1995; 15(10):6364–76.

22. Chen J, Zhu RL, Nakayama M, Kawaguchi K, Jin K, Stetler RA, et al. Expression of the apoptosis-effector gene, Bax, is up-regulated in vulnerable hippocampal CA1 neurons following global ischemia. J. Neurochem. 1996;67(1):64–71.

23. Cao G, Minami M, Yan C, Chen D, Pei W, O'Horo C, et al. Intracellular Bax translocation following transient cerebral ischemia: Implications for a role of the mitochondrial apoptotic-signaling pathway in ischemic neuronal death. J. Cerebral Blood Flow Metabol. 2001;(in press).

24. Gillardon F, Lenz C, Waschke KF, Krajewski S, Reed JC, Zimmermann M, et al. Altered expression of Bcl-2, Bcl-X, Bax, and c-Fos colocalizes with DNA fragmentation and ischemic cell damage following middle cerebral artery occlusion in rats. Brain Res Mol Brain Res 1996;40(2):254–60.

25. Martinou JC, Dubois-Dauphin M, Staple JK, Rodriguez I, Frankowski H, Missotten M, et al. Overexpression of BCL-2 in transgenic mice protects neurons from naturally occurring cell death and experimental ischemia. Neuron 1994;13(4):1017–30.

26. Linnik MD, Zahos P, Geschwind MD, Federoff HJ. Expression of bcl-2 from a defective herpes simplex virus-1 vector limits neuronal death in focal cerebral ischemia. Stroke 1995;26(9):1670–4.

27. Lawrence MS, McLaughlin JR, Sun GH, Ho DY, McIntosh L, Kunis DM, et al. Herpes simplex viral vectors expressing Bcl-2 are neuroprotective when delivered after a stroke. J Cereb Blood Flow Metab 1997;17(7):740–4.

28. Antonawich FJ, Federoff HJ, Davis JN. BCL-2 transduction, using a herpes simplex virus amplicon, protects hippocampal neurons from transient global ischemia. Exp Neurol 1999;156(1):130–7.

29. Chen J, Simon RP, Nagayama T, Zhu R, Loeffert JE, Watkins SC, et al. Suppression of endogenous bcl-2 expression by antisense treatment exacerbates ischemic neuronal death (rapid communication). J Cereb Blood Flow Metab 2000;20(7):1033–9.

30. Eldadah BA, Faden AI. Caspase pathways, neuronal apoptosis, and CNS injury. J Neurotrauma 2000;17(10):811–29.

31. Hara H, Friedlander RM, Gagliardini V, Ayata C, Fink K, Huang Z, et al. Inhibition of interleukin 1beta converting enzyme family proteases reduces ischemic and excitotoxic neuronal damage. Proc Natl Acad Sci U S A 1997;94(5):2007–12.

32. Ma J, Endres M, Moskowitz MA. Synergistic effects of caspase inhibitors and MK-801 in brain injury after transient focal cerebral ischaemia in mice. Br J Pharmacol 1998;124(4):756–62.

33. Endres M, Namura S, Shimizu-Sasamata M, Waeber C, Zhang L, Gomez-Isla T, et al. Attenuation of delayed neuronal death after mild focal ischemia in mice by inhibition of the caspase family. J Cereb Blood Flow Metab 1998;18(3):238–47.

34. Li H, Colbourne F, Sun P, Zhao Z, Buchan AM, Iadecola C. Caspase inhibitors reduce neuronal injury after focal but not global cerebral ischemia in rats. Stroke 2000;31(1):176–82.

35. Chen J, Nagayama T, Jin K, Stetler RA, Zhu RL, Graham SH, et al. Induction of caspase-3-like protease may mediate delayed neuronal death in the hippocampus after transient cerebral ischemia. J Neurosci 1998;18(13):4914–28.

36. Gillardon F, Kiprianova I, Sandkuhler J, Hossmann KA, Spranger M. Inhibition of caspases prevents cell death of hippocampal CA1 neurons, but not impairment of hippocampal long-term potentiation following global ischemia. Neuroscience 1999;93(4):1219–22.

37. Hara H, Fink K, Endres M, Friedlander RM, Gagliardini V, Yuan J, et al. Attenuation of transient focal cerebral ischemic injury in transgenic mice expressing a mutant ICE inhibitory protein. J Cereb Blood Flow Metab 1997;17(4):370–5.

38. Liu XH, Kwon D, Schielke GP, Yang GY, Silverstein FS, Barks JD. Mice deficient in interleukin-1 converting enzyme are resistant to neonatal hypoxic-ischemic brain damage. J Cereb Blood Flow Metab 1999;19(10):1099–108.

39. Friedlander RM, Gagliardini V, Hara H, Fink KB, Li W, MacDonald G, et al. Expression of a dominant negative mutant of interleukin-1 beta converting enzyme in transgenic mice prevents neuronal cell death induced by trophic factor withdrawal and ischemic brain injury. J Exp Med 1997;185(5):933–40.

40. Schielke GP, Yang GY, Shivers BD, Betz AL. Reduced ischemic brain injury in interleukin-1 beta converting enzyme- deficient mice. J Cereb Blood Flow Metab 1998;18(2):180–5.

41. u D, Bureau Y, McIntyre DC, Nicholson DW, Liston P, Zhu Y, et al. Attenuation of ischemia-induced cellular and behavioral deficits by X chromosome-linked inhibitor of apoptosis protein overexpression in the rat hippocampus. J Neurosci 1999;19(12):5026–33.

42. Bonfoco E, Krainc D, Ankarcrona M, Nicotera P, Lipton SA. Apoptosis and necrosis: two distinct events induced, respectively, by mild and intense insults with N-methyl-D-aspartate or nitric oxide/superoxide in cortical cell cultures. Proc Natl Acad Sci U S A 1995;92(16):7162–6.

43. Ankarcrona M, Dypbukt JM, Bonfoco E, Zhivotovsky B, Orrenius S, Lipton SA, et al. Glutamate-induced neuronal death: a succession of necrosis or apoptosis depending on mitochondrial function. Neuron 1995;15(4):961–73.

44. White MJ, Chen J, Zhu RL, Irvin S, Sinor A, DiCaprio MJ, et al. A bcl-2 antisense oligodeoxynucleotide increases AMPA toxicity in cultured cortical neurons. submitted 1996.

45. Massa SM, Swanson RA, Sharp FR. The stress gene response in brain. Cerebrovasc Brain Metab Rev 1996;8(2):95–158.

46. Nicotera P, Leist M, Manzo L. Neuronal cell death: a demise with different shapes. Trends Pharmacol Sci 1999;20(2):46–51.

47. Charriaut-Marlangue C, Margaill I, Represa A, Popovici T, Plotkine M, Ben-Ari Y. Apoptosis and necrosis after reversible focal ischemia: an in situ DNA fragmentation analysis. J Cereb Blood Flow Metab 1996;16(2):186–94.

48. Charriaut-Marlangue C, Aggoun-Zouaoui D, Represa A, Ben-Ari Y. Apoptotic features of selective neuronal death in ischemia, epilepsy and gp 120 toxicity. Trends Neurosci 1996; 19(3):109–14.

49. Charriaut-Marlangue C, Ben-Ari Y. A cautionary note on the use of the TUNEL stain to determine apoptosis. Neuroreport 1995;7(1):61–4.

50. Leist M, Single B, Castoldi AF, Kuhnle S, Nicotera P. Intracellular adenosine triphosphate (ATP) concentration: a switch in the decision between apoptosis and necrosis. J Exp Med 1997;185(8):1481–6.

51. Eguchi Y, Shimizu S, Tsujimoto Y. Intracellular ATP levels determine cell death fate by apoptosis or necrosis. Cancer Res 1997;57(10):1835–40.

52. Lorenzo HK, Susin SA, Penninger J, Kroemer G. Apoptosis inducing factor (AIF): a phylogenetically old, caspase- independent effector of cell death. Cell Death Differ 1999;6(6):516–24.

Cerebral Resuscitation from Temporary Complete Global Brain Ischemia

P. Safar

Introduction

The complete global brain ischemia of cardiac arrest (CA), potentially reversible by cardiopulmonary-cerebral resuscitation (CPCR) [1, 2] is the most common cause of sudden coma and death [1, 3]. Sudden CA kills about 400,000 persons each year in the U.S. In addition, in the over 100,000 accidental deaths each year, coma occurs as a result of trauma, intoxication, asphyxiation, severe shock, or other insults. This talk focused on CPCR research results by our teams, and mentioned only some of the important contributions made by others, most of which have been reviewed [4–7]. Epidemiologic studies suggest that the chance for conscious survival of normothermic CA decreases by about 10% for every minute of normothermic complete global brain ischemia (no-flow) [3].

Definitions. Resuscitation researchers need a common language. Here are some definitions, which our group of the Resuscitation Research Center of the University of Pittsburgh have recommended and used in the past 40 years: *Resuscitation research* concerns the study of the pathophysiology of acute terminal states (e.g., asphyxiation, severe shock, severe traumatic brain injury) and clinical death (i.e., potentially reversible CA). Studies should be conducted at multiple levels (from cell to community), by multidisciplinary teams, and encompass the sequence from insult via resuscitation and prolonged life support to outcome in terms of function and morphology. To reverse insults, *CPCR* is the sequence of basic, advanced, and prolonged life support (BLS-ALS-PLS) [1]. BLS consists of step A (airway control) [1, 8, 9], step B (breathing control starting with mouth-to-mouth ventilation [MMV]) [9], and step C (circulation control) [10]. Step C includes cardiac massage, external hemorrhage control, positioning, and other measures. In CA, sternal compressions alone (step C) cannot be relied upon to ventilate the lungs [11]. Since asphyxia as a result of airway obstruction in coma or apnea, when leading over 5–10 min to CA, is more injurious to the brain than the same duration of ventricular fibrillation (VF) CA [7], steps A-B-C must be taught to all people as a combined life-supporting first aid (LSFA) method [12]. Lay persons cannot diagnose the cause of sudden coma or pulselessness. ALS [1] is mostly meant for restoration of spontaneous circulation (ROSC) from CA, and in trauma cases for restoring blood volume while conducting hemostasis, including resuscitative surgery. Prolonged life support [13, 14] is primarily meant for mitigating the postresuscitation disease [15], which includes reperfusion injury [16]. After resuscitation from severe traumatic hemorrhagic shock (low flow), the post-resuscitation disease can lead to secondary multiple organ systems failure as a result of ischemia, release of cytokines (the systemic inflammatory response syndrome) and infection (septic shock). After shock the viscera are more likely permanently damaged than the brain, which protects itself during low perfusion pressure with vasodilation [2, 14].

Brain-oriented CPR BLS-ALS-PLS we call *CPCR* [1, 17], which is only as effective as the weakest of its nine steps, and as the weakest link in the life-support chain from scene via transport to the most appropriate hospital's emergency department, operating room, and intensive care unit (ICU) [18]. The combination of these two concepts is also called "chain of survival" [19].

For cerebral resuscitation [2], our CPCR diagram of 1961 [1, 17] labeled prolonged life support as steps G, H, and I – for gauged, humanized (brain-oriented with hypothermia), intensive care. CA includes complete temporary global brain ischemia, which differs from the incomplete temporary ischemia of shock, the (incomplete) temporary or permanent focal brain ischemia of stroke, and traumatic brain injury. As the pathophysiologies of these insults differ, so do the efficacies of treatments. This paper focuses on *resuscitation*, which is to reverse the insult and support recovery. We refer to treatment started before the insult as *protection*, which usually is continued during the insult for *preservation*. Treatments effective for protection-preservation may not be effective for resuscitation.

For *therapeutic hypothermia*, which at present is the most effective method for cerebral protection-preservation and resuscitation, we must differentiate between mild (about 34°C), moderate (30°C), deep (20°C), profound (10°C), and ultraprofound hypothermia (5°C) [2]. Sites for temperature measurements can be in brain tissue (Tb), epidural (Tep), at the tympanic membrane (Tty), in the nasopharynx (Tnp), and at sites within the core of the trunk such as the esophagus (Tes), pulmonary artery (Tpa), vena cava (Tcv), rectum (Tr), or urinary bladder (Tub) [2].

History. In the first half of the 20th century the brain was still in a "black box" [20]. Around 1950, when I was an anesthesiology resident at the University of Pennsylvania in Philadelphia, Seymour Kety [21] pioneered measurements of cerebral blood flow (CBF), cerebral oxygen uptake ($CMRO_2$), and cerebral glucose consumption (CMRG). Using Kety's method, Wechsler was the first to study the effects of a barbiturate on CBF and $CMRO_2$ [22]; and Stone studied CBF and $CMRO_2$ in prisoner volunteers exposed to total-body moderate hypothermia under anesthesia [23], or to hypovolemic hypotension without anesthesia [24]. These daring experiments gave the first such CBF data in humans; the volunteers suffered no injuries.

Between the two world wars, Guthrie was professor of pharmacology and physiology at the University of Pittsburgh. Already one century ago, he drew attention to the need for research into brain ischemia caused by CA [25]. During World War II, Negovsky of Moscow initiated the world's first resuscitation research laboratory, which in the 1980s became an Institute of the USSR Academy of the Medical Sciences [26]. Negovsky designed several dog models of sudden death, particularly one with exsanguination CA and resuscitation by intra-arterial pressure infusion plus artificial ventilation. We owe to Negovsky the concepts of "terminal state, clinical death, and the postresuscitation disease" [15]. He explored and documented effective protective-preservative (not resuscitative) cerebral hypothermia. In the late 1950s, at the Johns Hopkins University in Baltimore, investigators conducted some uncontrolled attempts at resuscitative cerebral hypothermia after CA in dogs and patients (see later). In summary – for cerebral resuscitation from CA, little was known in the 1960s, hopes were raised in the 1970s, much was learned about mechanisms in the 1980s; and clinically important breakthroughs were made in the 1990s.

Since the 1960s, our goal has been to maximize in humans the brain's tolerance of normothermic CA no-flow. If that can be extended from the so far documented limit of 5 min to 10 min, considering an urban mobile ICU ambulance response time of 8 min, the rate of conscious survival of CA-CPCR could be greatly enhanced. The treatments that could lead to such a breakthrough might come from pharmacologic and physical potentials. They should be ideally based on documented improvement in outcome and suspected (or documented) mechanisms of how cells die and how these mechanisms might be mitigated.

Pathophysiology

It has been known from clinical and experimental observations since the beginning of this century that complete occlusion of cerebral arteries in man causes unconsciousness within 15 s [27] and that the human brain can not recover fully after more than 4 or 5 min of normothermic CA without blood flow [28]. Standard external CPR produces unpredictably low total blood flow ("cardiac output") in animals [10, 29–33] and humans [34], which can at best deliver low CBF (about 20% normal) and often, after a prolonged no-flow period, only "trickle-flow" CBF (less than 10% normal). Trickle flow can be more injurious to the brain than no flow [5].

Open-chest CPR is physiologically more effective by producing higher perfusion pressures and cerebral and overall blood flows in animals [29–31, 35, 36] and man [34] and improved cerebral outcome in dogs [31]. Open-chest CPR for CA in operating rooms has been in occasional use for over one century with surprisingly good cerebral outcomes [37]. Open-chest CPR was explored in the pre-hospital setting [38]; it achieved ROSC when external CPR of 20–30 min had failed, but there was no enhanced cerebral recovery because of the preceding protracted low flow by external CPR. For brain recovery, the switch would have to be made in the first 5–10 min of ALS attempts at ROSC.

For VF, the first defibrillation in humans (via thoracotomy) was initiated by Beck of Cleveland in the 1940s [39]. Open-chest CPR was given up, even in hospitals around 1960 because of the advent of standard external CPR [10], which enabled initiation of some emergency oxygen delivery to brain and heart within seconds of collapse, even in the out-of-hospital arena [1, 3, 40]. For ROSC and reoxygenation and recovery of the brain, closed-chest emergency cardiopulmonary bypass (CPB) proved superior to closed-chest CPR-ALS, because CPB provides complete control over blood pressure, flow, composition, and temperature [41–48]. The clinical initiation of resuscitative CPB [49] is hampered by long delays due to procrastination and difficulty with vessel access.

Sudden deep coma in humans, irrespective of the cause, results in upper airway obstruction, unless the head is tilted backward [8, 9] or the trachea is intubated [1]. Complete airway obstruction or apnea under normothermia results in asphyxiation (decline of PaO_2 and pHa plus rise in $PaCO_2$), which causes CA within 5–10 min; even when 2 min later ROSC efforts were begun in dogs, slight histologic permanent brain damage was seen [7].

In sudden, complete normothermic global brain ischemia, brain oxygen stores become exhausted within 10–15 s [5, 27], and brain glucose and energy stores become exhausted in 4–5 min [50, 51]. This explains the CA duration limit for complete recovery of 4–5 min no-flow [28, 41, 42]. In the late 1960s we began exploring cerebral recovery after CA in dogs [52]. Around 1970, when I composed guidelines for brain-oriented prolonged life support [53], Hossmann's report that the majority of (but not all) cerebral neurons can recover protein synthesis and electric activity after up to 1 h of normothermic no-flow, inspired hope for more effective cerebral resuscitation [54, 55]. Over the past 30 years we and others have searched for novel CPCR methods to achieve long-term survival without brain damage after at least 10 min of complete normothermic global brain ischemia; we used mostly outcome models in monkeys and dogs [2]. Others have researched mechanisms and pharmacologic treatment potentials in rats [5, 6].

We began by hypothesizing that, after prolonged normothermic VF CA with no-flow over 5 min, normotensive reperfusion may not overcome the no-reflow phenomenon [56–58], and that there might be prolonged lower CBF than is needed to meet metabolic demands. In 1970/71, we therefore explored CBF and metabolism after CA [59, 60]. Using standard global CBF methods, we documented in dogs the now well-known hyperemia-hypoperfusion sequence. We also showed that CBF is inadequate to match the global $CMRO_2$, which recovers from ischemic silence over 1–2 hours post-CA. During CA of 15 min, cerebral impedance measurements suggested only temporary membrane depolarization and after ROSC there was no sustained intracranial pressure (ICP) increase, i.e., no evidence of gross brain swelling [59]. Others confirmed the post-global brain ischemia sequence of transient hyperemia followed by delayed hypoperfusion [5, 6, 15].

Right after our first CBF study after CA [59], coma pioneer Fred Plum hosted the Cornell Symposium concerning ischemic-anoxic brain injury [61]. There were stimulating discussions by GBI-focused basic scientists Fischer, Brierley, Cammermeyer, Hossmann, Myers, Siesjo, and others. In spite of much new knowledge acquired since then, the mechanisms by which only selectively vulnerable neurons in selectively vulnerable regions die after reperfusion from prolonged CA are still not known. Important for further cerebral resuscitation research was the recognition by Plum [62] that there are delayed derangements after reperfusion that lead to the postischemic encephalopathy.

After ROSC is achieved, which should be as quickly as possible, attempts to optimize CBF after CA must consider two different CBF derangements: 1) The immediate post-CA no-reflow phenomenon [15, 55–58]; and 2) the delayed protracted cerebral hypoperfusion, starting about 30 min after normotensive reperfusion and lasting for many hours, depending on the preceding arrest time and other factors [59, 60]. Both CBF reductions are quite inhomogeneous [63–70]. Although CBF measurements in humans during and early after CA are almost non-existent, the delayed cerebral hypoperfusion has been documented also in patients after CA [71, 72].

After prolonged CA in dogs, using the local (multifocal) CBF method by stable xenon-CT (which was pioneered by Pittsburgh radiologists and surgeons Yonas and Wolfson) we found reperfusion with low mean arterial pressure (MAP) by external or open-chest CPR to result in some no-reflow foci [64–66]. At 20–30 min reperfusion this is then followed for 2 h by a multifocal inhomogeneous cerebral hypoperfusion, in spite of controlled arterial normotension [64–68]. CMRO$_2$ recovered from metabolic silence to or above baseline values starting at 2 h. The resulting O$_2$ delivery/uptake mismatch is reflected in mixed cerebral venous blood PO$_2$ decrease [64–69] below the critical level of about 25 mm Hg [69, 70, 73]. Exact mechanisms have not been documented, but probably the initial no-reflow is mainly the result of blood sludging, while the delayed hypoperfusion is due at least in part to vasospasm. There is some evidence to suggest that intravascular coagulation might also play a role [74]. Tolerance thresholds of low-flow (CBF 10–20% normal) or trickle-flow (CBF <10% normal) have been documented in focal ischemia experiments [73]. When regional CBF is reduced to about 20–30% normal, EEG depression leads quickly to EEG silence, which is reversible.

During complete global brain ischemia, energy loss results in depolarization of membranes [75] with extra-intracellular shift of sodium and water and efflux of potassium. This triggers cascades over about 5 min that lead to irreversible damage after reperfusion. These cascades [2] include intracellular calcium loading and maldistribution [5, 76, 77]; brain tissue lactic acidosis [78]; and increase in brain free fatty acids and phospholipases [79], osmolality [80]; and nore-pinephrine [81]; and massive extracellular release of excitatory amino acids (particularly glutamate and aspartate) [5, 82–84]. All this sets the stage for cell damage starting with reperfusion and resulting in cytoskeletal damage generated by lipases, proteases and nucleases.

After complete global brain ischemia of longer than 5 min, even with optimal reperfusion, the highly complex chemical cascades that occur during ischemia flare up [16]. Reperfusion-reoxygenation is accompanied by relatively quick recovery from acidosis, increased glutamate, and cellular edema. Even if there is homogeneous reperfusion there is reoxygenation injury involving free iron and free radicals that result in lipid peroxidation of membranes [2, 16, 85–88]. Secondary delayed calcium shifts, and excitatory amino acids release are uncertain [89]. Increasing attention has been paid recently to the delayed damage to mito-chondria [90, 91]. After initial recovery from accumulated lactic acid, calcium shifts, and excitotoxicity, there might be a delayed postarrest increase in total brain calcium and glutamate release [90]. The encephalopathy "matures" over 3 days or longer to a plateau of scattered necrosis of selectively vulnerable neurons, predominantly in the hippocampus, neocortex, and cerebellum [92–96]. The role of subtle DNA damage during reperfusion from CA in possibly causing delayed apoptotic neuronal death has not yet been clarified [97, 98]. In DNA damage the repair enzyme PARP may lead to ATP exhaustion [99]. Changes in levels of cytokines or nitric oxide can be either good or bad, depending on the type and severity of the insult, when and where measured, and the degree of change in concentration of these molecular species. For partially proven and partially postulated complex cascades that occur in the brain during and after ischemia, see figure 4 of reference 2. Because of the complexity of these changes I predicted since 20 years ago that no single molecule-targeted drug will bring a breakthrough.

Animal Outcome Models

Mechanisms and effects of resuscitation potentials can be clarified only in controlled animal models with reproducible insult, resuscitation, life support, and long-term outcome [100, 101]. For studying the brain after CA and ROSC, we and others have used acute ($\leq$ 12 h), short-term (about 24 h), and long-term outcome experiments ($\geq$ 72 h). The latter should be with control of extracerebral variables that, when deranged, can influence the encephalopathy [41, 42, 92, 93–95, 100, 101].

Rats have been used extensively for modeling incomplete forebrain ischemia [102, 103]. This insult is not CA as it does not damage brainstem, medulla, and extracerebral organs, and usually does not cause postischemic coma. Although the model is not clinically realistic, it has been useful in studies of mechanisms and in preliminary evaluations of treatment potentials. It is also convenient, in that it does not require post-CA life support, which would be difficult in small animals. Unfortunately, the majority of treatments that led to a reduction in the loss of hippocampal neurons failed to produce a breakthrough effect in clinically realistic studies in higher species [2]. Measuring cerebral outcome after VF CA in rats proved to be difficult; the groups in Baltimore, Cologne, and Heidelberg found it possible [104]. Some have even succeeded with VF CA modeling in mice [105]. That opens the door for CA studies in genetically altered mice. Since 1980 we have searched for a practical CA model in rats for the screening of resuscitation potentials. After struggling with long-term survival [106, 107], Katz et al [95, 108–111] succeeded in firmly establishing the asphyxial CA rat model as a reproducible outcome model. It does cause postischemic coma for 12–24 h. Although it does not enable long-term life support, it has enabled fairly reproducible survival with brain damage in control groups after asphyxiation of 8 min and standard external CPR. Warner et al [6] succeeded with a rat CA-CPB model.

Monkeys and dogs can give clinically relevant answers. John Moossy, our neuropathologist of the 1970s and 1980s, and I agreed to avoid the "laborious climb up the phylogenetic ladder." We therefore started with monkey models of global brain ischemia by neck tourniquet [92], by hyperthermia-induced CA [112] and by severe hemorrhagic shock [113]. In the 1980s, for CA studies, I switched to dogs because affordable monkeys were inhomogeneous (caught in the wild), and showed behavior which was so human-like that shortening their lives, even when rationalizing it under the food chain, seemed not justified [114]. Using instead custom-bred hunting dogs (of the same subspecies, sex, age, and weight), the outcomes after the same insult, resuscitation, and life support have become reproducible [42, 93, 100, 101].

For the past 25 years, with a brief interruption in the 1990s, we have been developing, refining, and documenting cerebral resuscitation potentials with considerable clinical significance, using outcome experiments in dogs conducted in a research animal ICU. Prolonged life support, over as many days as needed, is provided there by a stable team of critical care physicians and technicians. Our prolonged CA dog models of greatest clinical value, in use since the late 1970s, produce VF by electric shock [2, 4, 41, 42, 93, 114] or asphyxia by airway obstruction and apnea [7, 93, 100, 115, 116], or exsanguination [100, 117–119], for no-flow periods ranging from 0 to 30 min [2, 41, 42]. Asphyxiation CA causes more brain damage than VF-CA [7, 93, 115, 116]. Exsanguination CA is equally injurious as VF-CA [119]. ROSC is by standard external CPR (which proved effective only up to 10 min normothermic no-flow) [42, 114]; or the more effective open-chest CPR [31]; or brief CPB (effective for the reversal of up to 30 min normothermic no-flow and up to 120 min profound-hypothermic no-flow) [41]. We have used CPB as an experimental tool, realizing that in clinical use for standard CPR-resistant cases outside of the hospital, vessel access time and CPB preparation time will require some other bridging method [48].

After life support for 3–7 days or longer, to let the encephalopathy mature, we evaluate outcome in terms of overall performance categories (OPC 1 = normal, 2 = moderate disability, 3 = severe disability, 4 = coma, and 5 = death or brain death); neurologic deficit (ND) scores (0–10% = normal, 100% = brain death); and scoring of histopathologic damage (HD) throughout the brain [92, 93]. While in the rat models, death of neurons in the hippocampus provided the most reliable target for evaluation [5, 6, 95], in monkeys and dogs, the neocortex, thalamus, cerebellum, and other areas proved as vulnerable as the CA-1 region of the hippocampus [92, 93]. Our pathologist Moossy [92] established a semi-quantitative scoring method, using standard light microscopy, for the scoring in about 20 brain regions of "ischemic neurons" (which on hematoxylin-eosin stain pink and are shrunken with pyknotic nuclei), microinfarcts, and edema. This method was modified by Radovsky [93]. Total HD scores correlated with ND scores [93]. Recently, even DNA damage scores (with TUNEL staining) correlated with ND scores [98].

During the past 25 years we learned about the requirements for clinically realistic outcome models in large animals [2]: 1) All animals should be of the same subspecies, sex, age, and weight. 2) The insult should be sufficiently moderate to allow mitigation of brain damage, e.g., by mild cooling. 3) Arrest reversal with controlled perfusion pressure should be possible without adding variable low-flow states. 4) Chance should be minimized by concurrent randomized controls for definitive treatment trials. 5) Life support post-CA should be standardized, using the same team, strains, and controls of the physiologic variables that can influence cerebral and overall outcome. 6) Brain temperature, or at least core temperature, should be controlled within ± 0.5°C before, during, and after the CA. 7) Intensive care for at least 72 h postarrest is needed to get reproducible final outcome evaluation data, by allowing maturation of cerebral changes while controlling extracerebral variables. 8) All control experiments should be within protocol and should result in survival with brain damage. 9) Postarrest deaths prior to 72 h should be excluded from neurologic outcome evaluation if they are the result of extracerebral complications, while primary brain death should be included. 10) To avoid bias, placebo controls, and blinded outcome evaluation by the same person or several persons with minimal inter-observer variability, are desirable.

Based on these criteria, we have developed and used carefully controlled dog models of VF, exsanguination, and asphyxiation-induced CA. These have produced acute pathophysiologic disturbances similar to each clinical condition, including postarrest coma, need for life support, etc. In addition, neurologic injury, in each case, mirrors the clinical condition as assessed by both functional tools and histopathology.

Cerebral Blood Flow Promotion

In 1974 I decided to explore the effect on outcome of CBF promotion after prolonged CA, using a dog VF CA model with 12 min normothermic no-flow [120]. Although the model then was rather crude, that study demonstrated for the first time that *any* treatment after CA can improve cerebral outcome. To treat both the immediate no-reflow [56–58], if any, and the delayed protracted hypoperfusion [59, 60, 63–72], the experimental group of dogs received a combination of post-CA hypertension by vasopressor (starting immediately after ROSC), normovolemic hemodilution by colloid plasma substitute, and heparinization [120]. When 10 years later we had established more reliable CA outcome models in dogs, we repeated the study with a clinically more realistic protocol and could confirm improved outcome with this treatment [121]. There was not only overall improvement in outcome, but also a correlation between a brief initial hypertension (the spontaneous or induced hypertensive bout) and improved outcome [121]. It is not clear whether that or the subsequent moderate hemodilution and hypertension by norepinephrine caused the improved outcome. In a parallel study we found normalization of global and multifocal CBF for the entire post-CA observation period with moderate hypertensive hemodilution [66]. Hypertensive reperfusion washed away no-reflow spots during the first 15 min of diffuse hyperemia [64–66]. Some brain regions need very high reperfusion pressures to restore normal tissue PO_2 [122]. Hypertensive hemodilution normalized global CBF and abolished the no-flow and trickle-flow foci [66]. There are many published animal studies which support the cerebral benefit of a high reperfusion pressure after prolonged CA [56–60, 120–127]. For clinical use, we could show in dogs that postarrest monitoring of mixed cerebral venous (sagittal sinus) PO_2 [68–70, 73], enabled prevention of a decrease of this variable below the critical level of about 25 torr [73] by titrating MAP, hematocrit, or $PaCO_2$ [127]. Animal studies also support CBF-promoting measures by vasodilators [114, 128–132].

The above animal data received strong support from the results of correlation statistics in clinical studies [132]. Two preliminary studies [133, 134] and two definitive studies [135, 136] showed strong association between early post-CA high blood pressure and good cerebral outcome, as well as between low blood pressure and poor cerebral outcome. The need for hypertensive reperfusion will be greater in some brain regions than others [66, 122], and after longer no-flow times [137]. A brief increase in systolic arterial pressure to about 150 mm Hg occurs either spontaneously, immediately after ROSC, as the result of the epinephrine given during CPR steps A-B-C, or should be controlled with vasopressor by titrated i.v. infusion. Further experimental and clinical clarifications are needed on the optimal level and duration of the initial hypertensive bout and its risks; and on what to do about the delayed protracted cerebral hypoperfusion.

Global CBF after prolonged CA seems to respond to changes in $PaCO_2$ [65, 127]. Very high $PaCO_2$ worsens tissue acidosis, and very low $PaCO_2$ can worsen brain ischemia and recovery [138]. Normalizing mixed cerebral venous (superior jugular bulb) PO_2 or SO_2 (reflecting cerebral O_2 delivery/demand relationships) is clinically possible with titration of blood pressure, hematocrit, arterial PCO_2, and/or a vasodilator. The cerebral effects of different post-insult levels of PaO_2 and $PaCO_2$ have been evaluated for TBI, not for CA. Low PaO_2 can worsen the injured brain [138]. High PaO_2 may [140, 141] or may not [142] worsen free radical damage. At present a reasonable recommendation for life support in coma after CA-ROSC would be to control PaO_2 at $\geq$ 100 torr and $PaCO_2$ at 35–45 torr.

Resuscitative Pharmacologic Strategies

Cerebral resuscitation potentials by pharmacologic strategies, which at first appeared promising, but later increasingly disappointing, have been reviewed [2, 6]. Drug effects have paled in comparison with the effects of hypothermia (see later). The first hope concerning pharmacologic cerebral resuscitation after CA came in the early 1970s about barbiturates, when others could reduce infarct size in dogs [143] and monkeys [144] given after middle cerebral artery occlusion, and show some (although uncontrolled) benefit after global ischemia in animals [145, 146]. It seemed logical that barbiturate loading after CA might be beneficial because barbiturates reduce O_2 demand [22], cerebral edema and ICP [147], seizures [148], and free radical effects [149].

Our first barbiturate study, using our neck tourniquet model in monkeys [92] was by Bleyaert et al [150]. It showed improved NDS and HDS in the treatment group. Since no one else had an intensive care outcome model, I decided to reproduce this study in our laboratory; Gisvold et al [151] could not reproduce statistically significant outcome benefit using the same monkey model, but with "tighter" blood pressure control. In the meantime, clinicians were using barbiturates (uncontrolled) in patients. We therefore decided to conduct preliminary trials [152], which gave promising results and led to the first randomized clinical outcome study [153]. The overall outcome results showed no statistically significant difference in the proportion of patients who achieved good cerebral outcome; but a numerically beneficial comparison was apparent in a subgroup with long arrest time. Thiopental loading (30 mg/kg i.v.) early postarrest also threatened the ability to maintain normotension in some patients. Recently, new exploratory experiments in dogs, with a combination drug cocktail, showed that the addition of thiopental suggests some slight improvement in outcome if one can avoid postarrest cardiovascular-pulmonary complications [154]. Since there was no breakthrough effect, we decided not to recommend barbiturate therapy after CA unless needed for seizure control or ICP control.

We conducted the second drug trial in the 1980s when others had shown that calcium entry blockers improved CBF after CA in dogs [128]. We evaluated the calcium entry blocker lidoflazine given after VF CA of 10 min in dogs and found it to give significant improvement in cerebral outcome, but not histologic normalization after CA [114]. The same distribution of outcome variables was achieved with use of our monkey GBI model after resuscitative administration of the calcium entry blocker nimodipine by our past fellow Gisvold in Michenfelder's laboratory [129]. We then took lidoflazine to a randomized clinical outcome study [155, 156]. Again, the overall proportion of patients who achieved good cerebral outcome was not significantly different in the lidoflazine group as compared to the control group [155], but when inadequate life support cases (with hypotension or re-arrest) were excluded in both groups, there was a significant improvement in the lidoflazine group [156]. Similar promising but inconclusive results in the clinical trial were found with nimodipine in a study in Scandinavia [157]. Neither lidoflazine nor nimodipine is available for i.v. use in patients in the U.S. In dogs we found that calcium entry blockers may be more effective after VF CA, while free radical scavengers may be more effective after asphyxial CA [116].

Some drug evaluations in rodents without accurate temperature control gave erroneous positive results with some pharmacologic cerebral resuscitation potentials that depress normothermic control mechanisms, resulting in unintentional mild hypothermia. After the NMDA antagonist MK-801 appeared promising in focal [158] and global brain ischemia rodent models [159] (without rigid temperature control), we tested its effect after CA in our dog outcome model (with rigid temperature control); we found no beneficial effect on outcome [160]. The AMPA antagonist NBQX was effective in the rat forebrain ischemia model with accurate temperature control [96, 161]. This drug does not seem to be useful for CA in large animals or patients because of severe side effects. The aminosteroid Trilazad, declared by its manufacturer to be effective in numerous brain-insult studies in rodents, was found to be ineffective after GBI in rats [162] and did not increase CBF after CA in dogs [67]. After the neuron-specific calcium entry blocker SNX-111 showed promise in its effect on the CA-1 region of rats after forebrain ischemia or in its influence on infarct size [96, 163], we evaluated it thoroughly in dogs, under most rigid temperature controls, using multiple CA durations, dosing, and timing; we found no benefit on brain outcome [164]. In recent studies in rodents, hormone therapy looks promising [165]. Some benefit of inhalation anesthetics such as isoflurane in brain slices and rodents [6] remain to be explored in outcome models. Delayed calcium accumulation in mitochondria and the discovery of the mitochondrial permeability transition pores led recently to the discovery by Siesjo et al [89–91] that immune suppressants such as cyclosporin-A and FK-506 can reduce the number of postischemic necrotic hippocampal neurons, but only when the blood-brain barrier is broken, which is the case in stroke but clinically not feasible to achieve after CA.

The optimal blood glucose level after CA is also in need of clarification [166]. Although hyperglycemia during CA worsens the cerebral insult [5, 6], glucose plus insulin with moderate hyperglycemia seems to reduce brain damage after asphyxial CA in rats [109]. As for other drug treatment potentials [6], some of which look promising in neuron cultures, hippocampal brain slices, or rodents, none have been documented to achieve our goal, namely achieving complete functional and morphologic normality after normothermic CA with 10 min no-flow in dog CA outcome models. Most of the above drugs, when explored in dogs for cerebral *preservation* during plus *resuscitation* after prolonged CA (preservation should be more effective than mere post-CA administration) have failed to give a break-through effect (see later "suspended animation").

Clinical Trials

In 1979, with Bleyaert's positive monkey data on thiopental available [150] and uncontrolled barbiturate trials in CA patients underway by others and us [152], I decided to initiate the first randomized clinical outcome study of CPCR after CA for patients inside or outside hospitals [153]. This Brain Resuscitation Clinical Trial (BRCT), supported for 15 years (1979–94) by the National Institute of Neu-rologic Diseases and Stroke (NINDS), ultimately included 20 study groups in 7 countries [152, 153, 155, 156, 167–175]. Because prospective informed consent is not possible in resuscitation research, institutional review boards and the NIH agreed to waive that requirement [172]. As soon as possible, we obtained consent from families to continue collecting data. Over 15 years, we collected data on about 4,000 cases, up to 200 pages of data per patient for 6-month survivors. When in 1994–98 agencies required prospective informed consent, clinical resus-citation research in the USA became impossible.

Our thiopental loading study during the first 5 years (BRCT I, 1979–84) [153], our calcium entry blocker lidoflazine study during the second 5 years (BRCT II, 1984–89) [155, 156], and our third 5-year study on escalating high-dose epinephrine (BRCT III, 1989–94) [167] taught us much beyond the difficulty in differentiating outcomes between treatment groups. We used the large database also for so far over 10 adjunctive studies of associations (statistical correlations, "clues") between outcomes to 6 months and a variety of disease and treatment factors. We added to the Glasgow overall performance categories 1–5, which were established for cases of TBI, the cerebral performance categories (CPC) 1–5, since post-CA patients may be physically handicapped with good brains or vice versa [1, 2, 153]. We compared good CPC (CPC 1 = normal, or CPC 2 = moderate dis-ability, but self-sustaining) with bad CPC (CPC 3 = severely impaired cerebral performance, or CPC 4 = coma, or CPC 5 = brain death). These adjunctive corre-lation studies included insult [168]; old age [169]; clinical outcome predictions [170–172]; outcome prediction by cytosolic enzymes leaking into the CSF after CA-CPR [173–175]; and other topics. Among long-term survivors, the proportion of patients who remained with CPC 3 (conscious but severely damaged, the most tragic outcome), were relatively few. Old age per se did not obviate good cerebral outcome provided there was adequate cardiovascular recovery [169]. Socio-eco-nomically most important (for discontinuing futile prolonged life support) was the discovery that at 3–7 days [170], and even at 12–24 h after resuscitation from CA [171], *all* patients with low Glasgow Coma Score and/or with absent corneal, pupillary, or gag reflex, achieved poor outcome.

We learned that multicenter randomized clinical outcome studies in resuscita-tion medicine are extremely difficult to control; and that all we can expect from the results are "clues," not documentation of pathophysiologic mechanisms nor of therapeutic benefit for individual cases. We learned about the limitations of randomized clinical trials for resuscitation research [2], such as the fact that patients must be selected within seconds, which gives insufficient time to select those who might be within the therapeutic window; that the treatment protocols although intended to be controlled are actually uncontrollable; and that numerous variables that influence outcome are either not known or not measurable. The most critical limitation is that arrest time and CPR time (no-flow and low-flow times), the main determinant of outcome, which can be fully controlled in large-animal ICU outcome experiments, can only be crudely estimated in clinical cases. Epidemiologic correlation statistics cannot give proof of therapeutic efficacy. I therefore do not consider randomized clinical outcome trials to be the gold standard. When a simple, inexpensive, and apparently safe novel CPCR treatment gives breakthrough effects in several clinically realistic outcome studies in large animals, only clinical feasibility and side-effect studies should be needed. They should not necessarily lead to randomized clinical outcome trials, which are wasteful of time and money, and proved unreliable not only for CA studies, but also for other resuscitation trials as after brain trauma, hemorrhagic shock, or stroke.

For complex, expensive, and risky treatments, controlled clinical randomized outcome studies might still be urged by some. For those we recommend to meet the following requirements [2]: 1) There should be a good question or hypothesis. 2) Inclusion and exclusion criteria should be clearly established for quick entry of patients into the study; sample size can be estimated only with assumptions. 3) Investigative groups in multicenter trials must have influence over the entire life-support chain of the EMS system, from prehospital through transportation to intrahospital emergency department, operating room, and ICU environments. 4) The institutional review board must give approval to start special vs control treatment under the emergency exception to prospective informed consent [172]. When feasible, consent to continue is obtained later. 5) There should be concurrent or immediate-retrospective estimation of arrest (no-flow) time, CPR (low-flow) time, and prearrest and postarrest hypoxia (hypotension) times. 6) CPCR BLS-ALS-PLS should be by protocol throughout the life-support chain. 7) Early recovery should be monitored with coma scoring. 8) Outcome to 6 months should be monitored by assessing overall performance category 1–5, and (separately) cerebral performance category 1–5 [1, 19, 155]. 9) Side effects should be monitored. 10) Overall data management, analysis, subgroup analysis, evaluation, and interpretation of the results should be by an expert team.

Resuscitative Hypothermic Strategies

Starting in the 1950s, Bigelow of Toronto [176] pioneered moderate protective-preservative hypothermia for open-heart surgery in patients (before CPB became available); and Rosomoff documented in dogs physiologic effects of hypothermia [177] and found even resuscitative hypothermia effective after focal ischemic or traumatic brain insults [178–180]. Protective-preservative (elective) moderate hypothermia for heart and brain surgery has been reviewed since the 1950s [181]. In the 1960s, Rosomoff and Safar [182] conducted uncontrolled patient trials of resuscitative moderate hypothermia after brain surgery. White of Cleveland [183, 184] and Wolfson of Pittsburgh [185] tried isolated brain cooling. White [186] preserved with hypothermia the isolated perfused monkey brain; he and Albin [187] mitigated with post-insult hypothermia the disability after experimental spinal cord trauma. Around 1960, my associates and I used a combination of prolonged controlled ventilation, osmotherapy, and moderate hypothermia in some cases after prolonged normothermic CA. In one case there was a dramatic result [188].

Accidental, uncontrolled cooling, with normothermic defenses intact, can be deleterious [189, 190]. Without poikilothermia, surface cooling provokes potentially deleterious defense mechanisms until they are overwhelmed and core temperature decreases to moderate levels (30°C) with the electrocorticogram depressed, and to deeper levels, which induce cortical silence. and CA. Therapeutic (controlled) cooling which requires poikilothermia without shivering, vasoconstriction, sympathetic discharge, and thermogenesis, controlled by ischemia, trauma, or drugs, can be protective-preservative as well as resuscitative for the brain [2] and other vital organs [181, 190].

Hibernating mammals, by spontaneously switching from self-controlled normothermia to poikilothermia, decrease oxygen requirement by decreasing metabolism and blood flow in parallel, without suffering tissue hypoxia [191]. "Hibernating" poikilothermic animals, like certain turtles, survive severe tissue hypoxia during profound hypothermia, by still-unclear mechanisms [192].

Resuscitative post-CA *moderate* hypothermia (30°C) after CA was explored around 1960 in dogs [193, 194] and patients [188, 195], with uncontrolled methods and encouraging results. It was then given up because of management difficulties, uncertain benefit, and complications (arrhythmias) – and remained dormant for two decades. In the early 1980s, disappointed with drugs as cerebral resuscitation potentials [2], our team (Safar, Brader, Gisvold, Leonov, Sterz, and Tisherman) talked and revived large animal studies first with *moderate* resuscitative hypothermia after prolonged normothermic CA [196–198]. Outcome results were statistically significant but clinically unimpressive. The outcome study in monkeys was the first combining hypothermia with drugs [196]. In large dogs, external head cooling was slow [197]. Blood cooling was fast and semi-invasive techniques were moderately fast [199]. Peritoneal cooling may be a clinically rapid method [200].

The breakthrough, namely resuscitative *mild* hypothermia (34°C) after prolonged CA, came around 1990. In 1987, at the time of the International Resuscitation Researchers' Conference in Pittsburgh [201], Hossmann reported that accidental *mild* hypothermia during acute GBI in cat experiments correlated with better EEG recovery [202]. Although we had earlier found no correlation between EEG recovery times and cerebral outcome in dog studies, I was curious and initiated exploration of pre- and intra-CA factors that might explain our variable outcomes in dogs after the same insult. The only variable that correlated significantly with unexpected OPC 1 outcomes after "normothermic" CA of 7, 10, or 15 min, was unintentional *mild* hypothermia (Tty 35–36°C) present at the start of VF [41, 42]. This discovery of protective-preservative mild hypothermia made us embark on a systematic series of dog outcome studies with *mild* resuscitative hypothermia *after* normothermic VF CA of 10 or 12.5 min no-flow [203–207]. If effective it could become a breakthrough since mild hypothermia is easy and safe, while moderate hypothermia is difficult and risky. In studies 1–4 [203–206], after mild hypothermia of about 2 hours postarrest, there was significant improvement of function and morphology, but not normalization of histology. Study 2 [204] used clinically realistic external CPR and cooling methods. Study 3 [205] showed to our surprise that deep hypothermia, which is more protective than mild hypothermia when induced before arrest, if induced after arrest gave worse histologic outcome than mild hypothermia. One possible explanation is more blood sludging and stasis in deep hypothermia. In study 4 [206] there was less benefit when the onset of cooling was delayed by as little as 15 minutes.

In study 5 [207], however, we achieved the best results so far: after normothermic VF CA of 11 min no-flow and clinically relevant reperfusion, the combination of mild hypothermia from reperfusion to 12 h, plus CBF promotion with hypertensive hemodilution and normocapnia, resulted not only in OPC 1 and NDS = 0, but also, in the majority of dogs, in zero or near-zero HDS. HDS was significantly lower than in previous studies with the use of mild hypothermia alone or CBF promotion alone after a similar insult.

Simultaneously and independently, colleagues in Miami, Lund, and Detroit, using mostly the incomplete forebrain ischemia rat models, discovered mild protective-preservative as well as resuscitative hypothermia effects [208–211]. These investigators confirmed the histologic outcome effects of mild cerebral temperature changes, which occur easier in rats than in dogs, and explored and documented multiple mechanisms of therapeutic mild hypothermia.

The mechanism of cerebral preservation-resuscitation by mild-to-moderate hypothermia has become increasingly better understood. There is synergism of many damage-mitigating effects. In normal brains, anesthetics can silence the EEG, but they reduce $CMRO_2$ only to about 50% (i.e., block active metabolism), while hypothermia can decrease $CMRO_2$ to near-zero, by also reducing basal metabolism [212]. It has been known for a long time that in normal brain, reduction of $CMRO_2$ occurs by about 7% per °C reduction in brain temperature between 38°C and 28°C, depressing "active metabolism" [176, 177]. Then $CMRO_2$ decreases from 50% at 28°C to 10% at 18°C, by depressing "basal metabolism." The same applies to whole-body O_2 consumption [176, 181]. The situation is quite different after prolonged normothermic CA, when cooling is superimposed on the postischemic hypoperfusion. We found in dogs that after normothermic VF CA 12 min, mild hypothermia is accompanied by the same CBF, $CMRO_2$, and cerebral O_2 utilization coefficient as in normothermic controls [68, 70]. Thus, the beneficial mechanisms must be synergism of other potentially beneficial effects [2, 203]. Hypothermia preserves ATP [50, 51]; and reduces ion fluxes [213], lactacidosis [214], free fatty acid production [79, 215], glutamate release [215], leukotrienes and edema [216], protein kinase [217], ICP [179, 181, 218, 219], free radical triggered lipid peroxidation [220]; and inflammation [221]. The latter is more important in TBI than in CA. Hypothermia slows enzymatic reactions by 1.5% per °C (Arrhenius) and might tighten membranes [16]. For maximal benefit one should explore optimal temperature levels and timing to suppress deleterious reactions but not beneficial ones.

Protective-preservative mild hypothermia is more effective than resuscitive mild hypothermia after normothermic CA [222]. Cooling should be initiated early – the earlier the better [206]. However, initiation of cooling, even if delayed by several hours, has been shown to give some benefit in rats [223–225]. Recently, Dietrich et al [226] found in a rat study that after normothermic GBI, short mild hypothermia of 4 hours merely postponed the loss of neurons. Colbourne et al [227], however, found that longer duration of mild hypothermia (24 h) indeed produces permanent benefit in salvaging neurons, even after normothermic GBI.

Mild hypothermia after prolonged normothermic CA has been recently found to be possibly beneficial in patients in uncontrolled clinical trials [228, 229]. Preliminary data from the first controlled randomized clinical outcome study of mild hypothermia after CA, a multicenter European study initiated and coordinated by our alumnus Sterz of Vienna, look promising [230]. Definitive data will be available soon. In this study surface cooling has been late and slow. Many patients arrive in the hospital mildly hypothermic. Some in the past were actively warmed; some even developed a fever. Even mild *hyperthermia* is deleterious [231]. Therefore, clinical hypothermia trials should begin with avoidance of warming the organism, particularly the brain, at least by noninvasive cerebral temperature monitoring (Tty, Tnp). Then aiming for Tty 33–35°C in any acutely comatose patient might be beneficial and without risks [232].

How can one rapidly induce cerebral mild hypothermia in humans? It should be easy to achieve with only exposure cooling. Clinical observations, the literature, and our own cooling studies in dogs and human corpses suggest at this time the following [2, 181, 183, 197–199, 232, 233]: 1) During circulatory arrest, even immersion in ice water cools the brain extremely slowly; carotid cooling, aortic cold flush, or CPB via heat exchanger are fastest, but require cannulation time. 2) During low flow produced by standard external CPR, cooling methods have not been studied in a systematic way; in hypovolemic shock often spontaneous cooling occurs with exposure. 3) During normal spontaneous circulation, blood cooling and peritoneal cooling are faster than ice application on head and trunk; nasopharyngeal and gastric cooling are adjunctive. Several companies are now developing and testing various cooling catheters inserted into the vena cava. We postulate that arterio-venous or arterio-arterial (carotid) shunt flow via a cooler may give more rapid induction of mild cerebral hypothermia; the latter perhaps even with a slightly lower temperature in the brain than the heart sustained. That would be important for victims of severe stroke (not a topic for discussion in this talk) in whom hypothermic preservation should be initiated within a few minutes after the onset of symptoms, outside the hospital, to "buy time" for neurons to survive until thrombolysis. Intravascular or perivascular application of ice slush may be more effective than saline at 2–4°C. Transfer of cold via respiratory gases, using the lungs as heat exchanger, is too slow, but liquid cooling via the respiratory route (e.g., ice slush in oxygenated fluorocarbon) is another possibility presently explored by others.

Complications of controlled *moderate* hypothermia have been known since the 1950s [2, 180, 189, 190, 233]. They include dysrhythmias (even a risk of VF with heart temperature below 30°C, particularly in sick hearts); increased blood viscosity; coagulopathy by platelet sequestration and suppression of coagulation cascades; and, if longer than 24 h, increased risk of pulmonary infection. *Mild* hypothermia, however, has not been shown to cause any of these complications, but coagulopathy has not been studied sufficiently to call this treatment 100% safe in cases of traumatic hemorrhage.

Therapeutic (preservative-resuscitative) mild-to-moderate hypothermia, triggered by the breakthrough effects on CA [2, 41, 42, 207], has recently received positive trials, in animals more than in patients, also for TBI [218, 219, 221, 232], stroke [2], and hemorrhagic shock [190, 234–238]. A recent study of moderate hypothermia induced many hours after TBI with no statistical benefit [232a] was flawed [232b]. In normothermic hypovolemic shock, the viscera are the most vulnerable organs because of vasoconstriction and other derangements, while the brain protects itself by vasodilation [24, 113, 239]. Titrated therapeutic hypothermia for depressing deleterious and beneficial reactions should be also explored for septic shock [240].

Unanswered questions concerning mild-to-moderate hypothermia after CA are many, but the clinical use should not wait for more research results. With the reproducible benefit demonstrated in controlled large-animal outcome studies [203–207], to withhold potentially neuron-saving therapy that is simple, cheap, and safe, might be considered unethical.

Suspended Animation

For (temporarily) unresuscitable CA, research into the rapid induction of "suspended animation," to buy time, was recommended in 1996 for a "mini-Manhattan project" [191]. "Suspended animation" we define as preservation of the organism during prolonged periods of CA for transport and repair, to be followed by delayed resuscitation with CPB [191, 241]. In 1984, Safar and Bellamy discussed the resuscitability of combat casualties without brain trauma who rapidly exsanguinate internally to CA [191]. In those cases the brain becomes the main target organ. CPR and i.v. infusions would be useless before surgical hemostasis. Civilian cases of traumatic exsanguination CA have a near 100% mortality, in spite of emergency room thoracotomy [242]. A totally new approach is needed, which we have called "suspended animation for delayed resuscitation" [191, 241]. This means preservation of the temporarily unresuscitable, clinically dead organism, before loss of brain viability (which means before 5 min normothermic no-flow), to enable transport and surgical hemostasis during CA of 1 or 2 hours, to be followed by resuscitation with CPB to survival without brain damage.

In the late 1980s, our group under Tisherman developed and used a new dog model of normothermic hemorrhagic shock followed by exsanguination to CA [243–248]. Cooling to profound hypothermia with CPB and heat exchanger (10°C) [244] gave better outcome than cooling to deep hypothermia (15°C) [243]. Profound hypothermia during CA of 2 h resulted in survival with brain damage, while profound hypothermia with CA of 1 h (after hemorrhagic shock) resulted in complete recovery of the brain in terms of function and histology [248]. Cerebral recovery was not influenced by lack of anticoagulant [245], use of the Wisconsin organ preservation solution [246], or moderate changes in diluted hematocrit [247] during hypothermic stasis of 1–2 hours.

Electively and slowly induced profound hypothermia followed by circulatory arrest of 1–2 h has been survived to consciousness before in dogs [249, 250] and patients for open-heart surgery [251]. Needed are rapid induction of hypothermic preservation and a systematic search for arrest time limits with reliable functional and histologic studies. After profound hypothermic CA of 1 h (not 2 h) with use of CPB in dogs we achieved survival with histologically normal brains [248].

CPB by field medics, however, is not feasible. We therefore explored the use of an aortic balloon catheter (which in patients might be inserted rapidly via thoracotomy, from the groin, or parasternally by methods yet to be developed) – to enable a cold flush with an appropriate solution, perhaps with enhancing medication. The objective is to immediately induce preserving hypothermia of brain and heart during the end stage of bleed-out and within 5 min no-flow. The ultimate goal is to preserve the organism, first by aortic cold flush for at least 30 min, during which time CPB could become available to lower Tty further to 10° or 5°C, to gain another 1 or 2 hours of preservation.

In exsanguination CA dog outcome experiments to 72 h, aortic arch flush preservation with normal saline solution (NSS) at ambient temperature at CA 2 min (Tty 36°C) achieved cerebral recovery after 15 min CA [252]. A flush of NSS at 4°C (Tty 34°C) achieved complete cerebral recovery after CA 20 min [253]. To achieve complete cerebral recovery after CA 30 min with histologically normal brain, Tty below 30°C was needed; this required flush of NSS at 4°C in very large volumes into the abdominal aorta, in order to also prevent ischemic damage to spinal cord and viscera [254]. We have recently achieved, in dogs, survival without neurologic deficit after exsanguination CA of 60, 90, and 120 min, using aortic cold saline flush to Tty 10°C [255]. Tty could be lowered by 3°C per minute with NSS flush at 2°C. That might become feasible, in trained hands, where electric power and cold storage for very large fluid volumes are available. Starting with exsanguination CA in the civilian setting, clinical feasibility trials are being planned for pulseless emergency department patients receiving emergency thoracotomy [255a]. Once CPB is available, preservation can be extended to over 3 h by asanguineous profound hypothermic low flow [256].

For combat medics, we tried to develop aortic flush induction of preservation with a CA 20 min no-flow model [253], using a portable volume of saline at ambient temperature (24°C). We systematically explored, in mini-series, 14 different drugs, one at a time, according to the following six pharmacologic strategies: delaying energy failure (adenosine, thiopental, fructose biphosphate), protecting ion exchange through depolarized membranes (phenytoin, MK-801, nimodipine), inhibiting proteases (no drug available), inhibiting apoptosis (cycloheximide, calmodulin antagonist W-7), protecting mitochondrial permeability pores (cyclosporin-A), and combating reoxygenation injury (Tempol). None of the 14 drugs, in various doses, gave consistent OPC 1 after CA 20 min at mild hypothermia, which without drugs led to survival with severe brain damage [257]. One anti-oxidant, Tempol, which in aqueous solution permeates the blood brain barrier, gave consistently better functional outcome than controls, but only when given by flush at the start of CA [258]; it did not improve histologic brain damage.

We wonder whether suspended-animation strategies might also help save some victims of normovolemic sudden cardiac death out-of-hospital [191, 241]. An estimated 50% of CPR attempts out-of-hospital in the U.S. (over 200,000 cases per year), are given up because ROSC is not achievable with standard external

CPR-ALS [3, 40]. Aortic cold flush to profound hypothermic CA by emergency physicians in the field, or mild-to-moderate hypothermia with continued CPR-BLS-ALS during transport, might bridge the patient over at least 30 min with cerebral viability not lost, to prolonged CPB initiated in the hospital emergency department. CPB could be continued for hours or days, with heparin-bonded equipment, to permit evaluation of brain and heart, and if indicated the heart could be repaired, assisted, or replaced.

Conclusions

Epidemiologic data clearly show that what now is known is not widely applied; that many victims of CA have not only "hearts too good to die" (to quote C. Beck), but also "brains too good to die"; and that the reversibility of increasingly longer CA to survival without brain damage in patients creates a challenge for systematic integrated laboratory and patient studies.

Among challenging questions for the near future are the following [259, 260]:

1. How can we achieve more rapid clinical implementation of knowledge gained in the laboratory?
2. How can lay persons and paramedics most rapidly induce controlled mild hypothermia?
3. How could one best make hypothermic strategies even more effective with new pharmacologic cocktails; by clarification of side-effects (e.g., is there coagulopathy with mild hypothermia ?); by titration to suppress deleterious but not beneficial cascades?
4. For temporarily unresuscitable normothermic, normovolemic CA, how can we most rapidly induce ultra-ALS in the field, such as open-chest CPR (perhaps with a minimally invasive technique), emergency CPB, or prolonged suspended animation?
5. How do cerebral neurons die after reoxygenation from CA, and what is the cause of selective vulnerability? Are the ones that die those that are more stimulated (excitotoxicity trigger), or the ones programmed to die soon anyhow (apoptosis trigger)? Or are they the ones injured by a still-unknown mechanism?

These and other advances in cerebral resuscitation from prolonged CA will require ongoing open communication and collaboration among rescuers, clinicians, laboratory researchers, and industry.

Ethical dilemmas of resuscitation medicine in general and resuscitation from CA (GBI) in particular require ongoing debate [1, 168–175, 261–265]. The topics range from definitions of death to expectations, limitations, and ethics of randomized clinical trials. When sudden CA occurs after the onset of severe senility, emergency resuscitation is hardly indicated. If, however, a life-threatening emergency occurs at any time before severe senility, an all-out resuscitation attempt is indicated. The goal is to bring the person's brain back to pre-arrest function, to achieve the ancient ideal of "mens sana in corpore sano." If this proves not possible, long-term life support should be stopped.

The human brain is the tip of the arrow of evolution, according to the philosopher Teilhard de Chardin. Medicine represents an imposition of the values of individual humans on a random universe. CPCR, if practiced with reason and compassion, and if focused on the brain, is a positive force in human evolution on earth [1].

Acknowledgements. Doctors Patrick Kochanek and Wilhelm Behringer made valuable suggestions. Ms. Patricia Boyle helped with editing. Ms. Fran Mistrick and Ms. Donna Gaspich helped with preparation of the manuscript.

References

1. Safar P, Bircher NG. Cardiopulmonary-Cerebral Resuscitation. An Introduction to Resuscitation Medicine. World Federation of Societies of Anaesthesiologists. 3rd ed. London: A Laerdal, Stavanger; WB Saunders; 1988.
2. Safar P. Resuscitation of the ischemic brain. In: Albin MS, editor. Textbook of neuroanesthesia with neurosurgical and neuroscience perspectives. New York: McGraw-Hill; 1997. p. 557–93.
3. American Heart Association (AHA). Guidelines for cardiopulmonary resuscitation and emergency cardiovascular care. Circulation. Suppl. Vol. 102/8, 2000. p. I–I–380
4. Safar P. Resuscitation from clinical death: pathophysiologic limits and therapeutic potentials. Crit Care Med 1988;16:923–41.
5. Siesjo BK, Siesjo P. Mechanisms of secondary brain injury. Eur J Anaesthesiol 1996; 13(3): 247–68.
6. Warner DS. Effects of anesthetic agents and temperature on the injured brain. In: Albin MS, editor. Textbook of neuroanesthesia with neurosurgical and neuroscience perspectives. New York: McGraw-Hill; 1997. p. 595–611.
7. Safar P, Paradis NA. Asphyxial cardiac death. In: Paradis N, Halperin HR, Nowak RM, editors. Cardiac arrest. The science and practice of resuscitation medicine. Philadelphia: Williams and Wilkins; 1996. p. 702–26.
8. Safar P, Aguto-Escarraga L, Chang F. Upper airway obstruction in the unconscious patient. J Appl Physiol 1959;14:760–4.
9. Safar P. Ventilatory efficacy of mouth-to-mouth artificial respiration. Airway obstruction during manual and mouth-to-mouth artificial respiration. JAMA 1958;167:335–41.
10. Kouwenhoven WB, Jude JR, Knickerbocker GG. Closed-chest cardiac massage. JAMA 1960;173:1064–7.
11. Safar P, Brown TC, Holtey WH, Wilder R. Ventilation and circulation with closed chest cardiac massage in man. JAMA 1961;176:574–6.
12. Eisenburger P, Safar P. Life supporting first aid (LSFA) training of the public. Review and recommendations. Resuscitation 1999;41:3–18.
13. Safar P, DeKornfeld TJ, Pearson JW, Redding JS. Intensive care unit. Anaesthesia 1961;16:275–84.
14. Grenvik A, Ayres SM, Holbrook PR, Shoemaker W, editors. Society of Critical Care Medicine. 4th ed. Philadelphia (PA): WB Saunders Publishers; 2000.
15. Negovsky VA, Gurvitch AM, Zolotokrylina ES. Postresuscitation Disease. Amsterdam: Elsevier; 1983.
16. Ernster L. Biochemistry of reoxygenation injury. Crit Care Med 1988;16:947–53.
17. Safar P. Community-wide cardiopulmonary resuscitation. J Iowa Med Soc 1964 Nov:629–35.
18. American Society of Anesthesiologists. Committee on Acute Medicine (Safar P, Chairman). Community-wide emergency medical services. JAMA 1968;204:595–602.
19. Cummins RO, Ornato JP, Thies WH, Pepe PE. Improving survival from sudden cardiac arrest: the "chain of survival" concept. Circulation 1991;83:1832–47.
20. Safar P. History of Cardiopulmonary-Cerebral Resuscitation. In: Kaye W, Bircher N, editors. Cardiopulmonary resuscitation. New York: Churchill Livingstone; 1989. p. 1–53.

21. Kety SS, Schmidt CF. The nitrous oxide method for quantitative determination of cerebral blood flow in man: theory, procedure, and normal values. J Clin Invest 1948;27:476–83.
22. Wechsler RL, Dripps RD, Kety SS. Blood flow and oxygen consumption of the human brain during anesthesia produced by thiopental. Anesthesiology 1951;12:308–14.
23. Stone HH, Donnelly C, Frobese AS. The effect of lowered body temperature on the cerebral hemodynamics and metabolism of man. Surg Gyn Obstec 1956;103:313–22.
24. Stone HH, MacKrell TN, Brandstater GL, Hardak BJ, Nemir P. The effect of induced hemorrhagic shock on the cerebral circulation and metabolism of man. Surg Forum 1954;789–803.
25. Stewart GN, Guthrie C, Burns RI. The resuscitation of the central nervous system of mammals. J Exper Med 1906;8:289.
26. Negovsky VA. Fifty years of the Institute of General Reanimatology of the USSR Academy of Medical Sciences. Crit Care Med 1988;16:287–91.
27. Rossen R, Cabat H, Anderson JP. Acute arrest of cerebral circulation in man. Arch Neurol 1943;50:510–28.
28. Cole S, Corday E. Four-minute limit for cardiac resuscitation. JAMA 1956;161:1454–8.
29. Redding JS, Cozine RA. A comparison of open and closed-chest cardiac massage in dogs. Anesthesiology 1961;22:280–5.
30. Bircher N, Safar P, Stewart R. A comparison of standard, "MAST"-augmented, and open-chest CPR in dogs. Crit Care Med 1980;8:147–52.
31. Bircher N, Safar P. Cerebral preservation during cardiopulmonary resuscitation. Crit Care Med 1985;13:185–90.
32. Schleien CL, Dean JM, Koehler RC, Michael JR, Chantarojanasiri T, Traystman R, et al. Effect of epinephrine on cerebral and myocardial perfusion in an infant animal preparation of cardiopulmonary resuscitation. Circulation 1986;73:809–17.
33. Brown CG, Werman HA, Davis EA, Hamlin R, Hobson J, Ashton JA. Comparative effect of graded doses of epinephrine on regional brain blood flow during CPR in a swine model. Ann Emerg Med 1986;15:1138–44.
34. del Guercio LRM, Feins NR, Cohn JD, Coomaraswamy RP, Wollman SB, State D. Comparison of blood flow during external and internal cardiac massage in man. Circulation 1965;32 (Suppl 1):I-172-I-180.
35. Stajduhar K, Safar P, Steinberg R, Sotosky M, McNulty P, Alifimoff J, et al. Cerebral blood flow and other benefits from wider use of open-chest cardiopulmonary resuscitation [abstract]. Crit Care Med 1983;11:226.
36. Sanders AB, Kern KB, Ewy GA, Atlas M, Bailey L. Improved resuscitation from cardiac arrest with open-chest massage. Ann Emerg Med 1984;13:672–5.
37. Stephenson HE Jr, Reid LC, Hinton JW. Some common denominators in 1200 cases of cardiac arrest. Ann Surg 1953;137:731–44.
38. Hachimi-Idrissi S, Leeman J, Hubloue Y, Huyghens L, Corne L. Open chest cardiopulmonary resuscitation in out-of-hospital cardiac arrest. Resuscitation 1997;35:151–6.
39. Beck CS, Pritchard H, Feil SH. Ventricular fibrillation of long duration abolished by electric shock. JAMA 1947;135:985.
40. Eisenberg MS, Horwood BT, Cummins RO, Reynolds-Haertle R, Hearne TR. Cardiac arrest and resuscitation: a tale of 29 cities. Ann Emerg Med 1990;19:179–86.
41. Safar P, Abramson NS, Angelos M, Cantadore R, Leonov Y, Levine R, et al. Emergency cardiopulmonary bypass for resuscitation from prolonged cardiac arrest. Am J Emerg Med 1990;8:55–67.
42. Safar P. Resuscitation from clinical death: patho-physiologic limits and therapeutic potentials. Crit Care Med 1988;16:923–41.
43. Pretto E, Safar P, Saito R, Stezoski W, Kelsey S. Cardiopulmonary bypass after prolonged cardiac arrest in dogs. Ann Emerg Med 1987;16:611–9.
44. Reich H, Angelos M, Safar P, Sterz F, Leonov Y. Cardiac resuscitability with cardiopulmonary bypass after increasing ventricular fibrillation times in dogs. Ann Emerg Med 1990;19:887–90.
45. Angelos M, Safar P, Reich H. External cardiopulmonary resuscitation preserves brain viability after prolonged cardiac arrest in dogs. Am J Emerg Med 1991;9:436–43.

46. Angelos M, Safar P, Reich H. A comparison of cardiopulmonary resuscitation with cardiopulmonary bypass after prolonged cardiac arrest in dogs. Reperfusion pressures and neurologic recovery. Resuscitation 1991;21:121–35.

47. Tisherman S, Chabal C, Safar P, Stezoski W. Resuscitation of dogs from cold-water submersion using cardiopulmonary bypass. Ann Emerg Med 1985;14:389–96.

48. Tisherman SA, Vandevelde K, Safar P, Morioka T, Obrist W, Corne L, et al. Future directions for resuscitation research. V. Ultra-advanced life support. Resuscitation 1997;34(Pt 5): 281–93.

49. Tisherman S, Safar P, Kormos R, Paris P, Peitzman A. Clinical feasibility of emergency cardiopulmonary bypass for external CPR-refractory prehospital cardiac arrest [abstract]. Resuscitation 1994;28:S5.

50. Michenfelder JK, Theye RA. The effects of anesthesia and hypothermia on canine cerebral ATP and lactate during anoxia produced by decapitation. Anesthesiology 1970;33:430–9.

51. Kramer RS, Sanders AP, Lesage AM, Woodhall B, Sealy WC. The effect of profound hypothermia on preservation of cerebral ATP content during circulatory arrest. J Thorac Cardiovasc Surg 1968;56:699–709.

52. Kampschulte S, Morikawa S, Safar P. Recovery from anoxic encephalopathy following cardiac arrest [abstract]. Fed Proc 1969;28:522.

53. Safar P. Introduction to chapters 27–29. Resuscitation of the arrested brain. In: Safar P, Elam I, editors. Advances in cardiopulmonary resuscitation. New York: Springer-Verlag; 1977. p. 177–81.

54. Hossmann K-A, Sato K. Recovery of neuronal function after prolonged cerebral ischemia. Science 1970;168:375–6.

55. Hossmann KA, Lechtape-Gruter H, Hossmann V. The role of cerebral blood flow for the recovery of the brain after prolonged ischemia. Z Neurol 1973;204:281–99.

56. Ames A III, Wright RL, Kowada M, Thurston JM, Majno G. Cerebral ischemia. II. The no–reflow phenomenon. Am J Pathol 1968;52:437–53.

57. Cantu R, Ames A, DiGiancinto G, Dixon J. Hypotension. A major factor limiting recovery from cerebral ischemia. J Surg Res 1969;9:525–9.

58. Fischer EG, Ames A III, Hedley-Whyte ET, O'Gorman S. Reassessment of cerebral capillary changes in acute global ischemia and their relationship to the "no-reflow phenomenon." Stroke 1977;8:36–9.

59. Lind B, Snyder J, Safar P: Total brain ischaemia in dogs. Cerebral physiological and metabolic changes after 15 minutes of circulatory arrest. Resuscitation 1975;4(2):97–113.

60. Snyder JV, Nemoto EM, Carroll RG, Safar P. Global ischemia in dogs: intracranial pressures, brain blood flow and metabolism. Stroke 1975;6:21–7.

61. Plum F, editor. The clinical problem: how much anoxia-ischemia damages the brain? Symposium on brain ischemia. Arch Neurol 1973;29:259–360.

62. Plum F, Posner JB. The Diagnosis of stupor and coma. Philadelphia: FA Davis, 1980.

63. Kagstroem E, Smith ML, Siesjo BK. Local cerebral blood flow in the recovery period following complete cerebral ischemia in the rat. J Cereb Blood Flow Metab 1983;3:170–82.

64. Wolfson SK, Safar P, Reich H, Clark JM, Gur D, Stezoski W, et al. Dynamic heterogeneity of cerebral hypoperfusion after prolonged cardiac arrest in dogs measured by the stable xenon/CT technique: a preliminary study. Resuscitation 1992;23:1–20.

65. Sterz F, Leonov Y, Safar P, Johnson D, Oku K, Tisherman S, et al. Multifocal cerebral blood flow by Xe-CT and global cerebral metabolism after prolonged cardiac arrest in dogs. Reperfusion with open-chest CPR or cardiopulmonary bypass. Resuscitation 1992;24:27–47.

66. Leonov Y, Sterz F, Safar P, Johnson DW, Tisherman SA, Oku K. Hypertension with hemodilution prevents multifocal cerebral hypoperfusion after cardiac arrest in dogs. Stroke 1992;23:45–53.

67. Sterz F, Safar P, Johnson DW, Oku K, Tisherman SA. Effects of U74006F on multifocal cerebral blood flow and metabolism after cardiac arrest in dogs. Stroke 1991;22:889–95.

68. Oku K, Sterz F, Safar P, Johnson D, Obrist W, Leonov Y, et al. Mild hypothermia after cardiac arrest in dogs does not affect postarrest multifocal cerebral hypoperfusion. Stroke 1993; 24:1590–8.

69. Oku K, Kuboyama K, Safar P, Obrist W, Sterz F, Leonov Y, et al. Cerebral and systemic arteriovenous oxygen monitoring after cardiac arrest. Inadequate cerebral oxygen delivery. Resuscitation 1994;27:141–52.

70. Kuboyama K, Safar P, Oku K, Obrist W, Leonov Y, Sterz S, et al. Mild hypothermia after cardiac arrest in dogs does not affect postarrest cerebral oxygen uptake/delivery mismatching. Resuscitation 1994;27:231–44.

71. Beckstead JE, Tweed WA, Lee J, MacKeen WL. Cerebral blood flow and metabolism in man following cardiac arrest. Stroke 1978;9:569–73.

72. Cohan SL, Mun SK, Petite J, Correia J, Tavelra Da Silva AT. Cerebral blood flow in humans following resuscitation from cardiac arrest. Stroke 1989;20:761–5.

73. Symon L. Flow thresholds in brain ischemia and the effects of drugs. Brit J Anaesth 1985;57:34–43.

74. Bottiger BW, Motsch J, Bohrer H, Boker T, Aulmann M, Nawroth PP, et al. Activation of blood coagulation after cardiac arrest is not balanced adequately by activation of endogenous fibrinolysis. Circulation 1995;92:2572–8.

75. VanHarreveld A, Ochs S. Cerebral impedance changes after circulatory arrest. Amer J Physiol 1957;187:180.

76. Schanne FA, Kane AB, Young EE, Farber JL. Calcium dependence of toxic cell death: a final common pathway. Science 1979;206:700–2.

77. Miller RJ. Multiple calcium channels and neuronal function. Science 1987;235:46–52.

78. Rehncrona S, Rosen I, Siesjo BK. Excessive cellular acidosis: an important mechanism of neuronal damage in the brain? Acta Physiol Scand 1980;110:425–7.

79. Nemoto EM, Evans RW, Kochanek PM. Free fatty acid liberation in the pathogenesis and therapeutic brain damage. In: Bazan NG, Braquet P, Ginsberg MD, editors. Advances in neurochemistry, neurochemistry correlates of cerebral ischemia. New York: Plenum Press; 1992. p. 183–218.

80. Bandaranayke NM, Nemoto EM, Stezoski SW. Rat brain osmolality during barbiturate anesthesia and global brain ischemia. Stroke 1978;9:249–54.

81. Globus MY, Busto R, Dietrich WD, Martinez E, Valdes I, Ginsberg MD. Direct evidence for acute and massive norepinephrine release in the hippocampus during transient ischemia. J Cereb Blood Flow 1989;9:892–6.

82. Rothman SM, Olney JW. Glutamate and the pathophysiology of hypoxic-ischemic brain damage. Review. Ann Neurol 1986;19:105–11.

83. Benveniste H. The excitotoxine hypotheses in relation to cerebral ischemia. Cer Vasc & Brain Metabolism Reviews 1991;3:213–45.

84. Globus MYT, Ginsberg MD, Busto R. Excitotoxic index – a biochemical marker of selective vulnerability. Neuroscience Letter 1991;127:39–42.

85. Fridovich I. Superoxide radical: an endogenous toxicant. Ann Rev Pharmacol Toxicol 1983;23:239–57.

86. McCord JM. Oxygen-derived free radicals in postischemic tissue injury. N Engl J Med 1985;312:159–63.

87. Kontos HA. Oxygen radicals in CNS damage. Review article. Chem Biol Interactions 1989;72:229–55.

88. Traystman RJ, Kirsch JR, Koehler RC. Oxygen radical mechanisms of brain injury following ischemia and reperfusion. J Appl Physiol 1991;71(4):1185–95.

89. Siesjo BK, Bengtsson F. Calcium fluxes, calcium antagonists, and calcium-related pathology in brain ischemia, hypoglycemia, and spreading depression: a unifying hypothesis. J Cereb Blood Flow Metab 1989;9:127–40.

90. Siesjo BK, Ouyuang YB, Kristian T, Elmer E, Li PA, Uchino H. Role of mitrochondria in immediate and delayed reperfusion damage. In: Ito U, Kirino T, Kuroiwa T, et al, editors. Maturation phenomenon in cerebral ischemia III. Berlin: Springer-Verlag; 1999.

91. Uchino H, Elmer E, Uchino K, Li PA, He QP, Smith ML, Siesjo BK. Amelioration by cyclosporin A of brain damage in transient forebrain ischemia in the rat. Brain Res 1998; 812:216–26.

128 P. Safar

92. Nemoto EM, Bleyaert AL, Stezoski SW, Moossy J, Rao GR, Safar P. Global brain ischemia: a reproducible monkey model. Stroke 1977;8(5):558–64.
93. Radovsky A, Safar P, Sterz F, Leonov Y, Reich H, Kuboyama K. Regional prevalence and distribution of ischemic neurons in dog brains 96 hours after cardiac arrest of 0 to 20 minutes. Stroke 1995;26:2127–34.
94. Jenkins LW, Povlishock JT, Becker DP, Miller JD, Sullivan HG. Complete cerebral ischemia: an ultrastructural study. Acta Neuropathol (Berl) 1979;48:113–25.
95. Radovsky A, Katz L, Ebmeyer U, Safar P. Ischemic neurons in rat brains after 6, 8, or 10 minutes of transient hypoxic ischemia. Toxicology 1997;25:500–5.
96. Colbourne F, Li H, Buchan AM, Clemens JA. Continuing postischemic neuronal death in CA1: influence of ischemia duration and cytoprotective doses of NBQX and SNX-111 in rats. Stroke 1999 Mar;30(3):662–8.
97. Nitatori T, Sato N, Waguri S, Karasawa Y, Araki H, Shibanai K, et al. Delayed neuronal death in the CA1 pyramidal cell layer of the gerbil hippocampus following transient ischemia is apoptosis. J Neuroscience 1995;15:1001–11.
98. Prueckner S, Clark R, Woods R, Behringer W, Khan L, Radovsky A, et al. Cold aortic arch flush decreases apoptosis after exsanguination cardiac arrest in dogs [abstract]. Crit Care Med 1999;27:A30.
99. Takahashi K, Greenberg JH, Jackson P, Maclin K, Zhang J. Neuroprotective effects of inhibiting poly(ADP-Ribose) synthetase on focal cerebral ischemia in rats. J Cereb Blood Flow Metab 1997;17:1137–42.
100. Safar P, Gisvold SE, Vaagenes P, Hendrickx HHL, Bar-Joseph G, Bircher N, et al. Long-term animal models for the study of global brain ischemia. In: Wauquier A, et al, editors. Protection of tissues against hypoxia. Amsterdam: Elsevier; 1982. p. 147–70.
101. Safar P. Long-term animal outcome models for cardiopulmonary-cerebral resuscitation research. Crit Care Med 1985;13:936–40.
102. Pulsinelli W, Brierley J, Plum F. Temporal profile of neuronal damage in a model of transient forebrain ischemia. Ann Neurol 1982;11:491–8.
103. Smith ML, Bendek G, Dahlgren N, Rosen I, Sieloch T, Siesjo BK. Models for studying long-term recovery following forebrain ischemia in the rat. A two vessel occlusion model. Acta Neurol Scand 1984;69:385–401.
104. Bottiger BW, Krumnikl JJ, Gass P, Schmitz B, Motsch J, Martin E. The cerebral "no-flow" phenomenon after cardiac arrest in rats – influence of low-flow reperfusion. Resuscitation 1997;34:79–87.
105. Bottiger BW, Teschendorf P, Krumnikl J, Vogel P, Galmbacher R, Schmitz B, et al. Global cerebral ischemia due to cardiocirculatory arrest in mice causes neuronal degeneration and early induction of transcription factor genes in the hippocampus. Molecular Brain Research 1999;65:135–42.
106. Hendrickx H, Safar P, Rao GR, Gisvold SE. Asphyxia, cardiac arrest and resuscitation in rats. Short-term recovery. Resuscitation 1984;12:97–116.
107. Hendrickx HHL, Safar P, Miller A. Long-term behavioral changes. Resuscitation 1984; 12:117–28.
108. Katz L, Ebmeyer U, Safar P, Radovsky A, Neumar R. Outcome model of asphyxial cardiac arrest in rats. J Cereb Blood Flow Metab 1995;15:1032–9.
109. Katz L, Wang Y, Ebmeyer U, Radovsky A, Safar P. Glucose plus insulin infusion improves cerebral outcome after asphyxial cardiac arrest. Neuroreport 1998;9:3363–7.
110. Katz LM, Callaway CW, Kagan VE, Kochanek PM. Electron spin resonance measure of brain antioxidant activity during ischemia/reperfusion. Neuroreport 1998;9:1587–93.
111. Neumar RW, Bircher NG, Sim KM, Xiao F, Zadach KS, Radovsky A, et al. Epinephrine and sodium bicarbonate during CPR following asphyxial cardiac arrest in rats. Resuscitation 1994;29:249–63.
112. Eshel G, Safar P, Radovsky A, Stezoski SW. Hyperthermia-induced cardiac arrest in monkeys: limited efficacy of standard CPR. Aviation, Space, and Environmental Med 1997; 68:415–20.

113. Bar-Joseph G, Safar P, Saito R, Stezoski SW, Alexander H. Monkey model of severe volume-controlled hemorrhagic shock with resuscitation to outcome. Resuscitation 1991 Aug; 22(1):27–43.

114. Vaagenes P, Cantadore R, Safar P, Moossy J, Rao G, Diven W, et al. Amelioration of brain damage by lidoflazine after prolonged ventricular fibrillation cardiac arrest in dogs. Crit Care Med 1984;12:846–55.

115. Vaagenes P, Safar P, Diven W, Moossy J, Rao G, Cantadore R, et al. Brain enzyme levels in CSF after cardiac arrest and resuscitation in dogs: markers of damage and predictors of outcome. J Cereb Blood Flow Metab 1988;8:262–75.

116. Vaagenes P, Safar P, Moossy J, Rao G, Diven W, Ravi C, et al. Asphyxiation versus ventricular fibrillation cardiac arrest in dogs. Differences in cerebral resuscitation effects – a preliminary study. Resuscitation 1997;35:41–52.

117. Kirimli B, Kampschulte S, Safar P. Resuscitation from cardiac arrest due to exsanguination. Surg Gynecol Obstet 1969;129:89–97.

118. Tisherman SA, Safar P, Sterz F, Leonov Y, Oku K, Stezoski W. Exsanguination cardiac arrest in dogs: physiology of dying [abstract]. Ann Emerg Med 1989;18:460.

119. Tisherman SA, Safar P, Sterz F, Leonov Y, Oku K, Stezoski W. Exsanguination versus ventricular fibrillation cardiac arrest in dogs: comparison of neurologic outcome – preliminary data [abstract]. Ann Emerg Med 1989;18:460.

120. Safar P, Stezoski SW, Nemoto EM. Amelioration of brain damage after 12 minutes cardiac arrest in dogs. Arch Neurol 1976;33:91–5.

121. Sterz F, Leonov Y, Safar P, Radovsky A, Tisherman S, Oku K. Hypertension with or without hemodilution after cardiac arrest in dogs. Stroke 1990;21:1178–84.

122. Nemoto EM, Erdmann NW, Strong E, Rao GRM, Moossy J. Regional brain PO_2 after global ischemia in monkeys: evidence for regional differences in critical perfusion pressures. Stroke1979;10(1):44–52.

123. Lin SR, O'Connor MJ, Fischer HW, King A. The effect of combined dextran and streptokinase on cerebral function and blood flow after cardiac arrest: an experimental study on the dog. Invest Radiol 1978 Nov-Dec;13:490–8.

124. Wise G, Sutter R, Burkholder J. The treatment of brain ischemia with vasopressor drugs. Stroke 1972 Mar-Apr;3(2):135–40.

125. Muizelaar JP, Becker DP. Induced hypertension for the treatment of cerebral ischemia after subarachnoid hemorrhage. Direct effect on cerebral blood flow. Surg Neurol 1986;25:317–25.

126. Ito U, Ohno K, Yamaguchi T, Tomita H, Inaba Y, Kashima M. Transient appearance of "no-reflow" phenomenon in Mongolian gerbils. Stroke 1980;11:517–21.

127. Ebmeyer U, Safar P, Radovsky A, Sharma C, Tanigawa K, Wang Y, Capone A, Xiao F, Bircher N, Stezoski W, Alexander H: Effective combination treatments for cerebral resuscitation from cardiac arrest in dogs. Exploratory studies [abstract]. Resuscitation 1994;28:S20.

128. White BC, Gadzinski DS, Hoehner PJ, Krome C, Hoehnert, White JD. Effect of flunarizine on canine cerebral cortical blood flow and vascular resistance post cardiac arrest. Ann Emerg Med 1982;11:119–26.

129. Steen PA, Gisvold SE, Milde JH, Newberg LA, Scheithauer BW, Lanier WL, et al. Nimodipine improves outcome when given after complete cerebral ischemia in primates. Anesthesiology 1985;62:406–14.

130. Takasu A, Matushima S, Takino M, Okada Y. Effect of endothelin-1 antagonist, BQ 485, on cerebral oxygen metabolism after complete global cerebral ischemia in dogs. Resuscitation 1997;34:65–9.

131. Krep H, Brinker G, Schwindt W, Hossmann K-A. Endothelin type A-antagonist improves long-term neurological recovery after cardiac arrest in rats. Crit Care Med 2000;28:2873–80.

132. Safar P, Kochanek P. Cerebral blood flow promotion after prolonged cardiac arrest. Editorial. Crit Care Med 2000;28:3104–6.

133. Spivey WH, Abramson NS, Safar P, Sutton-Tyrell K, Schoffstaff JM, BRCT II Study Group. Correlation of blood pressure with mortality and neurologic recovery in comatose postresuscitation patients [abstract]. Ann Emerg Med 1991;20:453.

134. Martin DR, Persse D, Brown CG, Jastremski M, Cummins RO, Pepe PE, et al. Relation between initial post-resuscitation systolic blood pressure and neurologic outcome following cardiac arrest [abstract]. Ann Emerg Med 1993;22:206.

135. Sasser HC, Safar P, Kelsey SF, Ricci EM, Sutton-Tyrrell KC, Wisniewski SR. Arterial hypertension after cardiac arrest is associated with good cerebral outcome in patients [abstract]. Crit Care Med 1999;27(12):A29.

136. Mullner M, Sterz F, Binder M, Hellwagner K, Meron G, Herkner H, et al. Arterial blood pressure after human cardiac arrest and neurologic recovery. Stroke 1996;27(1):59–62.

137. Lee SK, Vaagenes D, Safar P, Stezoski SW, Scanlon M. Effect of cardiac arrest time on the cortical cerebral blood flow during subsequent standard external cardiopulmonary resuscitation in rabbits. Resuscitation 1989;17:105–117.

138. Ishige N, Pitts LH, Berry I, Carlson SG, Nishimura MC, Moseley ME, et al. The effect of hypoxia on traumatic head injury in rats: alterations in neurologic function, brain edema, and cerebral blood flow. J Cereb Blood Flow Metab 1987;7:759–67.

139. Muizelaar JP, Marmarou A, Ward JD, Kontos HA, Choi SC, Becker DP, et al. Adverse effects of prolonged hyperventilation in patients with severe head injury; a randomized clinical trial. J Neurosurg 1991;75:731–9.

140. Liu Y, Rosenthal RE, Haywood Y, Miljkovic-Lolic M, Vanderhoek JY, Fiskum G. Normoxic ventilation after cardiac arrest reduces oxidation of brain lipids and improves neurological outcome. Stroke 1998;29:1679–86.

141. Zwemer CF, Whitesall SE, D'Alecy LG. Cardiopulmonary-cerebral resuscitation with 100% oxygen exacerbates neurological dysfunction following nine minutes of normothermic cardiac arrest in dogs. Resuscitation 1994;27:159–70.

142. Zwemer CF, Whitesall SE, D'Alecy LG. Hypoxic cardiopulmonary-cerebral resuscitation fails to improve neurologic outcome following cardiac arrest in dogs. Resuscitation 1995;29:225–36.

143. Smith AL, Hoff JT, Nielson SL, Larson CP. Barbiturate protection in acute focal cerebral ischemia. Stroke 1974;5(1):1–7.

144. Michenfelder JD, et al: Cerebral protection by barbiturate anesthesia. Use after middle cerebral artery occlusion in Java monkeys. Arch Neurol 1976;33:345.

145. Goldstein A Jr, Wells BA, Keats AS. Increased tolerance to cerebral anoxia by pentobarbital. Arch Int Pharmacodyn Ther 1966;161:138–43.

146. Yatsu FM, Diamond I, Graziano C, Lindquist P. Experimental brain ischemia: protection from irreversible damage with a rapid-acting barbiturate (methohexital). Stroke 1972;3:726–32.

147. Shapiro HM. Intracranial hypertension. Therapeutic and anesthetic considerations. Anesthesiology 1975;43:445–71.

148. Todd MM, Dunlop BJ, Shapiro HM, Chadwick HS, Powell HC. Ventricular fibrillation in the cat: a model for global cerebral ischemia. Stroke 1981;12:808–15.

149. Demopoulos HB, Flamm ES, Pietronigro DD, Seligman ML. The free radical pathology and the microcirculation in the major central nervous system disorders. Acta Physiol Scand 1980;492(suppl):91–119.

150. Bleyaert AL, Nemoto EM, Safar P, Stezoski SW, Mickell JJ, Moossy J, et al: Thiopental amelioration of brain damage after global ischemia in monkeys. Anesthesiology 1978;49:390–8.

151. Gisvold SE, Safar P, Hendrickx HHL, Rao G, Moossy J, Alexander H. Thiopental treatment after global brain ischemia in pigtail monkeys. Anesthesiology 1984;60:88–96.

152. Breivik H, Safar P, Sands P, Fabritius R, Lind B, Lust P, et al. Clinical feasibility trials of barbiturate therapy after cardiac arrest. Crit Care Med 1978;6:228–44.

153. Brain Resuscitation Clinical Trial I Study Group. Steering Committee: Kelsey SF, Abramson NS, Detre KM, Monroe J, Reinmuth O, Safar P (P.I.), Snyder JV. Investigators: Mullie A, et al.: A randomized clinical study of cardiopulmonary-cerebral resuscitation: Design, methods and patient characteristics. Am J Emerg Med 1986;4:72–86.

154. Ebmeyer W, Safar P, Radovsky A, Xiao F, Capone A, Tanigawa K, et al. Thiopental combination treatments for cerebral resuscitation after prolonged cardiac arrest in dogs. Exploratory outcome study. Resuscitation 2000;45;119–131.

155. Brain Resuscitation Clinical Trial II Study Group (Safar P, P.I.). A randomized clinical study of a calcium-entry blocker (lidoflazine) in the treatment of comatose survivors of cardiac arrest. N Engl J Med 1991;324:1225–31.

156. Abramson N, Kelsey S, Safar P, Sutton-Tyrrell K. Simpson's paradox and clinical trials: What you find is not necessarily what you prove. Ann Emerg Med 1992;21:1480–2.

157. Roine RO, Kaste M, Kinnamen A, Nikki P, Sarna S, Kajaste S. Nimodipine after resuscitation from out-of-hospital ventricular fibrillation: a placebo-controlled, double-blind randomized trial. JAMA 1990;264:3171–7.

158. Park CK, Nehls DG, Graham DI, Teasdale GM, McCulloch J. Focal cerebral ischemia in the cat: treatment with glutamate antagonist MK-801 after induction of ischemia. J Cereb Blood Flow Metab 1988;8:757–62.

159. Gill R, Foster AC, Woodruff GN. Systemic administration of MK-801 protects against ischemia induced hippocampal neuro-degeneration in the gerbil. J Neurosci 1987;7:3343–9.

160. Sterz F, Leonov Y, Safar P, Radovsky A, Stezoski W, Reich H, et al. Effect of excitatory amino acid receptor blocker MK-801 on overall, neurologic, and morphologic outcome after prolonged cardiac arrest in dogs. Anesthesiology 1989;71:907–18.

161. Buchan AM, Li H, Cho S, Pulsinelli WA. Blockade of the AMPA receptor prevents CA1 hippocampal injury following severe but transient forebrain ischemia in adult rats. Neurosci Lett 1991 Nov 11;132(2):255–8.

162. Buchan AM, Bruederlin B, Heinicke E, Li H. Failure of the lipid peroxidation inhibitor, U74006F, to prevent postischemic selective neuronal injury. J Cereb Blood Flow Metab 1992;12:250–6.

163. Buchan AM, Gertler SZ, Li H, Xue D, Huang ZG, Chaundy KE, et al. A selective N-type Ca^{2+}-channel blocker prevents CA1 injury 24 h following severe forebrain ischemia and reduces infarction following focal ischemia. J Cereb Blood Flow Metab 1994;14:903–10.

164. Xiao F, Sim K, Safar P, Radovsky A, Capone A, Ebmeyer U, et al. Beneficial effects of neuron-specific calcium entry blocker SNX-111 on cerebral outcome after forebrain ischemia in rats, but not after ventricular fibrillation (VF) cardiac arrest (CA) in dogs [abstract]. Resuscitation 1994;28:S36.

165. Toung TK, Traystman RJ, Hurn PD. Estrogen-mediated neuroprotection after experimental stroke in male rats. Stroke 1998;29:1666–70.

166. Sieber FE, Traystman RJ. Special issues, glucose and the brain. Crit Care Med 1991;20:104–14.

167. Abramson NS, Safar P, Sutton-Tyrrell, Craig MT, for the BRCT III Study Group: A randomized clinical trial of escalating doses of high dose epinephrine during cardiac resuscitation [abstract]. Crit Care Med 1995;23:A178.

168. Brain Resuscitation Clinical Trial I Study Group: Steering Committee: Abramson NS, Safar P, Detre KM, Kelsey SF, Monroe J, Reinmuth O, et al. Neurologic recovery after cardiac arrest: effect of duration of ischemia. Crit Care Med 1985;13:930–1.

169. Rogove HJ, Safar P, Sutton-Tyrrell K, Abramson NS. Old age does not negate good clinical trials. Crit Care Med 1995;23:18–25.

170. Edgren E, Hedstrand U, Kelsey S, Sutton-Tyrrell K, Safar P. Assessment of neurological prognosis in comatose survivors of cardiac arrest. Lancet 1994;343:1055–9.

171. Sasser HC, Safar P, BRCT Study Group: Clinical signs early after CPR predict neurologic outcome [abstract]. Crit Care Med 1999;27(12):A30.

172. Abramson NS, Meisel A, Safar P. Deferred consent. A new approach for resuscitation research on comatose patients. JAMA 1986;255:2466–71.

173. Vaagenes P, Mullie M, Fodstad DT, Abramson NA, Safar P, and the Brain Resuscitation Clinical Trial I Study Group. The use of cytosolic enzyme increase in cerebrospinal fluid of patients resuscitated after cardiac arrest. Am J Emerg Med 1994;12:621–4.

174. Mullie A, Lust P, Penninckx J, Vanhove L, Vandevelde K, Vanhoonacker G, et al. Monitoring of cerebro-spinal fluid enzyme levels in postischemic encephalopathy after cardiac arrest. Crit Care Med 1981;9:399–400.

175. Edgren E, Terent A, Hedstrand U, Ronquist G. Cerebral spinal fluid markers in relation to outcome in patients with global cerebral ischemia. Crit Care Med 1983;11:4–6.

176. Bigelow WG, Lindsay WK, Greenwood WF. Hypothermia: its possible role in cardiac surgery. An investigation of factors governing survival in dogs at low body temperature. Ann Surg 1950;132:849–66.

177. Rosomoff HL, Holaday BA. Cerebral blood flow and cerebral oxygen consumption during hypothermia. Am J Physiol 1954;179:85–8.

178. Rosomoff HL. Hypothermia and cerebral vascular lesions. I. Experimental interruption of the middle cerebral artery during hypothermia. J Neurosurg 1956;13:332–43.

179. Rosomoff HL. Protective effects of hypothermia against pathological processes of the nervous system. Ann NY Acad Sci 1959;80:475–86.

180. Rosomoff HL, Shulman K, Raynor R, et al. Experimental brain injury and delayed hypothermia. Surg Gynecol Obstet 1960;110:27–32.

181. Dripps RD, editor. The Physiology of Induced Hypothermia. Washington (DC): National Academy of Sciences; 1956.

182. Rosomoff HL, Safar P. Management of the comatose patient. In: Safar P, editor. Respiratory therapy. Philadelphia: FA Davis Co; 1965. p. 244–58.

183. White RJ. Cerebral hypothermia and circulatory arrest. Review and commentator. Mayo Clin Proc 1978;53:450–8.

184. White RJ, Brown HW, Albin MS, Verdura J. Rapid selective brain-cooling using head immersion and naso-oral perfusion in dogs. Resuscitation 1983;10:189–91.

185. Wolfson SK, Selker RG. Carotid perfusion hypothermia for brain surgery using cardiac arrest without bypass. J Surg Res 1973;14:449–58.

186. White RJ, Albin MS, Verdura J, Locke GE. Prolonged whole brain refrigeration with electrical and metabolic recovery. Nature 1966;209(30):1320–2.

187. Albin MS. Resuscitation of spinal cord. Crit Care Med 1978;5:270–6.

188. Ravitch MM, Lane R, Safar P, Steichen F, Knowles P. Lightning stroke. Recovery following cardiac massage and prolonged artificial respiration. N Engl J Med 1961;264:36–8.

189. Casey LC, Ballantyne HK, Fletcher JR, Chernow B, Lake CR. Development of a primate model of exposure hypothermia. Adv Shock Res 1983;9:233–7.

190. Tisherman SA, Rodriguez A, Safar P. Therapeutic hypothermia in traumatology. Chapter in Surgery Clinics of North America 1999;79:1269–89.

191. Bellamy R, Safar P, Tisherman SA, Basford R, Bruttig SP, Capone A, et al. Suspended animation for delayed resuscitation. Crit Care Med 1996;24(2 Suppl):S24–47.

192. Hochachka PW, Lutz PL, Sick T, et al (eds): Surviving hypoxia. Mechanisms of control and adaptation. Boca Raton: CRC Press, Inc; 1993.

193. Wolfe KB. Effect of hypothermia in cerebral damage resulting from cardiac arrest. Amer J Cardiol 1960;6:809–12.

194. Zimmerman JM, Spencer FC. The influence of hypothermia on cerebral injury resulting from circulatory occlusion. Surg Forum 1958;9:216–8.

195. Benson DW, Williams GR, Spencer FC, et al: The use of hypothermia after cardiac arrest. Anes Analg 1958;38:423–8.

196. Gisvold SE, Safar P, Rao G, Moossy J, Kelsey S, Alexander H. Multifaceted therapy after global brain ischemia in monkeys. Stroke 1984;15:803–12.

197. Brader E, Jehle D, Safar P. Protective head cooling during cardiac arrest in dogs [abstract]. Ann Emerg Med 1985;14:510.

198. Leonov Y, Sterz F, Safar P, Radovsky A. Moderate hypothermia after cardiac arrest of 17 min in dogs: effect on cerebral and cardiac outcome. A preliminary study. Stroke 1990;21:1600–6.

199. Safar P, Klain M, Tisherman S. Selective brain cooling after cardiac arrest (Editorial). Crit Care Med 1996;24:911–4.

200. Xiao F, Safar P, Alexander H. Peritoneal cooling for mild cerebral hypothermia after cardiac arrest in dogs. Resuscitation 1995;30:51–9.

201. Safar P, Grenvik A, Abramson N, Bircher N, editors. International resuscitation research symposium on the reversibility of clinical death. Crit Care Med 1988;16:919–1086.

202. Hossmann K-A. Resuscitation potentials after prolonged global ischemia in cats. Crit Care Med 1988;16:964–78.

203. Leonov Y, Sterz F, Safar P, Radovsky A, Oku K, Tisherman S, et al. Mild cerebral hypothermia during and after cardiac arrest improves neurologic outcome in dogs. J Cereb Blood Flow Metab 1990;10:57–70.

204. Sterz F, Safar P, Tisherman S, Radovsky A, Kuboyama K, Oku K. Mild hypothermic cardiopulmonary resuscitation improves outcome after prolonged cardiac arrest in dogs. Crit Care Med 1991;19:379–89.

205. Weinrauch V, Safar P, Tisherman S, Kuboyama K, Radovsky A. Beneficial effect of mild hypothermia and detrimental effect of deep hypothermia after cardiac arrest in dogs. Stroke 1992;23:1454–62.

206. Kuboyama K, Safar P, Radovsky A, Tisherman SA, Stezoski SW, Alexander H. Delay in cooling negates the beneficial effect of mild resuscitative cerebral hypothermia after cardiac arrest in dogs: a prospective, randomized, controlled study. Crit Care Med 1993;21:1348–58.

207. Safar P, Xiao F, Radovsky A, Tanigawa K, Ebmeyer U, Bircher N, et al. Improved cerebral resuscitation from cardiac arrest in dogs with mild hypothermia plus blood flow promotion. Stroke 1996;27:105–13.

208. Busto R, Deitrich WD, Globus MY, Valdes I, Scheinberg P, Ginsberg MD. Small differences in intra-ischemic brain temperature critically determine the extent of ischemic neuronal injury. J Cereb Blood Flow Metabol 1987;7:729–38.

209. Busto R, Dietrich WD, Globus MY, Ginsberg MD. Postischemic moderate hypothermia inhibits CA1 hippocampal ischemia neuronal injury. Neurosci Lett 1989;101:299–304.

210. Boris-Moller F, Smith ML, Siesjo BK. Effect of hypothermia on ischemic brain damage: a comparison between preischemic and postischemic cooling. Neurosci Res Comm 1989;5:87–94.

211. Chopp M, Chen H, Dereski MO, Garcia JH. Mild hypothermic intervention after graded ischemic stress in rats. Stroke 1991;22:37–43.

212. Nemoto EM, Klementavicius R, Melick JA, Yonas H. Effect of mild hypothermia on active and basal cerebral oxygen metabolism and blood flow. Adv Exp Med Biol 1994;361:469–73.

213. Astrup J, Rehncrona S, Siesjo BK. The increase in extracellular potassium concentration in the ischemic brain in relation to the preischemic functional activity and cerebral metabolic rate. Brain Res 1980;199:61–74.

214. Chopp M, Knight R, Tidwell CD, Helpern JA, Brown E, Welch KM. The metabolic effects of mild hypothermia on global cerebral ischemia and recirculation in the cat: comparison to normothermia and hyperthermia. J Cereb Blood Flow Metab 1989:9:141–8.

215. Busto R, Globus MY, Dietrich WD, Martinez E, Valdes I, Ginsberg MD. Effect of mild hypothermia on ischemia-induced release of neurotransmitters and free fatty acids in rat brain. Stroke 1989;20:904–10.

216. Dempsey RJ, Combs DJ, Maley ME, Cowen DE, Roy MW, Donaldson DL, et al. Moderate hypothermia reduces postischemic edema development and leukotriene production. Neurosurgery 1987;21:177–81.

217. Cardell M, Boris-Moller F, Wieloch T. Hypothermia prevents the ischemia-induced translocation and inhibition of protein kinase C in the rat striatum. J Neurochem 1991 Nov;57(5):1814–7.

218. Pomeranz S, Safar P, Radovsky A, Tisherman SA, Alexander H, Stezoski W. The effect of resuscitative moderate hypothermia following epidural brain compression on cerebral damage in a canine outcome model. J Neurosurg 1993;79:241–51.

219. Ebmeyer U, Safar P, Radovsky A, Obrist W, Alexander H, Pomeranz S. Moderate hypothermia for 48 hours after temporary epidural brain compression injury in a canine outcome model. J Neurotrauma 1998;15:323–36.

220. Baiping L, Xiujuan T, Hongwei C, et al: Effect of moderate hypothermia on lipid peroxidation in canine brain tissue after cardiac arrest and resuscitation. Stroke 1994;25:147–152.

221. Whalen MJ, Carlos TM, Clark RS, Marion DW, DeKosky ST, Heineman S, et al. The effect of brain temperature on acute inflammation after traumatic brain injury in rats. J Neurotrauma 1997;14:561–72.

222. Xiao F, Safar P, Katz L, Radovsky A, Ebmeyer U, Sim KM, Neumar R. Mild protective and resuscitative cerebral hypothermia improves outcome after asphyxial cardiac arrest in rats [abstract]. Resuscitation 1994;28:S21.

223. Coimbra C, Wieloch T. Hypothermia ameliorates neuronal survival when induced 2 hours after ischemia in the rat. Acta Physio Scand 1992;146:543–4.

224. Coimbra C, Boris MF, Drake M, Wieloch T. Diminished neuronal damage in the rat brain by late treatment with the antipyretic drug dipyrone or cooling following cerebral ischemia. Acta Neuropathol Berl 1996;92:447–453.

225. Hickey RW, Ferimer HN, Alexander HN, Garman RH, Callaway CL, Safar P, et al. Cerebral resuscitation with prolonged, delayed spontaneous hypothermia after asphyxial cardiac arrest in rats [abstract]. Soc Neurosci 1998;24:1506.

226. Dietrich WD, Busto R, Alonso O, Globus MY, Ginsberg MD. Intraischemic but not postischemic brain hypothermia protects chronically following global forebrain ischemia in rats. J Cereb Blood Flow Metab 1993;13:541–9.

227. Colbourne F, Li H, Buchan AM. Indefatigable CA1 sector neuroprotection with mild hypothermia induced 6 hours after severe forebrain ischemia in rats. J Cereb Blood Flow Metab 1999;19:724–49.

228. Bernard SA, Jones BM, Horne MK. Clinical trial of induced hypothermia in comatose survivors of out-of-hospital cardiac arrest. Ann Emerg Med 1997;30(2):146–53.

229. Yamashita C, Nakagiri K, Yamashita T, Matsuda H, Wakiyama H, Yoshida M, Ataka K, Okada M. Mild hypothermia for temporary brain ischemia during cardiopulmonary support systems: report of three cases. Surg Today 1999;29(2):182–5. Positive results of a subsequent randomized clinical outcome study of mild hypothermia after cardiac arrest have been submitted in 2001.

230. Zeiner A, Holzer M, Sterz F, Behringer W, Schorkhuber W, Mullner M, et al. For the Hypothermia after Cardiac Arrest (HACA) Study group: Mild Resuscitative Hypothermia to improve neurological outcome after cardiac arrest: a clinical feasibility trial. Stroke 2000;31:86–94.

231. Dietrich WD, Busto R, Valdes I, Loor Y. Effects of normothermic versus mild hyperthermic forebrain ischemia in rats. Stroke 1990;21:1318–25.

232. Marion DW, Penrod LE, Kelsey SF, Obrist WD, Kochanek PM, Palmer AM, et al. Treatment of traumatic brain injury with moderate hypothermia. New Engl J Med 1997; 336:540–6.

232a Clifton GL, Miller ER, Choi SC, et al: Lack of effect of induction of hyperthermia after acute brain injury. N Engl J Med 2001;344:556–563.

232b Safar P, Kochanek PM: Resuscitative hypothermia after acute brain injury. Letter to Editor. In press, N Engl J Med 2001.

233. Rupp SM, Severinghaus JW. Hypothermia. In: Miller RD, editor. Anesthesia. 2nd ed. New York: Churchill Livingstone; 1986. p. 1995–2022.

234. Capone AC, Safar P, Stezoski W, Tisherman S, Peitzman AB. Improved outcome with fluid restriction in treatment of uncontrolled hemorrhagic shock. J Am Coll Surg 1995; 180:49–56.

235. Crippen D, Safar P, Porter L, Zona J. Improved survival of hemorrhagic shock with oxygen and hypothermia in rats. Resuscitation 1991;21:271–81.

236. Kim SH, Stezoski SW, Safar P, Capone A, Tisherman S. Hypothermia and minimal fluid resuscitation increase survival after uncontrolled hemorrhagic shock in rats. J Trauma 1997;42:213–22.

237. Takasu A, Carrillo P, Stezoski SW, Safar P, Tisherman SA. Mild or moderate hypothermia, but not increased oxygen breathing, prolongs survival during lethal uncontrolled hemorrhagic shock in rats with monitoring of visceral dysoxia. Crit Care Med 1999;27:1557–64.

238. Prueckner S, Safar P, Kentner R, Stezoski J, Tisherman SA. Mild hypothermia increases survival from severe pressure controlled hemorrhagic shock in rats [abstract]. J. Trauma 1999;47:1172.

239. Carrillo P, Takasu A, Safar P, Tisherman S, Stezoski SW, Stolz G, et al. Prolonged severe hemorrhagic shock and resuscitation in rats does not cause subtle brain damage. J Trauma 1998;45:239–49.

240. Villar J, Slutsky AS. Effects of induced hypothermia in patients with septic adult respiratory distress syndrome. Resuscitation 1993;26:183–92.

241. Safar P, Tisherman S, Behringer W, Capone A, Prueckner S, Radovsky A, et al. Suspended animation for resuscitation from prolonged cardiac arrest. CPCR. Crit Care Med. 2000; 28:N214–N218 (Suppl.)

242. Rhee PM, Acosta J, Bridgeman A, Wang D, Jordan M, Rich N. Survival after emergency department thoracotomy: review of published data from the past 25 years. J Am Coll Surg 2000;190:288–98.

243. Tisherman SA, Safar P, Radovsky A, Peitzman A, Sterz F, Kuboyama K. Therapeutic deep hypothermic circulatory arrest in dogs: a resuscitation modality for hemorrhagic shock with 'irreparable' injury. J Trauma 1990;30:836–47.

244. Tisherman SA, Safar P, Radovsky A, Peitzman A, Marrone G, Kuboyama K, et al. Profound hypothermia (<10°C) compared with deep hypothermia (15°C) improves neurologic outcome in dogs after two hours' circulatory arrest induced to enable resuscitative surgery. J Trauma 1991;31:1051–62.

245. Tisherman S, Safar P, Radovsky A, Kuboyama K, Marrone G, Peitzman A. Heparin -bonded cardiopulmonary bypass without systemic anticoagulation does not diminish protection in hypothermic circulatory arrest after hemorrhagic shock in dogs [abstract]. Anesthesiology 1992;77:A285.

246. Tisherman SA, Safar P, Radovsky, Marrone G, Peitzman A, Kuboyama K. Profound hypothermia does, and an organ preservation solution does not, improve neurologic outcome after therapeutic circulatory arrest of 2 h in dogs [abstract]. Crit Care Med 1991;19:S89.

247. Tisherman S, Safar P, Radovsky A. "Suspended animation" research for otherwise infeasible resuscitative traumatologic surgery [abstract]. Prehosp Disaster Med 1993;8:S131.

248. Capone A, Safar P, Radovsky A, Wang Y, Peitzman A, Tisherman SA. Complete recovery after normothermic hemorrhagic shock and profound hypothermic circulatory arrest of 60 minutes in dogs. J Trauma 1996;40:388–94.

249. Rush, BF, Wilder RJ, Fishbein R, et al. Effects of total circulatory standstill in profound hypothermia. Surgery 1962;50:40-.

250. Popovic V, Popovic P. Survival of hypothermic dogs after 2-h circulatory arrest. Am J Physiol 1985;248(3 Pt 2):R308–11.

251. Livesay JJ, Cooley DA, Reul GJ, Walker WE, Frazier OH, Duncan JM. Resection of aortic arch aneurysms: a comparison of hypothermia techniques in 60 patients. Ann Thorac Surg 1983;36(1):19–28.

252. Woods RJ, Prueckner S, Safar P, Radovsky A, Takasu A, Stezoski SW, et al. Hypothermic aortic arch flush for preservation during exsanguination cardiac arrest of 15 minutes in dogs. J Trauma 1999;47:1028–38.

253. Behringer W, Prueckner S, Safar P, Radovsky A, Kentner, Stezoski SW, et al. Rapid induction of mild cerebral hypothermia by cold aortic flush achieves normal recovery in a dog outcome model with 20-minutes exsanguination cardiac arrest. Acad Emerg Med. In press 2000.

254. Behringer W, Prueckner S, Kentner R, Tisherman SA, Radovsky A, Clark R, et al. Rapid hypothermic aortic flush can achieve survival without brain damage after 30 min cardiac arrest in dogs. Anesthesiology. In press 2000.

255. Behringer W, Safar P, Kentner R, Wu X, Radovsky A, Stezoski SW, et al. Cold aortic flush can allow normal recovery after exsanguination cardiac arrest (CA) of 60 min in dogs [abstract]. Submitted to EAST meeting 2001.

256. Taylor MJ, Bailes JE, Elrifai AM, Shih SR, Teeple E, Leavitt ML, et al. A new solution for life without blood: asanguinous low flow perfusion of a whole-body perfusate during 3 hours of cardiac arrest and profound hypothermia. Circulation 1995;91:431–4.

257. Behringer W, Prueckner S, Kentner R, Safar P, Radovsky A, Stezoski W, et al. Exploration of pharmacologic aortic arch flush strategies for rapid induction of suspended animation (SA) (cerebral preservation) during exsanguination cardiac arrest (ExCA) of 20 min in dogs [abstract]. Crit Care Med 1999;27(12):A65.

258. Behringer W, Wu X, Radovsky A, Tisherman SA, Safar P. Tempol by aortic arch flush (AAF) for cerebral preservation during 20 min exsanguination cardiac arrest (CA) in dogs. Exploratory experiments [abstract]. Anesthesiology. In press 2000.

259. Safar P. Resuscitation medicine research: quo vadis. Ann Emerg Med 1996;27:542–52.
260. Safar P. On the future of reanimatology. Acad Emerg Med 2000;7:75–89.
261. Safar P. The physician's responsibility towards hopelessly critically ill patients. Ethical dilemmas in resuscitation medicine. Acta Anaesth Scand 1991;35 (Suppl 96):147–9.
262. Grenvik A, Powner DJ, Snyder JV, Jastremski MS, Babcock RA, Loughhead MG. Cessation of therapy in terminal illness and brain death. Crit Care Med 1978;6:284–91.
263. Wanzer SH, Adelstein SJ, Cranford RE, Federman DD, Hook ED, Moertel CG, et al. The physician's responsibility toward hopelessly ill patients. N Engl J Med 1984;310:955–9.
264. Wanzer SH, Federman DD, Adelstein SJ, Cassel CK, Cassem EH, Cranford RE, et al. The physician's responsibility toward hopelessly ill patients. A second look. N Engl J Med 1989;320:844–9.
265. Safar P, Winter P. Helping to die. Crit Care Med 1990;18:788–9.

The Ischemic Penumbra:
Pathophysiology and Therapeutic Implications

K.-A. Hossmann

Introduction

Under physiological conditions the brain covers its energy demands almost exclusively by oxidation of glucose. Opitz and Schneider [1] were the first to point out that an impairment of energy production induced by constrained oxygen supply affects the energy-consuming processes in a sequential way: first the functional activity of the brain is impaired followed, at a more severe degree of hypoxia, by the suppression of the metabolic activity required to maintain its structural integrity. The concept of two different thresholds of hypoxia for the preservation of functional and structural integrity was later refined by Symon et al. [2] who used a model of focal ischemia to establish the respective rates of blood flow. These studies revealed that EEG and evoked potentials are disturbed at substantially higher flow rates than the potassium gradient across the plasma membranes. Since the preservation of this gradient is a sign of cell viability, Symon and his colleagues proposed that neurons located in the flow range between "electrical" and "membrane" failure are functionally silent but structurally intact. In focal ischemia, this flow range corresponds to a coronal region intercalated between the necrotic infarct core and the normal brain; it has been termed "penumbra" in analogy to the partly illuminated area around the complete shadow of the moon in full eclipse [3].

The penumbra concept of focal ischemia had a considerable clinical impact because it was thought that this region remains viable and can be reactivated at any time after vascular occlusion by raising the blood flow above the threshold of electrical failure. Numerous studies have, therefore, been carried out to improve blood flow by the use of so-called vasoactive drugs, hemodilution or reconstructive surgery. Regrettably, most of these interventions did not lead to a major improvement of stroke outcome [4]. Studies of the reversibility of focal ischemia further revealed that the volume of brain infarct is the same after three hours temporary middle cerebral artery occlusion as after permanent ligation [5]. Lassen et al. [6], therefore, concluded that the penumbra remains viable for "only one or perhaps a few hours but not longer". These and similar observations dampened the hope to salvage the penumbra by improvement of blood flow and contributed to the nihilistic attitude in regard to the treatment of stroke.

During the past years two lines of research have rekindled the hope for a successful stroke treatment. Progression in molecular stroke research has led to the observation that ischemic injury can be substantially reduced by other means than flow improvement. A variety of drugs that interfere with signal transduction pathways are able to reduce the size of ischemic infarcts even though blood flow is not, or only marginally, altered [7]. Furthermore, the application of thrombolytic agents shortly after the onset of stroke results in neurological improvement, particularly in patients with mild degree of ischemia [8]. The concept of ischemic penumbra, therefore, had to be re-defined. In the following, the current state of this concept will be briefly reviewed.

Definition of Penumbra

In the original description by Astrup et al. [9], penumbra was characterized as a reduction of blood flow that led to electrical but not to membrane failure, as reflected by the suppression of spontaneous or evoked electrical activity on the one hand, and anoxic depolarization on the other (electrophysiological definition of the penumbra). In the monkey brain, these disturbances correspond to flow reductions to about 35% and 10% of control, respectively. The penumbra is, therefore, frequently defined as a reduction of blood flow to between these values (hemodynamic definition of the penumbra). Obviously the validity of this definition depends on stable thresholds which, however, may shift in different directions: hypothermia, anesthesia or various neuroprotective drugs cause a lowering, and hyperthermia or drugs that increase metabolic rate, a rise of these thresholds. The threshold of anoxic depolarization also rises with ongoing ischemia time, reflecting the time-limited viability of the penumbra (see below). A hemodynamic definition of the penumbra is, therefore, only possible if measurements are carried out shortly after the onset of ischemia, and if shifts of the ischemic thresholds by temperature or drugs can be excluded.

A more reliable characterization of the penumbra is, therefore, its association with biochemical alterations (Fig. 1). Anoxic depolarization is closely linked to the depletion of energy reserves which in rodents occurs at flow rates between 15% and 20%. The beginning suppression of spontaneous or evoked electrical activity correlates with molecular alterations that occur at flow values that are distinctly above the threshold of energy failure [10]. Examples of such biochemical alterations are the gradual inhibition of cerebral protein synthesis (CPS) which ceases at about 50% of control, the evolution of lactacidosis which develops as a result of anaerobic glycolysis at flow rates around 35%, or the upregulation of the heat stress protein 72 which colocalizes with the region of suppressed CPS but preserved ATP (molecular definition of the penumbra).

Anoxic depolarization causes ion- and water shifts between the extra- and intracellular compartments which, in turn, result in alterations of the diffusion properties of brain water that can be detected by diffusion weighted imaging. Correlation analysis revealed that energy failure is associated with a decline of the apparent diffusion coefficient (ADC) of water to below 80% of control [11]. Accordingly, the ADC range between 80% and normal can be defined as the NMR-detectable penumbra.

Finally, the penumbra has been defined by its viability characteristics. Kinouchi and associates [12] described it as the "area that can be rescued by phar-

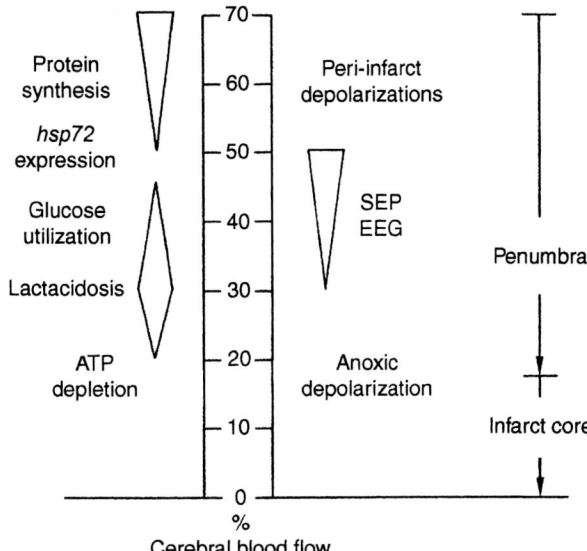

Fig. 1. Thresholds of biochemical *(left)* and physiological *(right)* disturbances during graded focal ischemia. The thresholds for ATP depletion and/or anoxic depolarization mark the border between infarct core and penumbra. Penumbral changes are characterized by multiple metabolic and physiological alterations such as inhibition of protein synthesis, lactacidosis or suppression of somatosensory evoked potentials (SEP) and spontaneous EEG activity. As these changes occur over a wide range of flow values, penumbra is defined as a region of constrained blood supply in which energy metabolism is preserved

macological agents". Hakim [13] characterized the penumbra as "fundamentally reversible" but he stressed that this reversibility is time-limited, and Memezawa et al. [14] defined the penumbra as the difference between the ischemic infarct developing after 1 and 24 h vascular occlusion. Other characterizations include intermediate staining with neutral red as an indicator of beginning acidosis [15], or the loss of calmodulin staining [16] as an indicator of increased intracellular calcium uptake.

The main denominators of these and the other definitions of the penumbra are a) the reduction in blood flow and b) preserved viability of the tissue. Since viability of brain tissue requires maintenance of energy-dependent metabolic processes, I proposed to define the penumbra as a region of constrained blood supply in which energy metabolism is preserved (operational definition of the penumbra) [17].

The postulation of a reduced flow rate as a necessary criterion for the definition of penumbra differentiates this pathophysiological situation from other disease states in which tissue viability is also at risk. In particular, selective vulnerability after brief episodes of global ischemia or delayed infarction after transient focal ischemia are heralded by a mismatch of protein synthesis and energy metabolism which is reminiscent of that observed in the peri-infarct penumbra. However, in these pathophysiologies blood flow is at or even above normal which clearly differs from the situation in permanent vascular occlusion. To avoid possible confusions, the term penumbra should therefore be reserved to the misery-perfused peri-infarct surrounding.

Imaging of Penumbra

According to the operational definition given above, the ischemic penumbra is a region of constrained blood supply in which the energy metabolism of the tissue is preserved. Under experimental conditions regional blood flow and energy state can be imaged by combining [14C] iodoantipyrine autoradiography with ATP-induced bioluminescence [18, 19]. An alternative way for detecting the penumbra is the combination of ATP bioluminescence with autoradiographic imaging of cerebral protein synthesis (CPS, Fig. 2) where the penumbra can be identified by the subtraction of the ATP-depleted core region from the area of suppressed protein synthesis. The functional relevance of this approach is exemplified by the comparison of the metabolic images with in situ hybridization autoradiograms. As shown in Fig. 2, the expression of hsp72 – which represents the cytosolic response to non-lethal ischemic stress – precisely colocalizes with the ATP/CPS mismatch whereas the upregulation of immediate-early genes – which is due to peri-infarct depolarizations – expands into the intact non-ischemic tissue.

The autoradiographic and bioluminescence approaches provide excellent regional resolution but do not allow repeated studies. Attempts have, therefore, been made to identify the penumbra by non-invasive means. In principle, this can be done by combining toposelective phosphorus NMR-spectroscopy with either PET or NMR imaging of blood flow. However, the resolution of phosphorus spectroscopy is still too low for a reliable differentiation, particularly in small brains of laboratory animals. Measurements of regional blood flow alone are not adequate to image the penumbra because volume elements with flow values that fall into the classical penumbra range, may include irreversibly damaged tissue in which spontaneous recirculation has occurred. PET imaging of glucose utilization is able to localize the core of the infarct in which metabolic activity is completely suppressed [20] but the penumbra cannot be identified because glucose utilization may be normal, increased or decreased, depending on the actual flow rate [21–23]. A more reliable PET parameter is the oxygen extraction ratio [24–26]. In the ischemic penumbra oxygen extraction is increased because the tissue is viable and continues to consume oxygen. As soon as metabolism ceases, the oxygen extraction declines.

A promising non-invasive approach which combines high resolution imaging with the possibility of repeated measurements, is diffusion-weighted NMR imaging [27–31]. Signal intensity in DWI increases at ADC levels that correspond to the beginning energy failure and, therefore, essentially co-localizes with the infarct core. The combination with perfusion-weighted imaging (PWI) therefore allows the identification of a perfusion/diffusion mismatch [32] in which – according to our operational definition – blood flow is reduced but ATP is preserved. A more precise allocation of the penumbra is thresholding of ADC maps between 100 and 80% of control [11] but due to the inherent scatter, the overall results do not differ much from the technically easier documentation of the perfusion/diffusion mismatch.

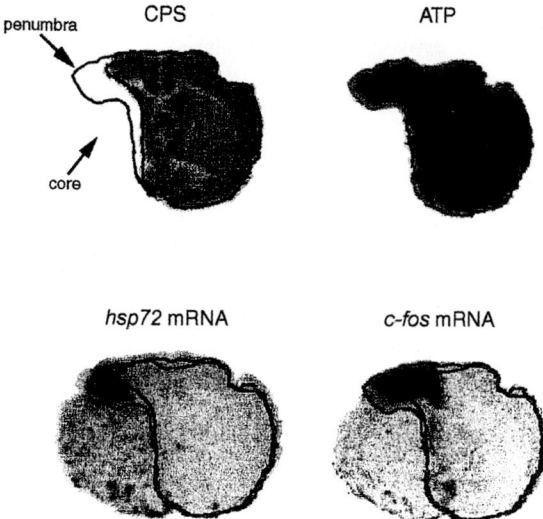

Fig. 2. Autoradiographic imaging of cerebral protein synthesis (CPS), bioluminescence imaging of ATP and *in situ* hybridization autoradiographs of *hsp72* and *c-fos* mRNAs on adjacent cryostat sections of mouse brain at the level of caudate/putamen after 2 hours middle cerebral artery occlusion. The outlines of preserved ATP and CPS are superimposed to demarcate the metabolic penumbra. Note precise allocation of *hsp72* mRNA to the penumbra in contrast to *c-fos* mRNA which is also upregulated in the normal peri-infarct tissue. (Modified from Hata [56])

Pathophysiology of Penumbra

Biochemical imaging of the developing infarct in mice after permanent occlusion of the middle cerebral artery revealed that the core region of the infarct gradually expands into the peri-infarct penumbra zone [33]. After 1 hour vascular occlusion, the outer margin of the penumbra visualized by autoradiography of cerebral protein synthesis encompasses a region that is about 50% larger than the area in which ATP is depleted. After 3–6 hours this difference declines to 20%, and after 1 day the CPS- and ATP-depleted regions become congruent (Fig. 3). Blood flow remains stable during the initial hours of ischemia which excludes the possibility that the growth of the infarct core is due to a progression of ischemia.

A possible reason for the expansion of tissue injury into the penumbra zone is the occurrence of peri-infarct spreading depression like depolarizations [34]. As first described by Nedergaard and Astrup [35], such depolarizations are generated by the infarct core from where they spread into the peripheral zone. During spreading depression the metabolic rate of the tissue markedly increases in response to the greatly enhanced energy demands of the activated ion exchange pumps [36, 37]. In the healthy brain the associated increase of glucose and oxygen demands are coupled to a parallel increase of blood flow which may rise to more than 200% of control [37–39]. This flow response is suppressed in the peri-infarct penumbra because the reduced hemodynamic capacity of the collateral system prevents the adequate coupling of blood supply to the metabolic needs of the tis-

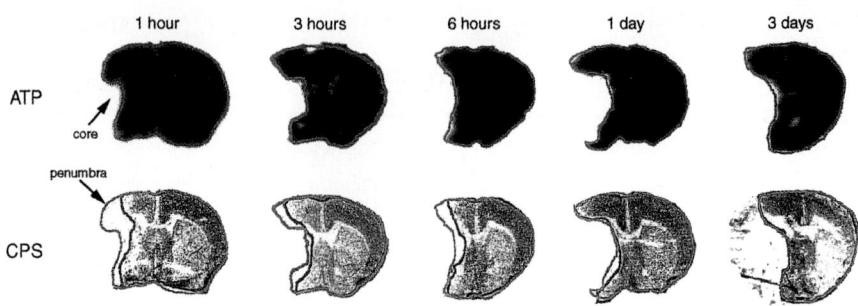

Fig. 3. Evolution of ischemic injury in mouse brain during permanent middle cerebral artery occlusion. Imaging of ATP and cerebral protein synthesis (CPS) on adjacent cryostat sections at the level of caudate/putamen. The areas of preserved ATP and CPS are outlined to differentiate between infarct core and penumbra. Note gradual expansion of the core region into the penumbra during the first day of ischemia. (Modified from Hata [33])

sue [40]. As a result, a misrelationship arises between the increased metabolic workload and the low oxygen supply. In fact, recordings of tissue oxygen pressure during KCl-induced spreading depression in intact animals and during peri-infarct depolarizations in MCA-occluded rats clearly demonstrate that the latter result in transient episodes of tissue hypoxia during the passage of each depolarization [26]. Evidence of tissue hypoxia has also been provided by biochemical and NMR spectroscopic studies which revealed substantial increase of lactate in the area of peri-infarct depolarizations [41, 42].

An alternative explanation for infarct expansion is apoptosis, as suggested by modulations of infarct size by pro- and anti-apoptotic drugs or mutations (for review see [43, 44]. However, labeling by the TUNEL method of cells undergoing DNA fragmentation clearly revealed that such alterations appear in the core rather than in the penumbra of the evolving infarct [33]. A contribution of apoptosis to cell death in the peri-infarct penumbra is, therefore, unlikely.

Therapeutic Implications

Based on the concept of viability thresholds, treatment of ischemic stroke may pursue different strategies: improvement of blood flow, lowering of the threshold for structural injury and prevention of the time-related rise of viability thresholds. Obviously, all three approaches should be combined to achieve the maximum effect but the relative efficacy of each of these interventions depends on the type of ischemia and the beginning of treatment.

The infarct core, defined as the region in which ATP is depleted, can only be salvaged if blood flow is restored before ischemic injury has become irreversible. A precise evaluation of the duration of focal ischemia following which ATP depletion can be reversed, requires repeated measurements. In principle, this is possible using spectroscopic phosphorus imaging but for most practical applications the sensitivity of this method is too low. However, available information on the flow thresholds of ATP depletion (see above) and the revival time of the brain after global ischemia [45] allow the prediction that at normothermia focal ATP depletion cannot be reversed after more than 1 or 2 h, at the most. Even within this time frame, ATP recovery would require full restoration of blood flow which under most clinical conditions can only be expected if a sudden embolic vascular occlusion is treated by thrombolysis or embolectomy. Case reports about improved neurological outcome by thrombolytic therapy after as late as 24 h following stroke [46] are, therefore, explained by the reversal of functional disturbances in the penumbra (in which ATP is preserved) rather than by a reduction of the volume of the infarct core.

Therapeutic lowering of the threshold of ATP depletion – and hence that of structural injury – is also unlikely unless the tissue is protected against ischemia by pre-ischemic hypothermia or other measures which reduce the metabolic rate of the tissue. However, a spectacular lowering of the threshold of protein synthesis from 50 to 19 ml/100 g/min has been reported by treating MCA-occluded rats with NMDA or non-NMDA glutamate antagonists [47, 48]. This effect has been linked to the inhibition of peri-infarct spreading depolarizations [40, 49] which provoke episodes of hypoxia, as described above [28, 50]. Since protein synthesis is particularly sensitive to hypoxia, the lowering of its threshold by glutamate antagonists may be due to the prevention of these hypoxic episodes rather than to an alleviation of excitotoxicity [51]. This could explain that glutamate antagonists do not or only marginally modify the threshold for ATP depletion [47, 48].

There are indications that the penumbral mismatch between oxygen supply and oxygen requirements can also be reduced by other means. Improvement of collateral blood supply following thrombolysis or reconstructive vascular surgery, inhibition of metabolic rate by neurodepressive agents or hypothermia, or the prevention of mitochondrial uncoupling with calcium blockers or free radical scavengers have the same effect (for reviews on stroke therapy see [52–54]). Similarly, the protective effect of anti-apoptotic interventions may be related to the penumbral energy state because the activation of the DNA repair enzyme, poly(ADP-ribose)polymerase (PARP) results in the consumption of NAD [55]. With the advent of non-invasive imaging techniques for the visualization of core and penumbra, it is now possible to test these concepts as well as their therapeutic implications under clinical conditions. The pathophysiological insight into the interrelationship between flow, metabolism and functional activation acquired in experimental animals will, therefore, be of great help for understanding the probably even more complicated situation of clinical stroke.

References

1. Opitz E, Schneider M. Über die Sauerstoffversorgung des Gehirns und den Mechanismus der Mangelwirkungen. Ergeb Physiol 1950;46:126–260.
2. Symon L, Branston NM, Strong AJ, Hope TD. The concepts of thresholds of ischaemia in relation to brain structure and function. Journal of Clinical Pathology 1977;30, Suppl.11:149–54.
3. Astrup J, Symon L, Siesjö BK. Thresholds in cerebral ischemia – The ischemic penumbra. Stroke 1981;12:723–25.

4. del Zoppo GJ. Why do all drugs work in animals but none in stroke patients? 1. Drugs promoting cerebral blood flow. J Intern Med 1995;237(1):79–88.

5. Kaplan B, Brint S, Tanabe J, Jacewicz M, Wang X-J, Pulsinelli W. Temporal thresholds for neocortical infarction in rats subjected to reversible focal cerebral ischemia. Stroke 1991; 22:1032–39.

6. Lassen NA, Fieschi C, Lenzi GL. Ischemic penumbra and neuronal death: comments on the therapeutic window in acute stroke with particular reference to thrombolytic therapy. Cerebrovasc Dis 1991;1,Suppl.1:32–35.

7. McCulloch J. Glutamate receptor antagonists in cerebral ischaemia. J Neural Transm 1994;43 (Suppl.):71–79.

8. Marler JR, Brott T, Broderick J, Kothari R, M OD, Barsan W, et al. Tissue plasminogen activator for acute ischemic stroke. N Engl J Med 1995;333:1581–87.

9. Astrup J, Symon L, Branston NM, Lassen NA. Cortical evoked potential and extracellular K+ and H+ at critical levels of brain ischemia. Stroke 1977;8:51–57.

10. Sharp FR, Lu AG, Tang Y, Millhorn DE. Multiple molecular penumbras after focal cerebral ischemia. J Cereb Blood Flow Metab 2000;20:1011–32.

11. Hoehn-Berlage M, Norris DG, Kohno K, Mies G, Leibfritz D, Hossmann K-A. Evolution of regional changes in apparent diffusion coefficient during focal ischemia of rat brain: The relationship of quantitative diffusion NMR imaging to reduction in cerebral blood flow and metabolic disturbances. J Cereb Blood Flow Metab 1995;15:1002–11.

12. Kinouchi H, Sharp FR, Koistinaho J, Hicks K, Kamii H, Chan PH. Induction of heat shock hsp70 messenger RNA and HSP70-kDa protein in neurons in the penumbra following focal cerebral ischemia in the rat. Brain Res 1993;619:334–38.

13. Hakim AM. The cerebral ischemic penumbra. Can J Neurol Sci 1987;14:557–59.

14. Memezawa H, Smith M-L, Siesjö BK. Penumbral tissues salvaged by reperfusion following middle cerebral artery occlusion in rats. Stroke 1992;23:552–59.

15. Selman WR, VanderVeer C, Whittingham TS, LaManna JC, Lust WD, Ratcheson RA. Visually defined zones of focal ischemia in the rat brain KW: Metabolic penumbra. Neurosurgery 1987;21:825–30.

16. Degraba TJ, Ostrow PT, Grotta JC. Threshold of calcium disturbances after focal cerebral ischemia in rats – Implications of the window of therapeutic opportunity. Stroke 1993; 24:1212–17.

17. Hossmann K-A. Viability thresholds and the penumbra of focal ischemia. Ann Neurol 1994;36:557–65.

18. Mies G, Ishimaru S, Xie Y, Seo K, Hossmann K-A. Ischemic thresholds of cerebral protein synthesis and energy state following middle cerebral artery occlusion in rat. J Cereb Blood Flow Metab 1991;11:753–61.

19. Hossmann K-A, Mies G, Paschen W, Csiba L, Bodsch W, Rapin JR, et al. Multiparametric imaging of blood flow and metabolism after middle cerebral artery occlusion in cats. J Cereb Blood Flow Metab 1985;5:97–107.

20. Heiss W-D, Podreka I. Role of PET and SPECT in the assessment of ischemic cerebrovascular disease. Cereb Brain Metab Rev 1993;5:235–63.

21. Paschen W, Mies G, Hossmann K-A. Threshold relationship between cerebral blood flow, glucose utilization, and energy metabolites during development of stroke in gerbils. Exp Neurol 1992;117:325–33.

22. Hossmann K-A, Schuier FJ. Experimental brain infarcts in cats. I. Pathophysiological observations. Stroke 1980;11:583–92.

23. Peek KE, Lockwood AH, Izumiyama M, Yap EWH, Labove J. Glucose metabolism and acidosis in the metabolic penumbra of rat brain. Metab Brain Dis 1989;4:261–72.

24. Jones T, Chesler DA, Ter-Pogossian MM. The continuous inhalation of oxygen-15 for assessing regional oxygen extraction in the brain of man. Br J Radiol 1976;49:339–43.

25. Kanno I, Uemura K, Higano S, Murakami M, Iida H, Miura S, et al. Oxygen extraction fraction at maximally vasodilated tissue in the ischemic brain estimated from the regional CO2 responsiveness measured by positron emission tomography. J Cereb Blood Flow Metab 1988;8:227–35.

26. Back T, Kohno K, Hossmann K-A. Cortical negative DC deflections following middle cerebral artery occlusion and KCl-induced spreading depression – Effect on blood flow, tissue oxygenation, and electroencephalogram. J Cereb Blood Flow Metab 1994;14:12–19.

27. Kohno K, Hoehn-Berlage M, Mies G, Back T, Hossmann K-A. Relationship between diffusion-weighted MR images, cerebral blood flow, and energy state in experimental brain infarction. Magn Reson Imaging 1995;13:73–80.

28. Back T, Hoehn-Berlage M, Kohno K, Hossmann K-A. Diffusion nuclear magnetic resonance imaging in experimental stroke – Correlation with cerebral metabolites. Stroke 1994; 25:494–500.

29. Kucharczyk J, Mintorovitch J, Asgari H, Tsuura M, Moseley M. In vivo diffusion-perfusion magnetic resonance imaging of acute cerebral ischemia. Can J Physiol Pharmacol 1991; 69:1719–25.

30. Minematsu K, Fisher M, Li L, Sotak CH, Davis MA, Fiandaca MS. Diffusion weighted MRI rapidly detects rat focal brain abnormalities induced by suture occlusion of the MCA. Neurology 1991;41:1162–62.

31. Roberts TPL, Vexler Z, Derugin N, Moseley ME, Kucharczyk J. High-speed MR imaging of ischemic brain injury following stenosis of the middle cerebral artery. J Cereb Blood Flow Metab 1993;13:940–46.

32. Neumann-Haefelin T, Wittsack HJ, Wenserski F, Siebler M, Seitz RJ, Modder U, et al. Diffusion-and perfusion-weighted MRI. The DWI/PWI mismatch region in acute stroke. Stroke 1999;30:1591–97.

33. Hata R, Maeda K, Hermann D, Mies G, Hossmann K-A. Dynamics of regional brain metabolism and gene expression after middle cerebral artery occlusion in mice. J Cereb Blood Flow Metab 2000;20:306–15.

34. Hossmann K-A. Periinfarct depolarizations. Cereb Brain Metab Rev 1996;8:195–208.

35. Nedergaard M, Astrup J. Infarct rim: effect of hyperglycemia on direct current potential and (14 C)- deoxyglucose phosphorylation. J Cereb Blood Flow Metab 1986;6:607–15.

36. Shinohara M, Dollinger B, Brown G, Rapoport S, Sokoloff L. Cerebral glucose utilization: local changes during and after recovery from spreading cortical depression. Science 1979;203: 188–90.

37. Kocher M. Metabolic and hemodynamic activation of postischemic rat brain by cortical spreading depression. J Cereb Blood Flow Metab 1990;10:564–71.

38. Mies G, Paschen W. Regional changes of blood flow, glucose, and ATP content determined on brain sections during a single passage of spreading depression in rat brain cortex. Exp Neurol 1984;84:249–58.

39. Duckrow RB. Regional cerebral blood flow during spreading cortical depression in conscious rats. J Cereb Blood Flow Metab 1991;11:150–54.

40. Iijima T, Mies G, Hossmann K-A. Repeated negative DC deflections in rat cortex following middle cerebral artery occlusion are abolished by MK-801. Effect on volume of ischemic injury. J Cereb Blood Flow Metab 1992;12:727–33.

41. Gyngell ML, Back T, Hoehn-Berlage M, Kohno K, Hossmann K-A. Transient cell depolarization after permanent middle cerebral artery occlusion: an observation by diffusion-weighted MRI and localized ^{1}H-MRS. Magn Reson Med 1994;31:337–41.

42. Takeda Y, Jacewicz M, Takeda Y, Nowak Jr. TS, Pulsinelli WA. DC-potential and energy metabolites in the focal ischemia. J Cereb Blood Flow Metab 1993;13:S450-S450.

43. Mattson MP, Culmsee C, Yu ZF. Apoptotic and antiapoptotic mechanisms in stroke. Cell Tissue Res 2000;301:173–87.

44. Lipton P. Ischemic cell death in brain neurons. Physiol Rev 1999;79:1431–568.

45. Hossmann K-A. Neuronal survival and revival during and after cerebral ischemia. Amer J Emerg Med 1983;1:191–97.

46. Von Kummer R, Holle R, Rosin L, Forsting M, Hacke W. Does arterial recanalization improve outcome in carotid territory stroke? Stroke 1995;26:581–87.

47. Kohno K, Mies G, Djuricic B, Hossmann K-A. NBQX reduces threshold of protein synthesis inhibition in focal ischaemia in rats. Neuroreport 1994;5:2342–44.

48. Mies G, Kohno K, Hossmann K-A. MK-801, a glutamate antagonist, lowers flow threshold for inhibition of protein synthesis after middle cerebral artery occlusion of rat. Neurosci Lett 1993;155:65–68.
49. Mies G, Kohno K, Hossmann K-A. Prevention of periinfarct direct current shifts with glutamate antagonist NBQX following occlusion of the middle cerebral artery in the rat. J Cereb Blood Flow Metab 1994;14:802–07.
50. Strong AJ, Harland SP, Meldrum BS, Whittington DJ. Imaging the origins, propagation and frequence of transient depolarisations in focal cerebral ischemia. J Cereb Blood Flow Metab 1995;15, Suppl. 1:S14-S14.
51. Hossmann K-A. Glutamate-mediated injury in focal cerebral ischemia: The excitotoxin hypothesis revised. Brain Pathol 1994;4:23–36.
52. Heiss W-D, Thiel A, Grond M, Graf R. Which targets are relevant for therapy of acute ischemic stroke? Stroke 1999;30:1486–89.
53. Grotta JC. Acute stroke therapy at the millennium: consummating the marriage between laboratory and bedside. The Feinberg lecture. Stroke 1999;30:1722–28.
54. Devuyst G, Bogousslavsky J. Recent progress in drug treatment for acute stroke. Journal of Neurology, Neurosurgery and Psychiatry 1999;67:420–25.
55. Pieper AA, Verma A, Zhang J, Snyder SH. Poly (ADP-ribose) polymerase, nitric oxide and cell death. Trends Pharmacol Sci 1999;20:171–81.
56. Hata R, Mies G, Wiessner C, Hossmann K-A. Differential expression of c-fos and hsp72 mRNA in focal cerebral ischemia of mice. Neuroreport 1998;9:27–32.

Section III:
Assessment of Cerebral Blood Flow

The Assessment of Determinants of Cerebral Oxygenation and Microcirculation

F.A. Pennings, G.J. Bouma, and C. Ince

Introduction

During recent decades, cerebral circulation and tissue oxygenation has been the subject of much clinical and basic research. Due to its complexity, the brain remains an area of research vastly unknown and challenging due to the very nature of its design: a closed box, thereby preventing the study of intraparenchymal function in vivo.

General parameters, like saturation and blood pressure are insufficient to provide information about the cerebral circulation and tissue oxygenation. Moreover, the brain circulation is tightly controlled by cerebral autoregulation, the intrinsic ability of the brain to maintain cerebral blood flow near constant within a range of perfusion pressures. Cerebral pathology can cause an impairment of the cerebral vasculature, which renders the brain at risk to secondary insults such as ischemia and intracranial hypertension.

Since systemic parameters of circulation and oxygen delivery to the brain fail to provide specific information about global and regional cerebral characteristics, there is a need for improvement in methods to monitor the cerebral circulation, metabolism and tissue oxygenation. In the last decades several monitoring instruments of cerebral circulation, such as Xenon techniques, jugular bulb oximetry and transcranial Doppler, have been applied successfully and have yielded a wealth of information about cerebral blood flow and metabolism and its regulation in health and disease. More recently, research interest has shifted towards the study of the cerebral microcirculation and local tissue oxygenation. The purpose of this chapter is to give an overview of available techniques and their clinical relevance and application in clinical situations. In this review we will focus on those techniques, that have been applied in humans.

Jugular Bulb Oximetry

The arteriovenous difference of oxygen ($AVDO_2$), the amount of oxygen extracted by the brain from each deciliter of blood supplied to it, is calculated from intermittent sampling of both arterial and jugular venous blood. Such intermittent measurements, however, are time consuming and present only a "snapshot" of the system. Therefore, transient ischemic insults can go undetected. This problem was solved by the introduction of the fiberoptic based jugular bulb oximetry in the mid- Eighties, which provided a continuous measurement of global cerebral oxygenation [13]. In jugular bulb venous oxygen saturation monitoring selected wavelengths of light are transmitted along fiberoptic cables, and the intensity of light reflected from red blood cells down the fibers is quantified by a photodetector. The intensity of the reflected light varies according to the relative concentrations of oxygenated and reduced hemoglobin. The measurement of jugular bulb oximetry is expressed as the percentage of oxygen saturation in venous blood of the jugular bulb (SjO_2). The jugular bulb is considered to be the cerebral venous outflow site, and therefore jugular bulb oximetry allows identification and correction of potential global ischemia. Currently, two commercial systems are available for continuous measurements of SjO_2, the Opticath Oximetrix catheter (Abbott, North Chicago, IL) and the Edslab SAT II (Baxter Edwards). Placement is relatively easy and with few complications and no effect on ICP has been demonstrated [31, 47, 63].

Normal jugular bulb SjO_2 values range from 55 to 71% [30]. A normal value does not exclude the presence of focal ischemia, and for this reason it is an insensitive monitor of regional ischemia. A value <50% ($AVDO_2$>7 ml O_2/ 100 ml blood) is considered the threshold below which the brain is ischemic [50]. At that point, oxygen demand is either not matched with an equivalent increase in CBF or an absolute decrease in CBF exists. As ischemia progresses, SjO_2 values may return to normal despite an insufficient blood flow caused by a decrease in viable brain tissue. The concomitant measurement of cerebral lactate in the SjO_2 may help to identify progressive ischemia accompanied with normal jugular bulb saturations [78]. If CBF declines further, the extracerebral portion of the venous blood sample may increase, thereby elevating jugular venous saturations values. An SjO_2 above 90% ($AVDO_2$<4 ml O_2/100 ml blood) reveals that cerebral blood flow (oxygen supply) exceeds the oxygen demand. However, SjO_2 alone cannot differentiate between relative and absolute hyperemia. The management of jugular bulb desaturation has been thoroughly described by Sheinberg et al. [83]. According to their protocol, exclusion of a poor catheter position and verification of the detected SjO_2 value with a co-oximetry analysis needs to be done prior to the interpretation of the measured saturation changes.

Accurate measurement of SjO_2 necessitates radiological confirmation of the position of the catheter tip high in the jugular bulb, a few millimeters away from its superior wall. Incorrect placement of the instrument below the jugular bulb can result in contamination with extracranial blood from the facial vein [50]. To keep accurate positioning of the catheter tip during the whole monitoring course in the Intensive Care Unit (ICU), appears to be a major difficulty and technical limitation of this type of monitoring. A slight change in positioning in head and neck may easily occur during nursing care, although with well-trained nursing personnel and careful patient selection this limitation can be minimized [12].

The accuracy of the jugular bulb monitoring catheters is dependent on the intensity of the reflected light [71]. This emphasizes the need for calibrating the jugular bulb oximetry device frequently (every 4 to 8 hours). If the quality of the light intensity is poor, the patient head or catheter needs to be repositioned. Accordingly, a co-oximetry analysis should be done with great attention for the way aspiration of blood is done to reduce the possibility of extracerebral contamination [47]. A difference exists in accuracy between ICU and intraoperative monitoring, which may be explained by the shorter length of use in the operating room and by the inability of the patient to move during surgery [12].

Although blood usually drains from both cerebral hemispheres into the right internal jugular vein, predominant drainage to the left also occurs [70]. This finding opens the discussion about the optimal side of the neck for catheter placement. Two different approaches currently exist. The first is to place the jugular bulb catheter ipsilateral to the lateralizing lesions [79]. With the second method, the dominant jugular foramen is identified either by neuroimaging or by determination of the greatest rise in intracranial pressure upon unilateral compression, when intracranial pressure monitoring is in situ [17, 86]. If equal rise is noted then the right side can be chosen for ease of access. Finally, bilateral catheterization studies suggest that a reliable method to determine which side will give the most abnormal values is not available and therefore the most practical solution is to insert the catheter on the dominant side, which is usually the right side [53, 86].

Jugular bulb oximetry has been used extensively in brain disease where global oxygenation may be periodically compromised. Most experience with this device has been gained in acute brain injury, where it seems promising for the management and outcome of this disorder. Bouma et al. [2] demonstrated the high incidence of very early cerebral ischemia after acute brain injury by Xenon CT CBF measurements. There results were verified with jugular venous saturation measurements in severe closed head injury patients, where especially in the initial phase of ICU management low saturation values were found [54, 77]. These desaturations were predominantly associated with low cerebral perfusion pressure (<70 mm Hg), hyperventilation, vasospasm, anemia, and hypoxemia [6, 82]. Also this instrument was able to identify patients with desaturations not detected by routine monitoring of CPP [14]. Therefore outcome could be improved if these factors were treated optimally. De Deyne et al. [16] were able to make a distinction in primary and secondary intracranial hypertension and adjusted the treatment strategies, which resulted in a more efficient use of intracranial pressure reducing agents.

Matta et al. [63] conclude that jugular bulb oximetry may be beneficial in detecting an increase in oxygen extraction during various neurosurgical procedures such as aneurysms and tumors, however with the exception of AVMs. Hirayama et al. [49] reported that changes in the shunt flow ratio as a whole in AVMs could be detected by jugular bulb oximetry. Even so, jugular saturations may add important bedside information to the diagnosis of brain death, where extremely high values indicate the complete cessation of cerebral metabolism [99].

In conclusion it can be said that jugular bulb saturation measurements accurately reflect global cerebral oxygenation and can be used as a bedside monitoring system in the ICU and during neurosurgical procedures to identify early transient ischemic insults. The use of SjO_2 monitoring may improve management and outcome, when treatable causes for desaturation are identified and corrected. On the other hand, regional ischemia can be present and not be detected by this instrument and as venous jugular outflow on one side may not represent the whole brain, ischemic insults can easily be missed.

Near-Infrared Spectroscopy (NIRS)

Near-infrared spectroscopy (NIRS) relies on the relative transparency of the head to near-infrared light and to the different absorption of this light by various components important for the oxygenation of the brain. It was first applied to the brain by Jöbsis and since then has been investigated in neonatal and adult medicine [3, 48, 65]. Near-infrared provides a continuous and non-invasive assessment of regional oxygen metabolism (rSO_2) and hemodynamics by measuring the different light absorption patterns of deoxyhemoglobin (Hb), oxyhemoglobin (HbO_2) and oxidized cytochrome oxidase (CytOx) in the near-infrared area (650–900 nm) [48, 65]. In the near-infrared region, the absorption of light by Hb peaks at ~760 nm and that of HbO_2 at ~ 900 nm. Total Hb can be calculated at ~ 800 nm, the peak where the attenuation of Hb and HbO_2 are equal. The oxidized copper center of cytochrome oxidase is responsible for a different absorption band (between 800 and 900 nm) than other cytochromes. Anoxia results in a quick reduction of this enzyme leading to a disappearance of this absorbance peak and therefore cellular oxidative metabolism can be assessed with NIRS [7].

NIRS can be used to measure cerebral oxygenation, cerebral blood flow (CBF) and cerebral blood volume (CBV). First clinical application of transmission NIRS involved mainly newborns, and changes in cerebral hemodynamics to alterations in arterial CO_2 and surfactant have been described [24, 97, 98]. Also absolute values of CBF and CBV can be calculated with NIRS, although measurements of cerebral oxygenation appears to be more accurate than estimation of CBF and CBV using NIRS [72, 96].

The main problem associated with the use and interpretation of data with the NIRS is explained with the Lambert-Beer equation, which relates the concentration of a solute to the intensity of light transmitted through the solution by an exponential function. The Lambert-Beer formula requires a known optical pathlength to calculate an absolute concentration of a substance from its baseline value. In NIRS this optical pathlength of the transmitted light is unknown due to scattering of light and unspecific light absorptions, making absolute quantification of the concentration of the chromophores difficult. This remains the major drawback of this monitoring system.

Different methods have been developed to determine the optical pathlength of the reflected light. The first, the "time of flight" method, calculates pathlength from the mean transit time of picosecond light pulses [18]. The second method uses the phase shift technique, which measures the phase shift of detected light, which is directly related to the pathlength [8]. The third method uses the measurable absorption peak of water. Since water is relatively well maintained in tissue and its concentration is known, the effective optical pathlength of the tissue can be measured by the strong absorption of light by water at 740, 820 and 970 nm [11, 61]. With this technique absolute values of chromophore concentrations have been described [25].

NIRS instruments may be categorized into non-quantitative measurements (INVOS; Somanetics, Troy, MI) and quantitative concentration measurements. The non-quantitative monitors measure the saturation ratio of oxygenated to deoxygenated hemoglobin and derive a value for the mean cerebral saturation. This technique uses a dual receiver probe set at different source –detector spacings allowing measurements of cerebral tissue and extracerebral components. Subtracting one from another gives an estimate of the regional tissue oxygenation [23, 65]. However, extracerebral contamination remains a problem even in the latest INVOS versions [28]. Moreover in a study by Colier et al. [10] it was shown that decreased CBF could only be detected with the conventional type of monitoring and not by the INVOS. The quantitative technique allows full quantification of changes in chromophore concentrations. In contrast to saturation monitors, this technique requires knowledge of the actual optical pathlength. McKeating et al. [66] compared these two categories of NIRS equipment and showed that neither gave reliable and consistent readings over time. Moreover, they concluded that the high failure rate of the Criticon 2020, a concentration monitor, probably prevents or limits its clinical use.

At least three more problems can be presented. First there is the intersubject variability and the lack of a definable threshold. Second, the influence of extracerebral contamination on the cerebral oxygenation values is unknown. Several investigators reported that the contribution of extracerebral tissues (skin, bone) remains a major problem despite an interoptode distance of 3–4 cm [29, 55]. The relative influence from the extracranial tissue could be reduced by optode separation and correction for an extracranial sample volume, or both [59]. However, the emitter-detector separation used by currently available cerebral oximeters is not large enough to provide optimal spatial resolution [27]. Finally, the NIRS measures hemoglobin in three different compartments: arterial, venous and microcirculatory. In the cerebral cortex the venous system predominates, and it is assumed that the tissue being monitored is approximately 70% venous blood [94]. However, a change in position in healthy subjects had no influence on NIRS measurements, in contrast to an increase in CBV by hypoventilation [75]. Recently though, a change in posture was correlated to a change in CBV [56]. This reflects the difficulty arising when NIRS is compared to other monitoring instruments such as jugular bulb oximetry, because it remains unclear which compartment is studied with NIRS. Heterogeneity exists in cerebral blood flow distributions and tissue oxygenation under pathological conditions. Therefore regional oxygenation saturation might be quite different from global oxygenation due to the difference in blood flow distributions and local metabolic activity. In this context NIRS tomography may prove to be a promising advancement in this technique [36, 92].

The comparison of NIRS derived cerebral saturation and jugular bulb oximetry has been made with the INVOS 3100 in the intensive care and during cardiac surgery [5, 15, 34, 55, 64, 87]. When jugular bulb and NIRS are compared, the first technique seems to be a better monitoring instrument for cerebral saturation. In comatose patients a poor correlation was observed, as NIRS over-read at low jugular bulb saturations and under-read at high jugular bulb saturations even during herniation and cerebral death [5, 55]. However, a closer relationship between SjO_2 and rSO_2 values was found in infants compared with older children. This might be explained by the increased spatial resolution achieved in infants due to the less contamination of extracerebral tissue [28].

Explanations for the poor correlation could be related to the NIRS type. The basic assumptions to quantify regional oxygen saturations by the INVOS 3100 i.e. hemoglobin from the jugular bulb as the calibration standard, and the assumption that path length and light scattering are constant in all individuals, might be incorrect. The lack of correlation could be explained by the different entities, which are measured. NIRS values are obtained from a mixture of arterial, microcirculatory and venous blood, although the largest contribution is considered to be venous. Other possible causes for the errors could be the contamination of extracerebral tissues and the absence of a "true" golden standard. This latter actually prevents the use of regression analyses [76]. The existing heterogeneity of CBF and metabolic activity following acute brain injury could be responsible [2]. Holzschuh et al. [42] compared NIRS favorably to brain tissue pO$_2$ monitoring in 10 patients suffering from acute brain injury.

In conclusion, the main problems are associated with the effect of the scattering of light on the interpretation of data, especially in adult medicine. If this difficulty can be resolved then NIRS has the potential to become a safe, non-invasive bedside monitoring device for cerebral oxygenation, CBF and CBV, although it remains an investigative tool in its present form. Because of the thin scalp and skull in the neonate and infant, it holds promise in this patient population.

Reflectance Spectrophotometry

Reflectance spectrophotometry uses light absorption of reflected visible light on the tissue to measure the intracapillary oxygen saturation of virtually any organ surface. The heights of the peaks of the characteristic absorption spectra of hemoglobin at 542, 556 and 577 nm are used for quantitative estimation of hemoglobin oxygenation. The Erlanger Microlightguide Photometer (Bodenseewerk Geratetechnik, Überlingen, Germany) is the most widely used monitor system, introduced in 1989 [26]. It consists of a flexible light guide to transmit light from a high pressure Xenon lamp to the tissue. The backscattered light is transmitted to a rotating interference band pass filter via six optical fibers, which are arranged in a hexagonal pattern around the illuminating fiber. The filter disc works in the reflectance spectra area of 502 to 630 nm, where the characteristic absorption spectra of oxygenated hemoglobin and deoxygenated hemoglobin dominate.

The high temporal and spatial resolution permits an easy scanning procedure of superficial capillaries by moving the light guide above an organ. Reflectance spectrophotometry has been applied in plastic surgery, thoracic surgery, gastroenterology and recently also in neurosurgery [43, 69]. In the brain, its lack of an exact validation may be a potential disadvantage of the reflectance spectrophotometry. However, this may only be a problem if absolute values of SO$_2$ are required. Although comparison of the EMPHO II with other systems used for intravital measurements demonstrated that even then the error for absolute SO$_2$ values may be minor [95]. Due to its invasive nature, this technique is only suitable for use in animal studies or during surgery.

Intracerebral Oxygen Microsensors

In recent years much experience has been gained with direct measurements of regional brain tissue oxygen tension pressure. This technique was first applied using a Clark type electrode in the 1950's and since then has been investigated by many clinicians [9].Two types of brain tissue monitoring pO_2 probes are currently available and used extensively: a Clark type electrode (Licox, GMS, Kiel-Mielkendorf, Germany) and a multiparameter sensor (Neurotrend, Diametrics Medical, High Wycombe, UK).

The Licox probe uses a precalibrated flexible Clark type electrode catheter to determine tissue pO_2. A Clark type electrode consists of a noble metal (e.g. silver, gold or platinum), which reduces oxygen due to a negative polarizing voltage [9]. The Neurotrend system was originally developed as an alternative to conventional ex-vivo arterial blood gas measurements (Paratrend, Diametrics Medical, High Wycombe, UK) and later applied to brain tissue [73, 100]. It consisted of two optical fibers for measurement of pCO_2 and pH, a miniaturized Clark electrode and a thermocouple for the determination of pO_2 and temperature respectively. In the Neurotrend, the Clark electrode has been replaced by an optical pO_2 sensor, which is based on fluorescence quenching. Before insertion, the multiparameter sensor is calibrated with sterile precision gases bubbled in sequence through the tonometer under microprocessor control for 30 minutes.

Dings et al. [21] studied the technical and diagnostic reliability of the Licox system. The catheter probes were tested *in vitro*, and clinically in 101 patients. They concluded that it is a safe and reliable method of monitoring regional cerebral oxygenation, excluding the first hour after insertion. Roth et al. [80] found a good correlation between tissue pO_2 and sagittal sinus blood in pigs during a forced inspiratory fraction of 100% (FiO_2 100%). Animal studies were done to validate the Paratrend probe [60, 67, 100]. During brain insults with hypoxia and hypotension in dogs McKinley et al. [67] found stable, reproducible values of pO_2, pCO_2 and pH for periods >8 h. In rabbits, the Paratrend system was able to register accurately the pO_2 decline during gradually induced hypoxemia [60].

Normal values and ischemic values have been evaluated in different clinical and experimental studies. A normal range of 25–45 mmHg has been suggested. The ischemic threshold for compromised brain tissue is still uncertain, although evidence is available that it is probably below 10–20 mm Hg. Doppenberg et al. [22], testing the Paratrend, found in patients with severe head injury that an ischemic CBF threshold of 18 ml100 g/min correlated with a pO_2 of 22 mm Hg. Hoffmann et al. [37] found a threshold of 10 mm Hg during temporary artery clipping and in cerebral bypass surgery using the Neurotrend system [39]. In head trauma studies done with the Licox monitor, a threshold of 5–6 mm Hg was associated with a significant injury [88, 91].

The lower values found with the Licox could be explained by the overestimation of low values with the Paratrend [88]. Possibly, the Neurotrend system, where an optical O2 sensor replaces the Clark-electrode, may not have this problem, although this has not yet been investigated.

Regional brain tissue pO_2 monitoring using oxygen electrodes has been investigated under various pathological conditions in the Intensive Care Unit as well as during neurosurgical procedures and can be used for a long period of time without complications [38, 52, 68, 90]. A relationship between pO_2 values and outcome has been investigated in several brain injury studies. Kiening et al. [51] reported a 78% incidence of lower pO_2 values in contused brain compared to the non-affected side.

They also suggested that the duration of pO_2 values below a critical level of 10 mm Hg would be a sensitive predictor of ischemic tissue injury. A poor outcome was associated with ischemic periods of <10 mm Hg for >10 min after the first week of injury. Dings et al. [19] reported that patients with a poor neurological outcome had a 35% incidence of episodes of pO_2 less than 10 mm Hg compared with 10% in patients with a good neurological outcome. Other investigators found in head trauma patients that the time that pO_2 was <15 mm Hg was significantly less in patients who survived compared with those who died [88]. The pathophysiological finding of a decreased CBF in the initial days after injury followed by a period of hyperemia is also confirmed with this type of monitoring: low pO_2 values in the initial days followed by a return to normal values [88, 90]. If low pO_2 values persisted this was often associated with a poor neurological outcome [4, 19, 88, 90].

Intraoperative monitoring of brain tissue pO_2 has been applied during aneurysm surgery, AVM resections and brain tumors [37, 40, 68, 74]. The effect of different brain protection regimes were investigated and the influence of several therapeutic interventions (increasing FiO_2 to 100%, hyperventilation and increase of blood pressure) on pO_2 were studied.

In a study done by our group with brain tumors, we found that hyperventilation decreases pO_2 below critical ischemic levels [74]. This phenomenon was also repeatedly found in head trauma patients [20, 81]. Increasing cerebral perfusion pressure led to an improvement of pO_2 in the peritumoral area, suggesting impairment in autoregulation. This observation was also encountered by Stocchetti et al. [85] in a study population with a variety of cerebral pathology.

When using regional tissue monitoring, several factors interfering with the obtained data should be accounted for. The calibration time has a median time of 1 hour but can be as long as 3.5 hours. This is a major drawback in trauma studies, where secondary ischemic events mainly occur during the first hours after the insult. With the Clark type electrode the area of pO_2 measurement, the catchment area, is 15–20 μm deep [46]. This area could potentially contain vessels with a higher oxygen concentration than the surrounding area and can mimic ischemia. These electrodes are therefore sensitive to changes in arterial pO_2 [84]. In addition, the O_2 consumption of the electrode should be small compared to microcirculatory pO_2 level to prevent interference with tissue oxygen concentration [57]. This influence on the local tissue concentration may not occur with the fiberoptic pO_2 because it is oxygen passive.

Heterogeneity of the brain for CO_2-reactivity exists in the normal brain but most often in the injured brain [1]. In several studies the response of brain tissue pO_2 to hyperventilation was variable. It is therefore possible to underestimate the severity of global ischemia with consequences for therapy installment and possibly outcome [32,35].

Oxygen electrodes do not represent the heterogeneity of the oxygen distribution in the microcirculation, because the needle tip of the probes measures at a single point [58]. Dings et al. [21] demonstrated the difference in white and gray matter pO_2 values. A 10 mm Hg increase occurred when the Licox probe was moved 1 cm towards cortex. When Neurotrend probes were placed 1 cm apart 8 mm Hg difference (40%) existed with lesser variability in pH and pCO_2 between local sites [41]. This illustrates the importance of the accuracy of sensor placement in studies where O_2 values are compared with each other. Computer assisted stereotaxy could be an option to overcome this problem if accurate placement is demanded [74].

In hyperoxia, local tissue monitoring displayed a steeper increase than that would be expected from the arterial saturation, which suggested a contribution of the arterial pO_2 to the brain tissue pO_2 values [32]. This observation opens the discussion as to what the pO_2 sensor is actually measuring: the brain tissue pO_2, microcirculatory intravascular pO_2 or both? In addition, in our study in brain tumors brain swelling was associated with an attenuation of the pO_2 in response to raising FiO_2 to 100% (Fig. 1). We believe that the changes observed in brain tissue pO_2 with variations in FiO_2 represent the intravascular compartment in the monitored tissue volume. Maybe a correction for arterial pO_2 values needs to be integrated in the analysis of obtained pO_2 data.

Evidence exists that mechanical forces produced by tip and shaft of needle electrode cause micro-hemorrhages (tissue damage) as well as alterations in microvascular flow leading to low pO_2 values [58, 89, 93]. In addition, sensor malfunction occurs and may account for false pO_2 readings [32]. Solutions to reduce sensor malfunction could be improvement in insertion techniques to avoid catheter bending and calibration of the monitoring instruments before and after the procedure in a zero oxygen solution and in standard blood gas analysis solutions.

When tissue pO_2 monitoring is compared to jugular bulb oximetry, the most striking difference is the ability of the former to detect regional ischemia [32, 35]. On the other hand, local tissue monitoring may underestimate the severity of ischemia elsewhere in the brain. Brain tissue pO_2 monitoring may provide a less artifact prone method of cerebral oxygenation monitoring for a longer period of time, as jugular bulb oximetry requires constant care and recalibration. Simultaneous use of both these instruments may improve detection of cerebral ischemia.

In conclusion, monitoring of regional brain tissue by use of oxygen microsensors is a quantitative, safe tool with the advantage of the ability to detect regional ischemia. In the future, additional product refinements will hopefully lead to a further decrease in failure rate. A clinical indication for the routine use of oxygen electrodes in neuromonitoring needs to be established in prospective studies.

Orthogonal Polarization Spectral Imaging (OPS Imaging)

Microcirculatory function of the brain is essential for providing adequate oxygen to the tissue cells. Much insight has been obtained into the properties of brain microcirculation in animal experiments using intravital microscopy but methods to observe this microcirculation in humans had as yet not been achieved [44]. Recently OPS imaging was introduced for observation of the microcirculation and we have developed its use during neurosurgical procedures [33, 62]. OPS imaging is an optical technique using green polarized light that allows on-line microscopic observation of the microcirculation [38]. This optical technology has been implemented in a small probe that can be mounted conventionally or hand-held. The advantage of this imaging system is that it provides high contrast real-time images of the microcirculation from the surfaces of virtually any organ up to 500 µm tissue depth, with the ability to determine parameters such as: red blood cell velocity and direction, mi-

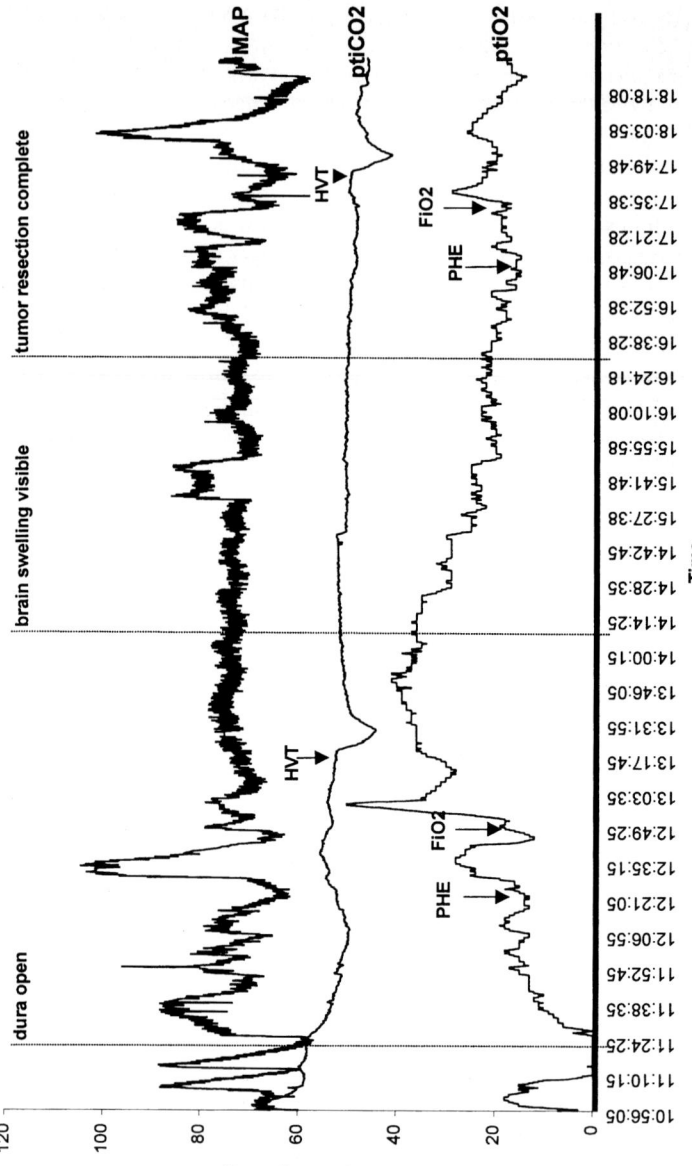

Fig. 1. The reaction of brain tissue pO_2 and pCO_2 to brain swelling during resection of a malignant brain tumor. Before the development of brain swelling, a gradual increase is seen of brain tissue pO_2 with a good response to raising blood pressure (PHE), increasing forced inspiratory oxygen fraction to 100% (FiO_2) and hyperventilation (HVT). Brain swelling causes a decline in pO_2 with an attenuation of the responses

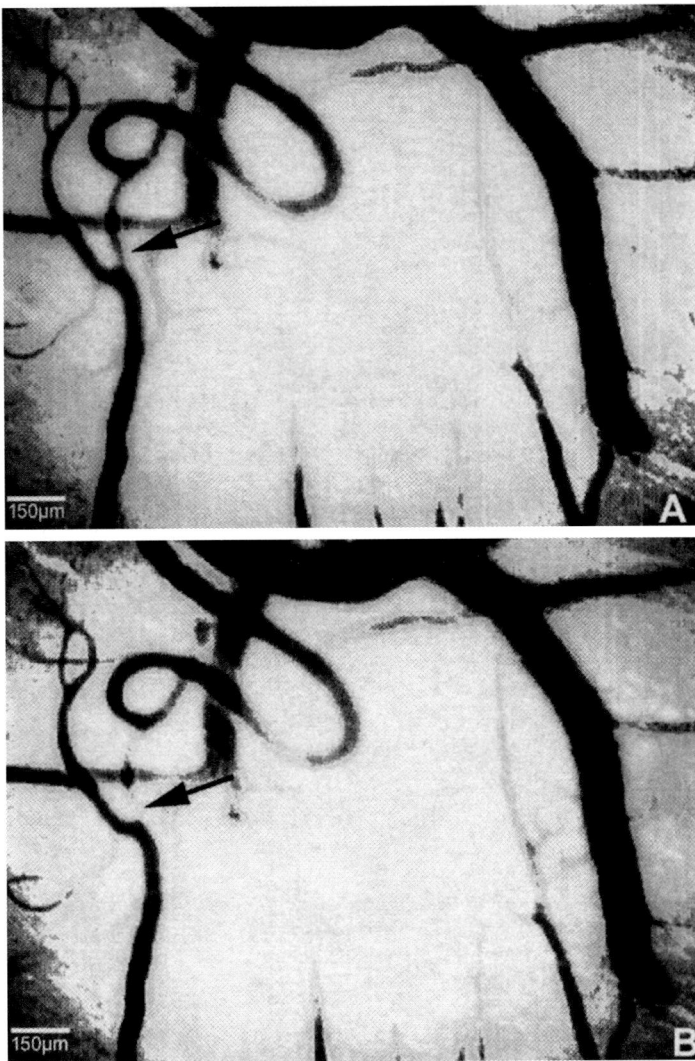

Fig. 2A, B. Example of vascular spasm as a result of hyperventilation

crocirculation morphology and capillary density. Because the chosen wavelength of light is within the hemoglobin absorption spectrum, the red blood cells can be clearly observed as they flow through the microcirculation. White blood cells too are observed by OPS imaging [62]. Indications for the use of this system could be neurological diseases, where the above-mentioned parameters are disturbed due to and may be responsible for the development of (regional) cerebral ischemia such as in subarachnoid hemorrhages, AVMs and neurotrauma. Altered vessel diameter and blood flow velocities as a result of CO_2-reactivity to hyperventilation could be readily observed (Fig. 2). In a recent study we observed microcirculatory abnormalities in human brain tumors [45]. It is expected that this new and exciting technique will provide the neurosurgeon a sensitive tool to observe the nature of brain microcirculation during various neurosurgical interventions.

References

1. Bouma GJ, Muizelaar JP: Cerebral blood flow, cerebral blood volume, and cerebrovascular reactivity after severe head injury. J. Neurotrauma 9 Suppl 1:S333-S348, 1992
2. Bouma GJ, Muizelaar JP, Choi SC, et al: Cerebral circulation and metabolism after severe traumatic brain injury: the elusive role of ischemia. J. Neurosurg. 75:685–693, 1991
3. Brazy JE: Cerebral oxygen monitoring with near infrared spectroscopy: clinical application to neonates. J. Clin.Monit. 7:325–334, 1991
4. Bruzzone P, Dionigi R, Bellinzona G, et al: Effects of cerebral perfusion pressure on brain tissue PO2 in patients with severe head injury. Acta Neurochir.Suppl (Wien) 71:111–113, 1998
5. Buunk G, van der Hoeven JG, Meinders AE: A comparison of near-infrared spectroscopy and jugular bulb oximetry in comatose patients resuscitated from a cardiac arrest. Anaesthesia 53:13–19, 1998
6. Chan KH, Miller JD, Dearden NM, et al: The effect of changes in cerebral perfusion pressure upon middle cerebral artery blood flow velocity and jugular bulb venous oxygen saturation after severe brain injury. J. Neurosurg. 77:55–61, 1992
7. Chance B: Mitochondrial redox state as a "gold standard" of tissue hypoxia. Adv.Exp.Med.Biol. 361:226, 1994
8. Chance B: Near-infrared images using continuous, phase-modulated, and pulsed light with quantitation of blood and blood oxygenation. Ann.N.Y.Acad.Sci. 838:29–45, 1998
9. Clark LC: Monitor and control of blood and tissue oxygen tension. Trans Am Soc Artif Intern Org 2:41–46, 1956
10. Colier WN, van Haaren NJ, Oeseburg B: A comparative study of two near infrared spectrophotometers for the assessment of cerebral haemodynamics. Acta Anaesthesiol.Scand.Suppl 107:101–105, 1995
11. Cope M, Delpy DT, Wray S, et al: A CCD spectrophotometer to quantitate the concentration of chromophores in living tissue utilising the absorption peak of water at 975 nm. Adv.Exp.Med.Biol. 248:33–40, 1989
12. Cruz J: Jugular venous oxygen saturation monitoring. J. Neurosurg. 77:162–163, 1992
13. Cruz J, Miner ME: Modulating cerebral oxygen delivery and extraction in acute traumatic coma, in Miner ME, Wagner KA (eds): Neurotrauma. Treatment, Rehabilitation, and Related Issues. Boston: Butterworths, 1986, pp 55–72
14. Cruz J, Miner ME, Allen SJ, et al: Continuous monitoring of cerebral oxygenation in acute brain injury: injection of mannitol during hyperventilation. J. Neurosurg. 73:725–730, 1990
15. Daubeney PE, Pilkington SN, Janke E, et al: Cerebral oxygenation measured by near-infrared spectroscopy: comparison with jugular bulb oximetry. Ann.Thorac.Surg. 61:930–934, 1996
16. De Deyne C, Vandekerckhove T, Decruyenaere J: Implementation of jugular bulb oximetry in the management of intracranial hypertension. Intensive Care Med. 21 (suppl. 1):S153, 1995
17. Dearden NM: Jugular bulb venous oxygen saturation in the management of severe head injury. Curr Opin Anaesth 4:279–286, 1991
18. Delpy DT, Cope M, van der ZP, et al: Estimation of optical pathlength through tissue from direct time of flight measurement. Phys.Med.Biol. 33:1433–1442, 1988
19. Dings J, Jager A, Meixensberger J, et al: Brain tissue pO2 and outcome after severe head injury. Neurol.Res. 20 Suppl 1:S71-S75, 1998
20. Dings J, Meixensberger J, Amschler J, et al: Brain tissue pO2 in relation to cerebral perfusion pressure, TCD findings and TCD-CO2-reactivity after severe head injury. Acta Neurochir.(Wien.) 138:425–434, 1996

21. Dings J, Meixensberger J, Jager A, et al: Clinical experience with 118 brain tissue oxygen partial pressure catheter probes. Neurosurgery 43:1082–1095, 1998
22. Doppenberg EM, Zauner A, Watson JC, et al: Determination of the ischemic threshold for brain oxygen tension. Acta Neurochir.Suppl (Wien.) 71:166–169, 1998
23. Dujovny M, Ausman JI, Stoddart H, et al: Somanetics INVOS 3100 cerebral oximeter. Neurosurgery 37:160, 1995
24. Edwards AD, McCormick DC, Roth SC, et al: Cerebral hemodynamic effects of treatment with modified natural surfactant investigated by near infrared spectroscopy. Pediatr.Res. 32:532–536, 1992
25. Ferrari M, Wilson DA, Hanley DF, et al: Determination of cerebral venous hemoglobin saturation by derivative near infrared spectroscopy. Adv.Exp.Med.Biol. 248:47–53, 1989
26. Frank KH, Kessler M, Appelbaum K, et al: The Erlangen micro-lightguide spectrophotometer EMPHO I. Phys.Med.Biol. 34:1883–1900, 1989
27. Germon TJ, Evans PD, Barnett NJ, et al: Cerebral near infrared spectroscopy: emitter-detector separation must be increased. Br. J. Anaesth. 82:831–837, 1999
28. Germon TJ, Kane NM, Manara AR, et al: Near-infrared spectroscopy in adults: effects of extracranial ischaemia and intracranial hypoxia on estimation of cerebral oxygenation. Br. J. Anaesth. 73:503–506, 1994
29. Germon TJ, Young AE, Manara AR, et al: Extracerebral absorption of near infrared light influences the detection of increased cerebral oxygenation monitored by near infrared spectroscopy. J. Neurol.Neurosurg.Psychiatry 58:477–479, 1995
30. Gibbs EL, Lennox WG, Nims LF, et al: Arterial and cerebral venous blood. Arterial-venous differences in man. J. Biol Chem 144:325–332, 1942
31. Goetting MG, Preston G: Jugular bulb catheterization does not increase intracranial pressure. Intensive Care Med. 17:195–198, 1991
32. Gopinath SP, Valadka A, Contant CF, et al: Relationship between global and cortical cerebral blood flow in patients with head injuries. Neurosurgery 44:1273–1278, 1999
33. Groner W, Winkelman JW, Harris AG, et al: Orthogonal polarization spectral imaging: a new method for study of the microcirculation. Nat.Med. 5:1209–1212, 1999
34. Grubhofer G, Lassnigg A, Manlik F, et al: The contribution of extracranial blood oxygenation on near-infrared spectroscopy during carotid thrombendarterectomy. Anaesthesia 52:116–120, 1997
35. Gupta AK, Hutchinson PJ, Al Rawi P, et al: Measuring brain tissue oxygenation compared with jugular venous oxygen saturation for monitoring cerebral oxygenation after traumatic brain injury. Anesth.Analg. 88:549–553, 1999
36. Hock C, Muller-Spahn F, Schuh-Hofer S, et al: Age dependency of changes in cerebral hemoglobin oxygenation during brain activation: a near-infrared spectroscopy study. J. Cereb.Blood Flow Metab 15:1103–1108, 1995
37. Hoffman WE, Charbel FT, Edelman G: Brain tissue oxygen, carbon dioxide, and pH in neurosurgical patients at risk for ischemia. Anesth.Analg. 82:582–586, 1996
38. Hoffman WE, Charbel FT, Edelman G, et al: Brain tissue response to CO_2 in patients with arteriovenous malformation. J. Cereb.Blood Flow Metab 16:1383–1386, 1996
39. Hoffman WE, Charbel FT, Edelman G, et al: Brain tissue oxygen pressure, carbon dioxide pressure, and pH during hypothermic circulatory arrest. Surg.Neurol. 46:75–79, 1996
40. Hoffman WE, Charbel FT, Edelman G, et al: Brain tissue oxygenation in patients with cerebral occlusive disease and arteriovenous malformations. Br. J. Anaesth. 78:169–171, 1997
41. Hoffman WE, Charbel FT, Portillo GG, et al: Regional tissue pO_2, pCO_2, pH and temperature measurement. Neurol.Res. 20 Suppl 1:S81-S84, 1998
42. Holzschuh M, Woertgen C, Metz C, et al: Dynamic changes of cerebral oxygenation measured by brain tissue oxygen pressure and near infrared spectroscopy. Neurol.Res. 19:246–248, 1997
43. Hoper J, Gaab MR: Intraoperative monitoring of local Hb-oxygenation in human brain cortex. Adv.Exp.Med.Biol. 361:483–489, 1994
44. Hudetz AG: Blood flow in the cerebral capillary network: a review emphasizing observations with intravital microscopy. Microcirculation. 4:233–252, 1997

45. Ince C, Mathura K R, Bouma G J: The microcirculation of the human brain and its tumours compared using OPS imaging. J. Vasc.Res 2000 (Abstract). 37:51:54

46. Ince C, Sinaasappel M: Microcirculatory oxygenation and shunting in sepsis and shock. Crit Care Med. 27:1369–1377, 1999

47. Jakobsen M, Enevoldsen E: Retrograde catheterization of the right internal jugular vein for serial measurements of cerebral venous oxygen content. J. Cereb.Blood Flow Metab 9:717–720, 1989

48. Jobsis FF: Noninvasive, infrared monitoring of cerebral and myocardial oxygen sufficiency and circulatory parameters. Science 198:1264–1267, 1977

49. Katayama Y, Tsubokawa T, Hirayama T, et al: Continuous monitoring of jugular bulb oxygen saturation as a measure of the shunt flow of cerebral arteriovenous malformations. J. Neurosurg. 80:826–833, 1994

50. Kety S, Schmidt C: The nitrous oxide method for the quantitative determination of cerebral blood flow in man: Theory, procedure, and normal values. J. Clin Invest476–483, 1948

51. Kiening KL, Schneider GH, Bardt TF, et al: Bifrontal measurements of brain tissue-PO2 in comatose patients. Acta Neurochir.Suppl (Wien.) 71:172–173, 1998

52. Kiening KL, Unterberg AW, Bardt TF, et al: Monitoring of cerebral oxygenation in patients with severe head injuries: brain tissue PO2 versus jugular vein oxygen saturation. J. Neurosurg. 85:751–757, 1996

53. Latronico N, Beindorf AE, Rasulo FA, et al: Limits of intermittent jugular bulb oxygen saturation monitoring in the management of severe head trauma patients. Neurosurgery 46:1131–1138, 2000

54. Lewis SB, Myburgh JA, Reilly PL: Detection of cerebral venous desaturation by continuous jugular bulb oximetry following acute neurotrauma. Anaesth.Intensive Care 23:307–314, 1995

55. Lewis SB, Myburgh JA, Thornton EL, et al: Cerebral oxygenation monitoring by near-infrared spectroscopy is not clinically useful in patients with severe closed-head injury: a comparison with jugular venous bulb oximetry. Crit Care Med. 24:1334–1338, 1996

56. Lovell AT, Marshall AC, Elwell CE, et al: Changes in cerebral blood volume with changes in position in awake and anesthetized subjects. Anesth.Analg. 90:372–376, 2000

57. Lubbers DW: Oxygen electrodes and optodes and their application in vivo. Adv.Exp.Med.Biol. 388:13–34, 1996

58. Lubbers DW, Baumgartl H, Zimelka W: Heterogeneity and stability of local PO2 distribution within the brain tissue. Adv.Exp.Med.Biol. 345:567–574, 1994

59. Madsen PL, Secher NH: Near-infrared oximetry of the brain. Prog.Neurobiol. 58:541–560, 1999

60. Martinez-Tica JF, Berbarie R, Davenport P, et al: Monitoring brain PO2, PCO2, and pH during graded levels of hypoxemia in rabbits. J. Neurosurg.Anesthesiol. 11:260–263, 1999

61. Matcher SJ, Cope M, Delpy DT: Use of the water absorption spectrum to quantify tissue chromophore concentration changes in near-infrared spectroscopy. Phys.Med.Biol. 39:177–196, 1994

62. Mathura K R, Ince C: First clinical use of OPS imaging, in Messmer K (ed): Progress in applied Microcirculation. Basel: Karger, 2000, vol 24:94–101

63. Matta BF, Lam AM, Mayberg TS, et al: A critique of the intraoperative use of jugular venous bulb catheters during neurosurgical procedures. Anesth.Analg. 79:745–750, 1994

64. McCormick PW, Stewart M, Goetting MG, et al: Regional cerebrovascular oxygen saturation measured by optical spectroscopy in humans. Stroke 22:596–602, 1991

65. McCormick PW, Stewart M, Goetting MG, et al: Noninvasive cerebral optical spectroscopy for monitoring cerebral oxygen delivery and hemodynamics. Crit Care Med. 19:89–97, 1991

66. McKeating EG, Monjardino JR, Signorini DF, et al: A comparison of the Invos 3100 and the Critikon 2020 near-infrared spectrophotometers as monitors of cerebral oxygenation. Anaesthesia 52:136–140, 1997

67. McKinley BA, Morris WP, Parmley CL, et al: Brain parenchyma PO2, PCO2, and pH during and after hypoxic, ischemic brain insult in dogs. Crit Care Med. 24:1858–1868, 1996

68. Meixensberger J, Dings J, Kuhnigk H, et al: Studies of tissue PO2 in normal and pathological human brain cortex. Acta Neurochir.Suppl (Wien.) 59:58–63, 1993

69. Meyer B, Schaller C, Frenkel C, et al: Distributions of local oxygen saturation and its response to changes of mean arterial blood pressure in the cerebral cortex adjacent to arteriovenous malformations. Stroke 30:2623–2630, 1999

70. Nylin G, Helund S, Regnstrom O: Cerebral circulation studied with labelled red cells in healthy males. Acta Radiol 55:281, 1961

71. Olsen KS, Madsen PL, Borme T, et al: Evaluation of a 7.5 French pulmonary catheter for continuous monitoring of cerebral venous oxygen saturation. J. Neurosurg.Anesthesiol. 6:233–238, 1994

72. Owen-Reece H, Elwell CE, Goldstone J, et al: Investigation of the effects of hypocapnia upon cerebral haemodynamics in normal volunteers and anaesthetised subjects by near infrared spectroscopy (NIRS). Adv.Exp.Med.Biol. 361:475–482, 1994

73. Pappert D, Rossaint R, Lewandowski K, et al: Preliminary evaluation of a new continuous intra-arterial blood gas monitoring device. Acta Anaesthesiol.Scand.Suppl 107:67–70, 1995

74. Pennings F A, Bouma G J, Kalkman C, et al: Intraoperative monitoring of brain tissue pO2 and pCO2 in peritumoral edema by stereotactic placement of Neurotrend® probes. Zentralbl Neurochir 60:37, 1999 (Abstract)

75. Pollard V, Prough DS, DeMelo AE, et al: The influence of carbon dioxide and body position on near-infrared spectroscopic assessment of cerebral hemoglobin oxygen saturation. Anesth.Analg. 82:278–287, 1996

76. Prough DS, Pollard V: Cerebral near-infrared spectroscopy: ready for prime time? Crit Care Med. 23:1624–1626, 1995

77. Robertson CS, Contant CF, Gokaslan ZL, et al: Cerebral blood flow, arteriovenous oxygen difference, and outcome in head injured patients. J. Neurol.Neurosurg.Psychiatry 55:594–603, 1992

78. Robertson CS, Grossman RG, Goodman JC, et al: The predictive value of cerebral anaerobic metabolism with cerebral infarction after head injury. J. Neurosurg. 67:361–368, 1987

79. Robertson CS, Narayan RK, Gokaslan ZL, et al: Cerebral arteriovenous oxygen difference as an estimate of cerebral blood flow in comatose patients. J. Neurosurg. 70:222–230, 1989

80. Roth S, Menzel M, Rieger A, et al: Continuous pO2 and pCO2 measurement in brain tissue and cerebrovenous blood during different inspired oxygen settings. A porcine model. Acta Chir Hung. 36:289–291, 1997

81. Schneider GH, Sarrafzadeh AS, Kiening KL, et al: Influence of hyperventilation on brain tissue-PO2, PCO2, and pH in patients with intracranial hypertension. Acta Neurochir.Suppl (Wien.) 71:62–65, 1998

82. Schneider GH, von Helden A, Lanksch WR, et al: Continuous monitoring of jugular bulb oxygen saturation in comatose patients–therapeutic implications. Acta Neurochir.(Wien.) 134:71–75, 1995

83. Sheinberg M, Kanter MJ, Robertson CS, et al: Continuous monitoring of jugular venous oxygen saturation in head- injured patients. J. Neurosurg. 76:212–217, 1992

84. Sinaasappel M, van Iterson M, Ince C: Microvascular oxygen pressure in the pig intestine during haemorrhagic shock and resuscitation. J. Physiol (Lond) 514 (Pt 1):245–253, 1999

85. Stocchetti N, Chieregato A, De Marchi M, et al: High cerebral perfusion pressure improves low values of local brain tissue O2 tension (PtiO2) in focal lesions. Acta Neurochir.Suppl (Wien.) 71:162–165, 1998

86. Stocchetti N, Paparella A, Bridelli F, et al: Cerebral venous oxygen saturation studied with bilateral samples in the internal jugular veins. Neurosurgery 34:38–43, 1994

87. Tateishi A, Maekawa T, Soejima Y, et al: Qualitative comparison of carbon dioxide-induced change in cerebral near-infrared spectroscopy versus jugular venous oxygen saturation in adults with acute brain disease. Crit Care Med. 23:1734–1738, 1995

88. Valadka AB, Gopinath SP, Contant CF, et al: Relationship of brain tissue PO2 to outcome after severe head injury. Crit Care Med. 26:1576–1581, 1998

89. van den Brink WA, Haitsma IK, Avezaat CJ, et al: Brain parenchyma/pO2 catheter interface: a histopathological study in the rat. J. Neurotrauma 15:813–824, 1998

90. van den Brink WA, van Santbrink H, Steyerberg EW, et al: Brain oxygen tension in severe head injury. Neurosurgery 46:868–876, 2000
91. van Santbrink H, Maas AI, Avezaat CJ: Continuous monitoring of partial pressure of brain tissue oxygen in patients with severe head injury. Neurosurgery 38:21–31, 1996
92. Villringer A, Planck J, Hock C, et al: Near infrared spectroscopy (NIRS): a new tool to study hemodynamic changes during activation of brain function in human adults. Neurosci.Lett. 154:101–104, 1993
93. Wagner K, Bossen W, Schramm U: Tissue alterations by the penetration of a pO2 sensing needle probe. Adv.Exp.Med.Biol. 317:639–644, 1992
94. Wahr JA, Tremper KK, Samra S, et al: Near-infrared spectroscopy: theory and applications. J. Cardiothorac.Vasc.Anesth. 10:406–418, 1996
95. Watanabe M, Harada N, Kosaka H, et al: Intravital microreflectometry of individual pial vessels and capillary region of rat. J. Cereb.Blood Flow Metab 14:75–84, 1994
96. Wyatt JS, Cope M, Delpy DT, et al: Quantitation of cerebral blood volume in human infants by near-infrared spectroscopy. J. Appl.Physiol 68:1086–1091, 1990
97. Wyatt JS, Cope M, Delpy DT, et al: Quantification of cerebral oxygenation and haemodynamics in sick newborn infants by near infrared spectrophotometry. Lancet 2:1063–1066, 1986
98. Wyatt JS, Edwards AD, Cope M, et al: Response of cerebral blood volume to changes in arterial carbon dioxide tension in preterm and term infants. Pediatr.Res. 29:553–557, 1991
99. Zarzuelo R, Castaneda J: Differences in oxygen content between mixed venous blood and cerebral venous blood for outcome prediction after cardiac arrest. Intensive Care Med. 21:71–75, 1995
100. Zauner A, Bullock R, Di X, et al: Brain oxygen, CO2, pH, and temperature monitoring: evaluation in the feline brain. Neurosurgery 37:1168–1176, 1995

Computed Tomography Angiography and Perfusion Imaging of Acute Stroke

G. Hunter, L. Hamberg, M.H. Lev, and R.G. González

The traditional thrust of diagnostic radiology has been in the evaluation of tissue structure and the changes in structure that may result from a variety of pathologies. However, with increasing sophistication and power of digital computers coupled with technological advances in imaging methods, it has become routinely possible to image organ function, and in particular vascular physiology, at the same time as providing traditional anatomical information. These developments have brought a wholly new dimension to the practice of neurology, neuroradiology and neurosurgery. We can now routinely investigate the fundamental changes underlying cerebrovascular disease; that is we can demonstrate vascular physiology as exemplified by bulk blood flow and parenchymal or tissue perfusion.

When a patient presents to a hospital with signs and symptoms suggesting they are suffering from a cerebral ischemia related event, it is computed tomography (CT) that is utilized as the first imaging resource. A potent reason for taking CT seriously as a tool for the immediate imaging evaluation of potential stroke victims is its ubiquitous availability. Furthermore, among all the different available imaging modalities it is still computed tomography that is the most common neurological imaging study. In the early 1970s, CT was perceived as a revolution in medicine – today it remains a revolution in medicine; the current generation of multi slice, helical CT scanners is able to scan from the aortic arch to the cranial vertex in approximately 40 seconds and provide images of this region with slice thicknesses approaching 0.5 mm and freely chosen, overlapping image intervals of as little as 0.1 mm. Our task has been to leverage this availability of information to provide true physiological or functional data about the state of the large vessels supplying blood to the brain and the status of the arteriolar and capillary microvasculature delivering that blood, and the nutrients it carries, to brain parenchyma. CTA provides the large vessel information, CT perfusion delivers the physiological evaluation of the parenchymal microvasculature.

Helical CT Imaging

Rotation of the X-ray tube during translation of the patient through the X-ray beam results in a helical beam path through the patient. The use of the term "spiral" CT should be avoided, as the mathematical difference between a spiral and a helix is that the radius of a spiral decreases with increasing distance along its long axis, while the radius of a helix remains constant; clearly with CT we are dealing with a helix, not a spiral. The movement of blood along vessels and through brain parenchyma defines the physiological function that we need to measure. In order to adequately identify this movement and extract accurate parametric information from the process, repeated snapshots of the vascular state of the brain and its supplying vessels need to be obtained sufficiently rapidly to identify any time dependent changes that occur; speed of data acquisition is of the essence. The development of single detector ring helical CT and more recently the extension of this technology to a multislice detector array has made truly rapid CT imaging a reality and thus we are able to measure vascular physiological function. An alternative way of obtaining vascular physiological data is to keep the patient stationary during tube rotation, and generate a series of images at a single location. In such a cine acquisition the same slice location can be repeatedly imaged at short intervals, typically every second. Provision of additional timing information allows flow related parameters of cerebrovascular physiology to be measured.

The movement of flowing blood can be identified with CT by using a contrast agent which remains localized in the cerebrovascular space during the time that we image the brain (Fig. 1). Such an agent is conventional iodinated X-ray contrast material. A typical molecule of such an agent has a molecular weight of approximately 770 Daltons and contains 3 iodine atoms attached to a benzene ring stabilized with three side chains. Modern contrast media are non-ionic and iso-osmolar to blood. A single molecule of contrast material is small in comparison with the size of the membrane channels that exist in the endothelial cells of the capillary circulation. Contrast material would move between the intravascular and extravascular spaces relatively freely, as it does for instance in the myocardi-

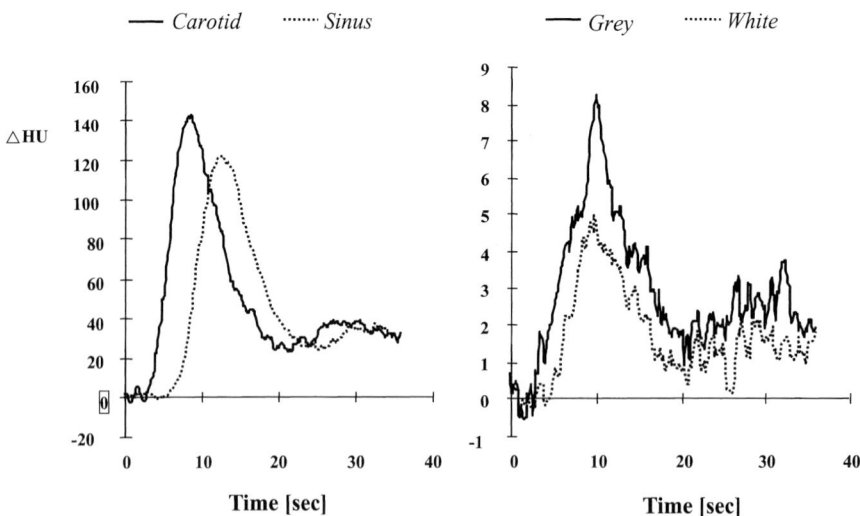

Fig. 1. Sample time density curves for cerebral structures. Graphs show the change in CT attenuation (measured in Hounsfield units) versus time during the dynamic, intravenous administration of nonionic CT contrast material

um, were it not for the presence of the blood brain barrier. It is the tight junctions of the blood brain barrier, that reduce the size of the membrane channels such that contrast material is retained in the cerebral capillary circulation; this allows us to measure vascular physiological function in the capillary circulation of the brain using mathematical modeling applicable to a restricted, single compartment or intravascular agent. Freely diffusible markers of cerebral blood flow, such as xenon gas, can also be used with computed tomography but require different imaging and mathematical modeling paradigms to obtain physiological data. There are two main ways of obtaining cerebrovascular physiological data by using a helical CT scanner with iodinated contrast material. These are the first pass bolus tracking technique and the constant infusion, steady state technique.

The Role of Noncontrast CT in Acute Stroke

Computed tomography (CT) is a very important component of clinical management for patients presenting with signs and symptoms of stroke during the hyperacute phase of its evolution. Here, "hyperacute" means less than 6 hours after the event which triggered stroke symptoms. This early period after stroke onset is important because it represents the accepted time window for the deployment of thrombolytic treatment [1–8]. Thrombolytic, or "clot-busting" therapy, can improve the outcome of embolic-type strokes, but it carries with it a high risk of intraparenchymal hemorrhage, and treatment failure, in patients with prolonged, severe ischemia [3, 8, 9].

In the treatment of stroke originating from the anterior circulation (MCA and ACA branches), current guidelines support the use of intravenous reverse tissue plasminogen activator (IV rt-PA) administered within 3 hours of symptom onset [7, 8]. Intraarterial (IA) thrombolysis, which has a longer treatment window, can be administered within 6 hours of anterior circulation stroke ictus [4]. In the case of brainstem (posterior circulation) stroke, the treatment window for thrombolysis is longer than 6 hours, partly because of increased resistance of the posterior circulation to hemorrhage and partly because there is a uniformly poor outcome in untreated cases [5]. Until recently, intraarterial thrombolysis has been performed with urokinase (UK), which has been supported by the results of the PROACT study [10]. Currently, however, due to the unavailability of urokinase, IA thrombolysis is being performed using rt-PA.

Typically, a patient demonstrating acute ischemic stroke symptoms will undergo a noncontrast CT (NCCT) scan of the head to determine if contraindications to thrombolytic treatment are present. Such contraindications include hemorrhage (absolute contraindication) or a "large" parenchymal hypodensity (indicating already infarcted brain, a relative contraindication) [8, 9]. At most centers, the involvement of CT scanning in the workup of hyperacute stroke patients ends at this point. There is considerable lack of agreement, however, in recognizing and quantifying early NCCT changes of stroke, and in using NCCT to determine appropriate candidates for thrombolysis [11]. In one study, only 45% of patients were identified correctly for inclusion in a hypothetical acute stroke treatment trial [12]. In the PROACT study, 294 of 474 patients (62%) who were screened with catheter arteriography in anticipation of IA thrombolysis were found to have normal middle cerebral arteries; that is there was no lesion present amenable to thrombolytic therapy. Improved methods of recognizing and measuring early cerebral ischemia were needed and have been developed [13].

The Role of Contrast CT in Acute Stroke

The "ideal" imaging test for hyperacute stroke patients should provide clinically relevant data to assist in the following actions:
- Rapid triage to appropriate stroke treatment
- Assessment of prognosis
- Assessment of hemorrhagic risk
- Rapid patient subtyping of stroke type for inclusion in clinical trials

Non-enhanced CT scanning together with whole brain helical CT imaging during contrast infusion has the potential to address each of these clinical issues, as it is by nature a multiparametric study that provides large-vessel angiograms as well as whole brain perfusion information.

Combined CT Angiogram and Steady State CT Perfusion Imaging

A three dimensional helical study is performed by simultaneously rotating the X-ray tube and translating the patient through the x-ray beam. This generates a stream of data along a single helical trajectory or multiple intertwined overlapping helical trajectories through the patient for single or multislice acquisition methods respectively. From these data, continuous and/or overlapping axial sections can be reconstructed through the brain. If such helical data are acquired through the whole brain during infusion of X-ray contrast material, the vasculature becomes visible throughout the volume imaged and a volumetric, multiparametric study of the cerebral vasculature is obtained. From these image data, morphologic evaluation of large vessels can be made by using 3D reconstruction of CT angiograms and physiological, quantitative evaluation of tissue perfusion can be visualized by calculating voxel-by-voxel maps of absolute perfused cerebral blood volume (CBV) [14]. Both angiographic and tissue perfusion images are typically created on an off-line workstation, thus releasing the scanner for the next patient.

To perform whole brain evaluation of the microvasculature, an 18-gauge antecubital cannula is inserted prior to the patient's entry into the scanner, and the patient's head is immobilized in a head-holder by forehead and chin straps. First a non-contrast study is acquired with contiguous 5-mm sections from the foramen magnum to the vertex. Then, twenty-five seconds after the start of a power infusion of 120 ml of nonionic, iso-osmolar contrast material at 3 ml/sec, a helical scan is obtained from the foramen magnum to the vertex. The scanning parameters are 140 kVp, scanner optimized mA, a 512 by 512 image matrix and a 25 cm acquisition field of view. The timing of the delay from the start of infusion is optimized so that contrast has filled the cerebral vasculature before imaging starts, and the infusion rate is optimized to maintain a steady contrast concentration in the cerebral vasculature during the time that the brain is imaged. In patients with atrial fibrillation, the delay of 25 seconds should be prolonged to account for the reduced cardiac output and consequent delay in filling of the cerebral vasculature before imaging. For production of CT angiograms, data from this helical acquisition are reconstructed at 0.5 mm intervals onto a 512 by 512 matrix and manipulated by using multiprojection volume reconstruction (MPVR) or maximum intensity projection (MIP) algorithms (Figs. 2, 3). The tissue perfusion data are immediately evaluated at the time of scanning by visual interpretation, which is sufficient to triage the patient, and then by offline post processing to gather quantitative information about regional cerebral perfusion (perfused cerebral blood volume) in the whole brain (Fig. 4).

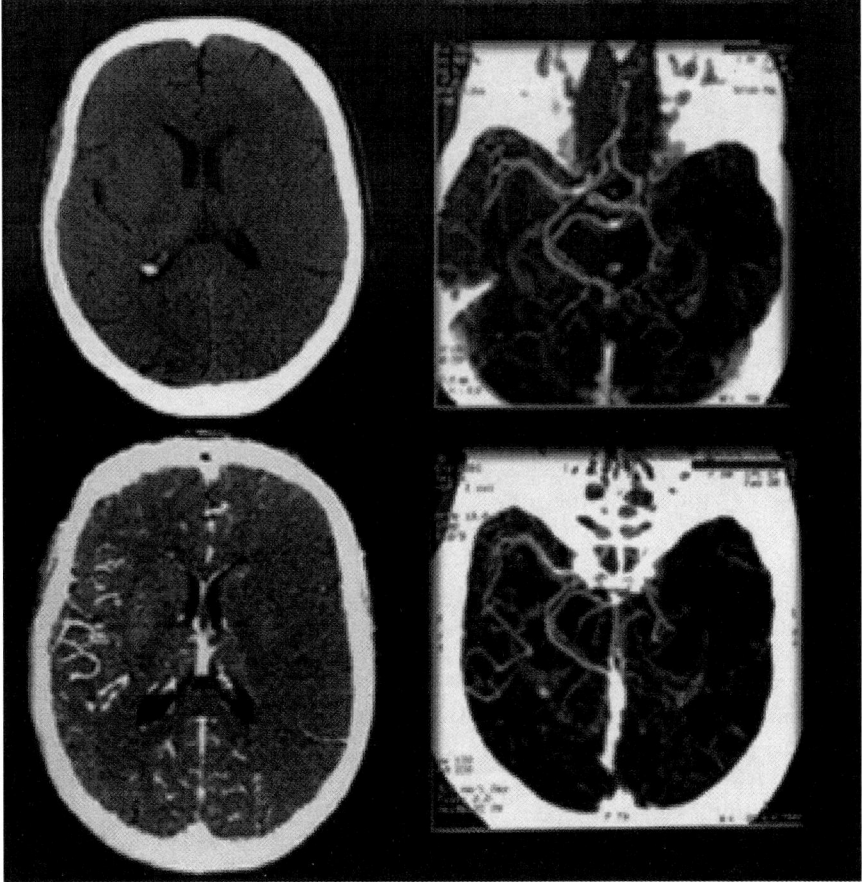

Fig. 2. "Collapsed MIP" reformatted images from a CT angiogram, viewed from superiorly, shows absence of contrast filling in the left middle cerebral artery (MCA) stem, compared to the normal filling on the right. This is an example of an acute proximal MCA embolus

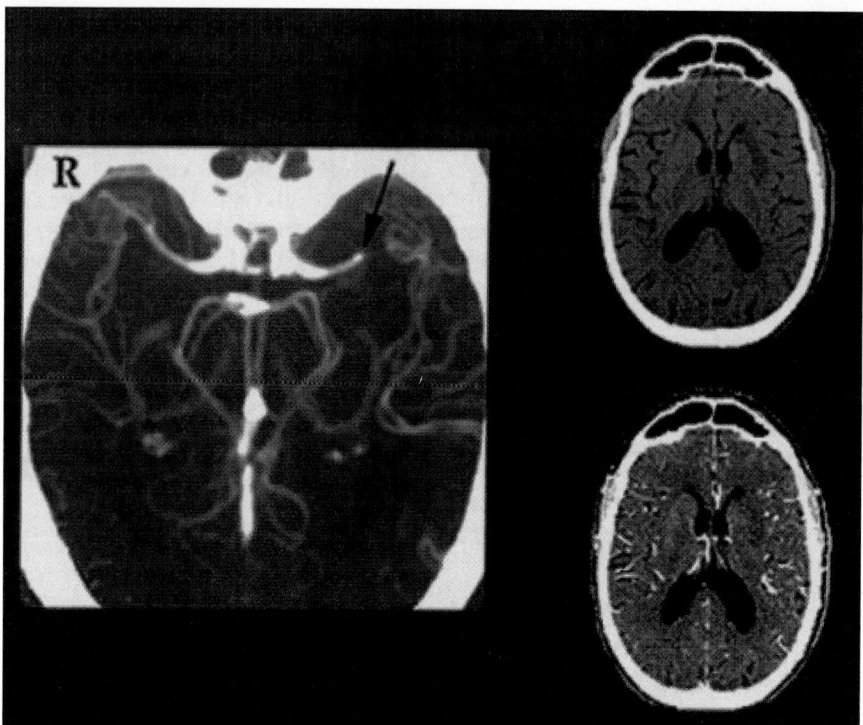

Fig. 3. "Collapsed MIP" reformatted images from a CT angiogram, superior view, shows absence of contrast filling in the left middle cerebral artery M1-M2 bifurcation, compared to the normal filling on the right. This is an example of a more distal MCA embolus than is shown in the previous case. Note the presence of extensive collateral filling of the sylvian branches on the left

First Pass CT Perfusion Imaging

First pass CT perfusion imaging is a different contrast CT technique capable of measuring tissue level perfusion [15, 16]. The protocol for a first pass bolus study is as follows: a 16-gauge cannula is inserted into the basilic or cephalic vein, and the patient is positioned supine in the helical CT scanner with head immobilized in the headholder using forehead and chin straps. The cine mode paradigm is used in this technique. With a single slice CT scanner only one slice location can be studied, while with multislice scanners, currently up to 4 adjacent slices can be imaged simultaneously. Once the slice location(s) are chosen, image data acquisition is initiated using 140 kVp, scanner optimized mA, a 512 by 512 display matrix, 5 or 10 mm slice thickness, and a 25 cm acquisition field of view. Imaging is started at one frame per second simultaneously with the injection of 80 ml of non-ionic contrast agent at a maximal possible rate (typically 10 ml/sec, although rates between 3 ml/sec and 15 ml/sec have been reported from different institutions) by using a power injector. Image data acquisition is continued until the

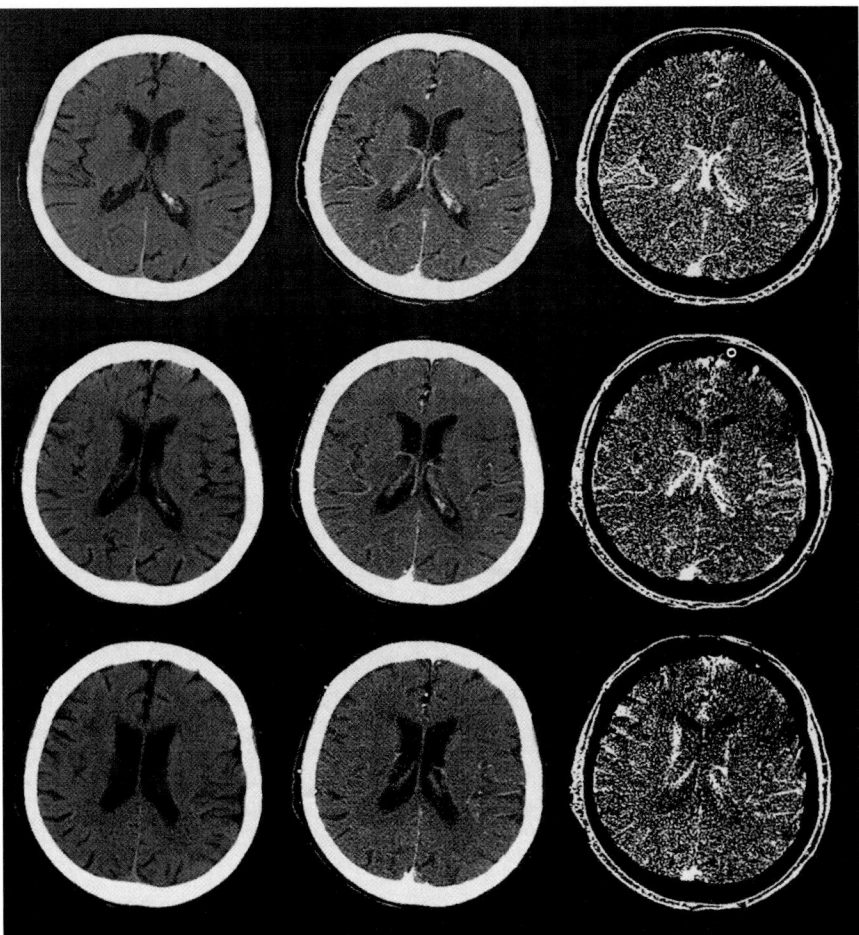

Fig. 4. Example of image coregistration and subtraction used to create fractional CT cerebral blood volume maps. Noncontrast CT images are in the first column and coregistered dynamic contrast enhanced CTP source images are in the second column. The noncontrast images are subtracted from the coregistered CTP images to form true cerebral blood volume maps, shown in the third column. Such maps may increase infarct conspicuity. *(Figure courtesy of IMIPS Inc., Boston, MA)*

whole of the first passage of contrast through the brain has been recorded, usually a total acquisition time of 50 seconds suffices. Image post-processing is applied to the reconstructed, axial CT images comprising the timed series of data in order to create voxel-by-voxel maps of cerebral blood volume (CBV), blood flow (CBF) and contrast mean transit time (MTT) (Figs. 5–7). The analysis uses mathematical modeling and function fitting to eliminate the effects of recirculation and noise in the time-density curves observed as the contrast material passes through the cerebral vasculature [17]. Currently the first pass technique is capable of imaging either a single slice or a small contiguous volume with a multislice CT scanner.

CT Perfusion
CBV

MR Perfusion
CBV

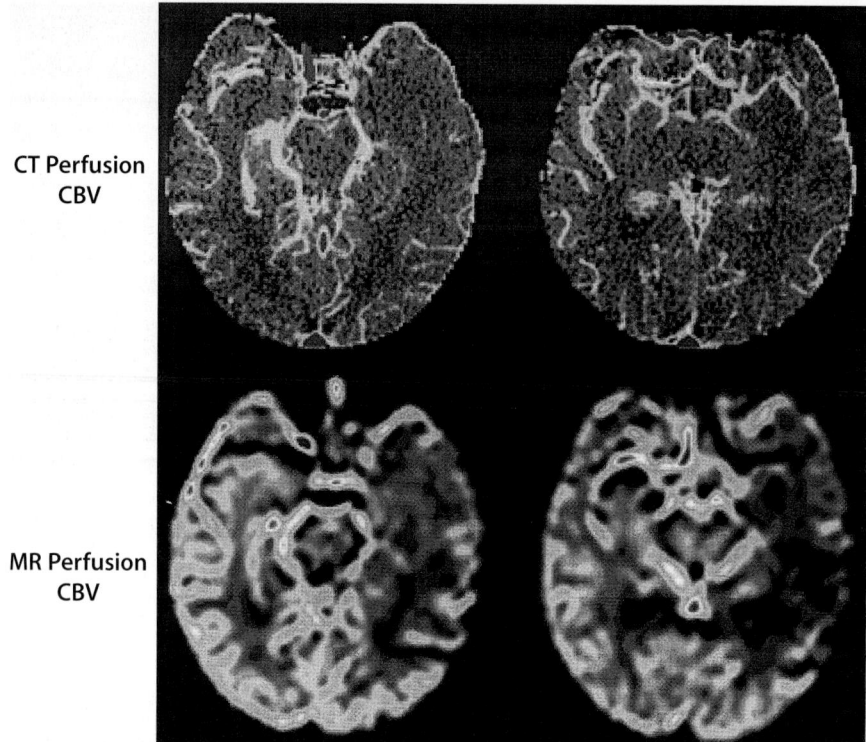

Fig. 5. Sample CT and MR cerebral blood volume (CBV) maps. Cerebral blood volume is measured in ml of blood per 100 gm brain tissue. Note the decreased *(black, dark blue)* cerebral blood volume in the left compared to the right hemisphere, in this patient who is approximately 12 hours status post a left MCA embolus

Rapid Triage to Appropriate Treatment

Because recanalization of proximal large vessel occlusions is more likely to be successful when treated by intraarterial (IA) thrombolysis than when treated by intravenous (IV) thrombolysis, it is important to identify such large vessel occlusions with CTA. Data supporting this view comes from a study in which angiographically proven recanalization 60 minutes after the administration of IV rt-PA was recorded. Recanalization rates with IV rt-PA were much higher for distal MCA occlusions than for ICA occlusions at the skull base [13]. In another study, CTA predicted little benefit from IV rt-PA in cases that had poor collaterals, autolyzed thrombi, or "top of carotid" saddle emboli [18].

The value of performing CT angiography in acute stroke patients might be especially important at centers which perform IV, but not IA, thrombolysis. CTA can be used as a triage tool to identify patients that would be better treated by transfer to a medical center at which IA thrombolysis is performed.

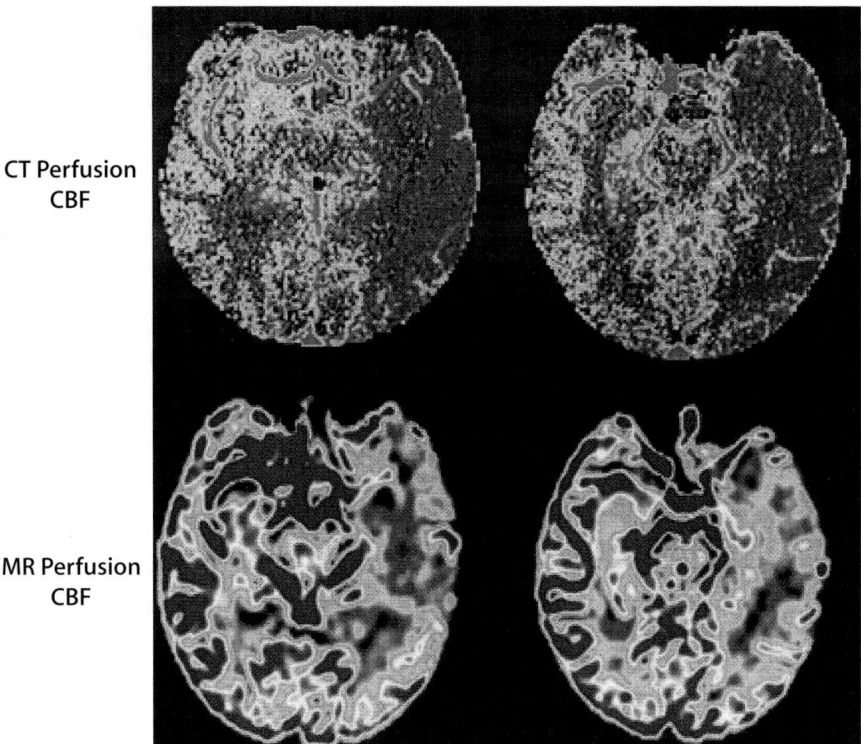

Fig. 6. CT and MR perfusion maps from the same patient as in Figure 5, showing quantitative CT cerebral blood flow (CBF). The units are ml blood per 100 gm brain tissue per minute. Note the marked decreased blood flow throughout the left hemisphere *(dark blue, green)* compared to the right hemisphere. There is also decreased collateral circulation seen in the sylvian vessels on the left (normal sylvian branch flow is shown in *orange on the right*)

Whole brain CT perfusion paradigms allow combined large vessel CTA and capillary level perfusion to be evaluated in order to identify intravascular clot (most commonly in the middle cerebral artery, which is involved in over 60% of all embolic strokes), and underperfused areas of the brain delineated as they have diminished contrast staining compared to adjacent normal regions. A combined CTA – steady state perfusion study can therefore be a valuable tool to help exclude patients with stroke 'mimics', such as transient ischemic attacks (TIAs), complex migraine headaches and seizures, from consideration for thrombolysis or other stroke treatments. CTA can be used to identify large vessel occlusions with high sensitivity and specificity (Figs. 2, 3). In addition the perfusion component can assist in identifying subtle parenchymal ischemic changes which facilitate the detection of distal embolic occlusions, and, potentially, identifying tissue that may be salvaged with thrombolytic treatment (Fig. 4).

Several studies have confirmed the value of CTA in detecting intracranial vascular occlusions in hyperacute stroke patients [19–22]. In a study of 53 consecutive

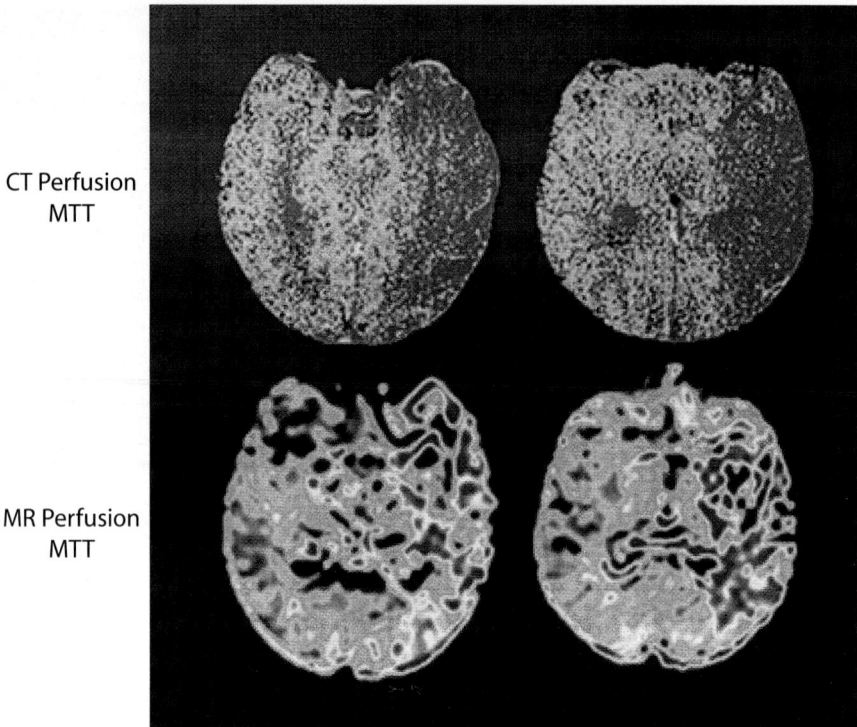

CT Perfusion
MTT

MR Perfusion
MTT

Fig. 7. CT and MR perfusion mean transit time (MTT) maps from the same patient as in Figs. 5 and 6. The units are seconds. Again, in this patient with a left MCA embolus, there is marked increase in mean transit time of the left *(orange, yellow)*, compared to the right *(blue)* hemisphere

patients presenting with stroke like symptoms CTA correctly identified the site of vessel occlusion in all patients (n=21) with proven large vessel occlusion (100% sensitivity). Of the patients (n=13) ultimately identified as suffering distal embolic or lacunar infarctions, CTA correctly demonstrated patent first and second order branches of Circle of Willis and skull base vessels. The remaining patients (n=19) without evidence of infarction on follow-up studies had either transient ischemic attacks (TIA) or non-stroke mimics [22]. In none of the cases without vessel occlusion did CTA falsely suggest thrombosis of a major intracranial vessel (100% specificity). CTA added about 11 minutes to scanner table time over that required for NCCT alone. Thus CTA is both specific and sensitive in the detection and exclusion of large vessel occlusion, making it a valuable first line test in the rapid triage of such patients to appropriate thrombolytic therapy [22]. Other studies have shown that the CTA component of whole brain CT perfusion imaging is useful in the evaluation of collateral circulation distal to an occlusion, and that the parenchymal phase of contrast staining improves the conspicuity of regions of the brain undergoing acute cerebral ischemia [23, 24]. The combination of optimized window and level review of both whole brain precontrast and contrast scans

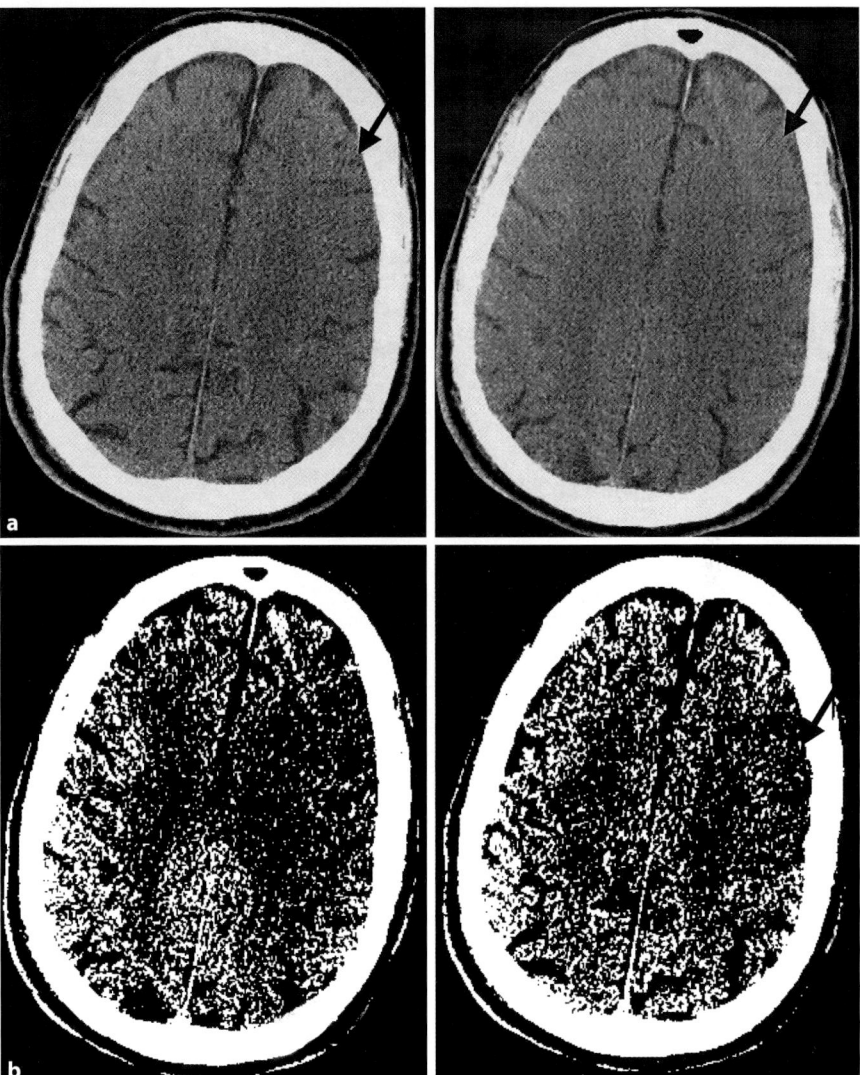

Fig. 8a–d. 65-year-old man with left hemispheric stroke, presenting 2 hours post ictus. **a** NCCT viewed with standard window width and center level settings. There is subtle ischemic hypodensity and loss of gray matter-white matter differentiation of the left, compared to the right, hemisphere. **b** NCCT viewed with narrowed window width and optimized center level settings. The ischemic hypodensity is more conspicuously identified than in Fig. 8A, because the minimal drop in CT attenuation caused by acute edema is accentuated.

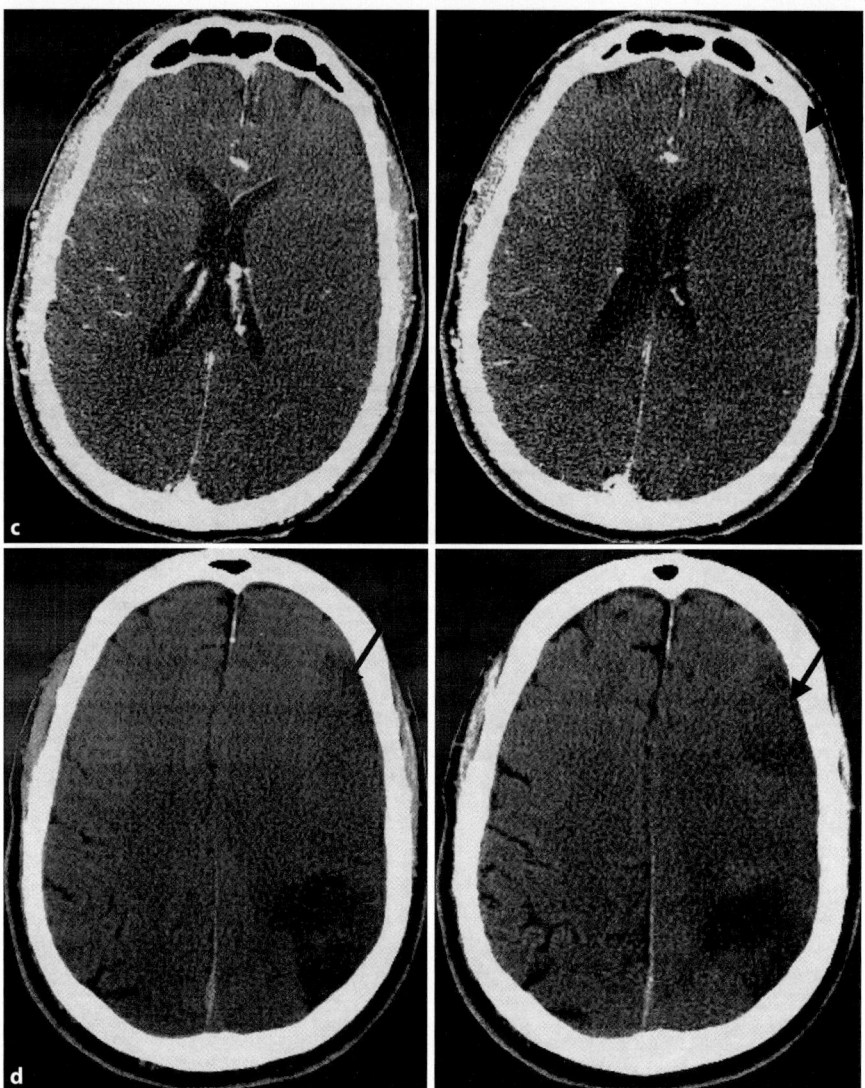

Fig. 8a–d. 65-year-old man with left hemispheric stroke, presenting 2 hours post ictus. **c** CT perfusion source images from the same level. Again, the left hemispheric ischemic hypodensity is more conspicuously identified than in Fig. 8A. **d** Follow-up NCCT scan at 5 days post ictus

improves sensitivity for identification of early infarction from 70% to almost 90% [25, 26] (Fig. 9). The whole brain contrast images are of particular value in identifying otherwise unsuspected regions of hypoperfusion; for instance, perfusion deficits can be present in multiple vascular territories, suggesting systemic emboli as a cause and prompting a search for a third and fourth order branch occlusions that might otherwise have been overlooked on the CTA images.

In addition to the more accurate detection of early ischemia, we have also found the whole brain CT perfusion study to be useful in the prediction of both final infarct size and patient outcome. By coregistering and subtracting, on a slice by slice basis, the precontrast from the postcontrast axial source images, fractional whole brain cerebral blood volume maps can be created [27] (Fig. 5).

A study assessing 22 consecutive patients with angiographically proven middle cerebral artery stem occlusion who received intraarterial thrombolytic treatment within 6 hours of stroke onset, showed a strong correlation between the volume of the initial CT perfusion deficit and both final infarction volume on follow-up imaging and clinical outcome. This suggests that the size of the initial, CT determined perfusion deficit predicts both final infarct size and clinical outcome [28].

Conclusion

The widespread availability of helical CT in most hospital emergency departments allows the routine acquisition of advanced angiographic and perfusion imaging of the acute stroke patient. Performance of whole brain CT perfusion and CTA is a quick and natural extension of the noncontrast head CT exam. The addition of a CT angiographic study adds about ten minutes of scanner table time to that of the conventional CT examination. All required post processing can typically be rapidly performed off-line, during which time the patient can be prepared for thrombolysis, should the decision to proceed with such treatment be made. CTA may become more important as the successful trial of intraarterial thrombolysis (PROACT) impacts on the national stroke treatment trends [10]. As intra-arterial thrombolysis becomes more widespread, CTA may prove useful to screen patients for large vessel occlusions prior to proceeding to more invasive, risky and expensive arteriography [29].

References

1. Alberts M. tPA in acute ischemic stroke- United States experience and issues for the future. Neurology 1998;51:S53–55.
2. Caplan L, Mohr J, Kistler P, al. e. Should thrombolytic therapy be the first-line treatment for acute ischemic stroke? New England Journal of Medicine 1997;337:1309–1310.
3. del Zoppo G, Poeck K, al e. Recombinant tissue plasminogen activator in acute thrombotic stroke. Ann Neurol 1992;32:78–86.
4. del Zoppo G, Higashida R, Furlan A, Pessin M, Rowley H, Gent M. PROACT: a phase II randomized trial of recombinant pro-urokinase by direct arterial delivery in acute middle cerebral artery stroke. Stroke 1998;29(1):4–11.
5. Hacke W, Zeumer H, Ferbert A, al. e. Intra-arterial thrombolytic therapy improves outcome in patients with acute vertebrobasilar occlusive disease. Stroke 1988;19:1216–212.
6. Hacke W, Kaste M, Fieschi C, et a. Intravenous thrombolysis with recombinant tissue plasminogen activator for acute hemispheric stroke: the European Cooperative Acute Stroke Study (ECASS). JAMA 1995;274:1017–1025.
7. National Institute of Neurological Disorders and Stroke rt-PA Stroke Study Group T. Tissueplasminogen activator for acute ischemic stroke. New England Journal of Medicine 1995;333:1581–1587.
8. NINDS SSG. Effect of rt-PA on ischemic lesion size by computed tomography. Preliminary results from the NINDS rt-PA Stroke Trial. Stroke 1997;28:2109–2118.

9. von Kummer R, Allen K, Holle R, et a. Acute stroke: Usefulness of early CT findings before thro-mobolytic therapy. Radiology 1997;205:327–333.

10. Furlan A, Higashida R, Wechsler L, et al. Intra-arterial prourokinase for acute ischemic stroke. JAMA 1999;282:2003–2011.

11. von Kummer R, Holle R, Grzyska U, Hofmann E, et a. Interobserver agreement in assessing early CT signs of middle cerebral artery infarction. American Journal of Neuroradiology 1996;17:1743–1748.

12. Wardlaw J, Dorman P, Lewis S, Sandercock P. Can stroke physicians and neuroradiologists identi-fy signs of early cerebral infarction on CT? J Neurol Neursosurg Psychiatry 1999;67:651–653.

13. Grotta J, Chiu D, Lu M, al e. Agreement and variability in the interpretation of early CT changes in stroke patients qualifying for intravenous rtPA therapy. Stroke 1999;30:1528–1533.

14. Hamberg LM, Hunter GJ, Kierstead D, Lo EH, Gonzalez RG, Wolf GL, Measurement of Cerebral Blood Volume with Subtraction Three-dimensional Functional CT, AJNR AM J Neuroradiol 17: 1861–1869, 1996.

15. Hamberg LM, Salonen OL, Hunter GL, Vuorela J, Kaste M, Wolf GL, Determination of Perfusion Deficits in Ischemic Patients by Using First Pass CT, 80th Scientific Assembly and Annual Meeting, November, Volume 193 (P), Supplement to Radiology, p 123, Chicago 1994.

16. Hunter GJ, Hamberg LM, Morris PP, Maynard K, Lo EH, Owen C, Debros FM, Choid IS, Tatter S, Gonzalez RG, Wolf GL, Ogilvy C, Demonstration of the cerebrovascular physiology of acute stroke using high resolution first pass slip-ring CT. Proceedings of the American Society of Neuroradi-ology, 33rd Annual Meeting, April 23–27, Chicago, p38, 1995

17. Hamberg LM, Hunter GJ, Halpern EF, Hoop B, Gazelle GS, Wolf GK, Quantitative High-Resolution Measurement of Cerebrovascular Physiology with Slip-Ring CT, AJNR Am J Neuroradiol 17:639–650, 1996.

18. Wildermuth S, Knauth M, Brandt T, Winter R, Sartor K, Hacke W. Role of CT Angiography in Patient Selection for Thrombolytic Therapy in Acute Hemispheric Stroke. Stroke 1998;29:935–938.

19. Knauth M, R. v, Jansen O, Hahnel S, Dorfler A, Sartor K. Potential of CT angiography in acute ischemic stroke [see comments]. American Journal of Neuroradiology 1997;18(6):1001–10.

20. Shrier D, Tanaka H, Numaguchi Y, Konno S, Patel U, Shibata D. CT angiography in the evaluation of acute stroke. American Journal of Neuroradiology 1997;18(6):1011–20.

21. Kendell B, Pullicono P. Intravascular contrast injection in ischemic lesions, II. Effect on prognosis. Neuroradiology 1980;19:241–243.

22. Farkas J, Lev M, Schwamm L, et al. The diagnostic value of CT angiography in hyperacute stroke. In: Stroke: Proceedings of the 23rd International Conference on Stroke and Cerebral Circulation, Orlando, FL 1998;

23. Ponzo J, Hunter G, Hamburg L, et al. Evaluation of collateral circulation in acute stroke patients using CT angiography. In: Stroke: Proceedings of the 23rd International Conference on Stroke and Cerebral Circulation, Orlando, FL 1998;

24. Barest G, Hunter G, Hamberg L, et al. Dynamic contrast enhanced helical CT improves conspicu-ity of acute cerebral ischemia. In: Proceedings of the 83nd Scientific Assembly and Annual Meet-ing of the Radiological Society of North America, (Hot topics), Chicago, IL 1997.

25. Lev M, Farkas J, Gemmete J, et al. Acute stroke: Improved nonenhanced CT detection- Benefits of soft-copy interpretation by using variable window width and center level settings. Radiology 1999;213:150–155.

26. Lev M, Farkas J, Gemmete J, et al. Improved CT detection of hyperacute stroke: the benefits of heli-cal CT perfusion imaging and soft copy interpretation. In: Proceedings of the 84th Scientific Assembly and Annual Meeting of the Radiological Society of North America, Chicago, IL 1998.

27. Hunter GJ, Hamberg LM, Ponzo JA, et al. Assessment of cerebral perfusion and arterial anatomy in hyperacute stroke with three-dimensional functional CT: Early clinical results. American Jour-nal of Neuroradiology 1998;19:29–37.

28. Lev M, Segal A, Farkas J, et al. CT perfusion imaging of hyperacute middle cerebral artery stroke predicts outcome of intraarterial thrombolytic treatment. In: Annual Meeting of the America Society of Neuroradiology, San Diego, CA 1999; 258–9.

29. Koroshetz WJ, Gonzalez RG. Imaging stroke in progress: magnetic resonance advances but com-puted tomography is poised for counterattack. Annals of Neurology 1999;46:556–558.

The Use of Xenon/CT Cerebral Blood Flow Studies in Acute Stroke

H. Yonas

Whether ischemic stroke is due to an embolus from the heart or to closure of a perforating vessel due to chronic hypertension, the final common pathway is a compromise of blood flow. While there is a complex system of hemodynamic mechanisms intended to protect neuronal tissue from less severe reductions of cerebral blood flow (CBF), it is the location, duration and severity of the compromise of CBF that determines the onset of a neurological deficit as well as the transition from reversible to irreversible ischemia [1]. While technologies that examine other physiological variables are all interesting and potentially useful, during the initial hours after an ischemic event the pathophysiology is flow driven with other variables being secondary events. Thus, it should follow that rapidly accessible, quantitative, high resolution CBF information should play a central role in the diagnosis and management of acute ischemic stroke.

The measurement of CBF with stable Xenon/CT (Xe/CT) was developed at the University of Pittsburgh in the early 1980's. It involves a series of CT images of 4–8 head levels obtained immediately prior to (N=2) and during (N=6) 4.3 minutes of stable xenon inhalation. The arterial input function is obtained indirectly by measuring "end tidal" xenon. The Kety Schmidt equation is solved utilizing iterative mathematics assuming a single compartment for each CT voxel ($1 \times 1x10mm^3$). Because a partition coefficient measurement is derived with each flow value, Xe/CT CBF information assesses and integrates changes of tissue solubility and thereby is likely to be valid even in disease states.

It took until the late 1990's for the technologies upon which Xe/CT CBF is directly dependent (CT scanners, computers, and computer networks) to evolve sufficiently for Xe/CT CBF to become a rapidly accessible and useful clinical instrument. Modern CT scanners have made it possible to study more levels of the brain at lower xenon concentration. Modern networking systems and rapid computers have made it possible to provide the flow data for clinical review within three minutes of study completion. Lastly, modern computer power has made it possible to provide more reliable data by using numerical integration. This mathematical approach that requires only a few seconds with modern computers to calculate the flow of 24,000 pixels per CT level would have required hours only a few years ago. The end result is a CT coupled, quantitative map of CBF that has equally high resolution within all brain regions except for those "hidden" by CT artifact. Xenon/CT CBF also integrates a measure of the quantitative reliability of the study so that a reader can better interpret the data for integration into clinical management. A phantom for Xe/CT CBF has been created so that all systems can be calibrated and standardized. Only in this way can flow values generated by one center be compared and or merged with flow values from another.

This article will review the insights obtained with stable Xe/CT CBF in experimental and clinical acute ischemic stroke. Our initial studies with xenon/CT involved a model of focal ischemia of the baboon that involved permanent or temporary occlusion of the lateral striate vessels [2, 3]. This work not only provided the information needed to fine tune the methodology but also the understanding that Xe/CT provided quantitative CBF information even when there was very low flow levels deep within the brain.

Since 1985 over 15,000 Xe/CT CBF studies have been performed at our institution in a wide range of disorders with over 150 papers documenting the broad utility of this kind of information. Since 1997 members of the University of Pittsburgh Stroke Institute have studied over 350 stroke victims with Xe/CT CBF as part of their acute evaluation. The triage capability of a CT based stroke assessment has recently been enhanced by the addition of information about vascular anatomy obtained with CT angiography. The ability to obtain within 20 minutes anatomy from the CT image, physiology from the Xe/CT CBF study and vascular patency from CT angiography makes the modern CT scanner a powerful instrument for acute stroke assessment.

Key Questions in Acute Stroke Care

There is a logical sequence of questions that must be answered when assuming the emergent care of a stroke victim.
1. Is the patient having a hemorrhagic or ischemic stroke?
2. Does the patient have a region of the brain that is either reversibly or irreversibly ischemic?
3. Is the patient no longer at risk from ischemia due to vascular occlusion? Has the embolic material already fragmented allowing reperfusion to occur?

The initial question is most often answered with a CT scan and the remaining questions can be answered with Xe/CT derived quantitative CBF information combined with CT angiography. Thus, within 15 to 20 minutes of arrival within a standard CT scanner all vital information needed for guiding acute stroke management can be in the hands of the treating physician.

Currently, there is hesitancy to treat ischemic stroke victims with thrombolytic therapy, in part, because of a ten-fold increase in the rate of clinically significant hemorrhagic conversion. The increased risk of hemorrhagic conversion occurs even when therapy is given in a timely manner to patients that meet current criteria [4]. Presumably, the highest incidence of significant hemorrhagic complications have occurred in older patients following reperfusion of large regions of already irreversibly ischemic tissue [5]. Xe/CT CBF studies have been shown to be capable of defining large brain regions with near absent flow that do predict an increased hemorrhage incidence [6].

The challenge in acute stroke management is to be able to provide patient specific care. From the examination of 56 acute CBF studies obtained in patients with major hemispheric ischemic events, we were able to distinguish three groups of patients. 25% had a major territorial region with essentially no flow (<7 ml/100 g/min) and 25% had normal (>30 ml/100 g/min) flow levels. Theoretically, reperfusion would harm one group by inducing hemorrhage or accelerated edema [6] and the other group would be exposed to the risks and expense of thrombolytic therapy without potential benefit. 50%, however, had MCA territorial flow levels between 6 and 30 ml/100 g/min and presumably constitute a subgroup most likely to benefit from reperfusion therapy. While these flow thresholds are arbitrary they provide a reasonable platform for future studies. These studies provide a rationale for "splitting" subgroups rather than "lumping" all stroke victims into the same treatment paradigm.

Reversible Ischemia

The critical question is whether a study can identify patients that have reversible ischemia as a cause of a new neurological deficit? This is the group that should receive maximal benefit of reperfusion therapy and for whom reperfusion efforts may be able to be extended beyond the current three-hour limit.

Brain tissue normally supplied by an occluded proximal vessel becomes dependent upon the collateral potential of the distal vasculature. While cervical internal carotid artery occlusion can receive collateral blood supply from vessels of the Circle of Willis, proximal middle cerebral artery (MCA) occlusion makes the distal vasculature dependent upon the far less predictable, leptomeningeal collateral network. In some individuals the leptomeningeal system can maintain normal flow levels while in others flow levels can acutely fall to zero (Figs. 1, 2). The goal of thrombolytic therapy must be to identify those individuals that have ischemic but reversible levels of flow when they present for medical care.

Jones et al. [1] based upon focal CBF measurements made by the hydrogen clearance technique in a primate stroke model published the hallmark experimental study that examined the time depth relationship of ischemic stroke. In that study flow levels near zero were tolerated for only a few minutes before irreversible ischemia occurred while levels of flow above 20 ml/100 g/min were tolerated indefinitely. Flow values between zero and 20 were tolerated for up to three hours before becoming infracted with a tendency for converting to an irreversible injury with longer and, or lower flow levels. An identical time depth relationship was reported for patients undergoing intra-arterial thrombolytic therapy for whom Xe/CT CBF studies were obtained prior to arterial therapy [7].

Clinical studies at the University of Pittsburgh have also demonstrated that patients with "penumbral" levels of perfusion, i.e. 7–20 ml/100 g/min have responded favorably to the timely introduction of effective reperfusion therapy. We have observed that penumbral levels of perfusion were consistent with clinical improvement with a lower incidence of hemorrhage complications following intra arterial thrombolysis (Fig. 3) [5, 8]. Because all of these patients began intra arterial therapy beyond three hours, and many were not reperfused until six or

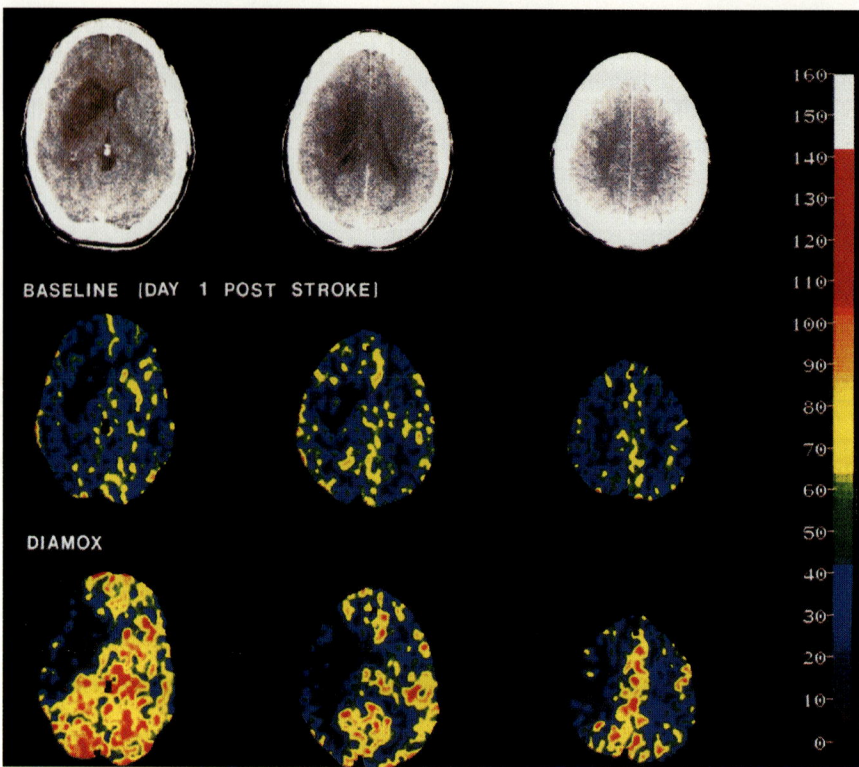

Fig. 1. Xe/CT CBF provides a quantitative CBF map with 24,000 calculations of flow per CT level. Direct correlation of the baseline CBF study with the CT scan demonstrates that the region of lowest flow is in the region of infarction within the basal ganglion of the right hemisphere. The second study was obtained 20 minutes after the administration of 1 g IV acetazolamide. Note the increase in all vascular regions except for the right distal middle cerebral distribution. The ability to repeat the study provides the opportunity to exam the response of blood flow to an alteration of acid base balance and thereby gain insight into the underlying physiological compromise. The fixed color scale on the right is in ml/100 g/min

seven hours after stroke onset, these reports strongly suggest that the window for reversible ischemia in some individuals may extend well beyond the three hour window suggested by the IV tPA stroke trial [9]. In a separate analysis we have also shown that the level of flow was statistically predictive of infarction while the time to treatment was not [10].

Although not the same insult, the delayed territorial ischemia that can follow subarachnoid hemorrhage (SAH) due to vasospasm does produce a potentially reversible ischemic injury that also responds to reperfusion therapy. Increased perfusion can be accomplished with hypertensive therapy, papaverine or angioplasty to either chemically or mechanically induce vasodilatation. In patients that developed delayed neurological deficits due to vasospasm a decrease of flow to between 10–15 ml/100 g/min was recorded within the MCA territory within an hour of

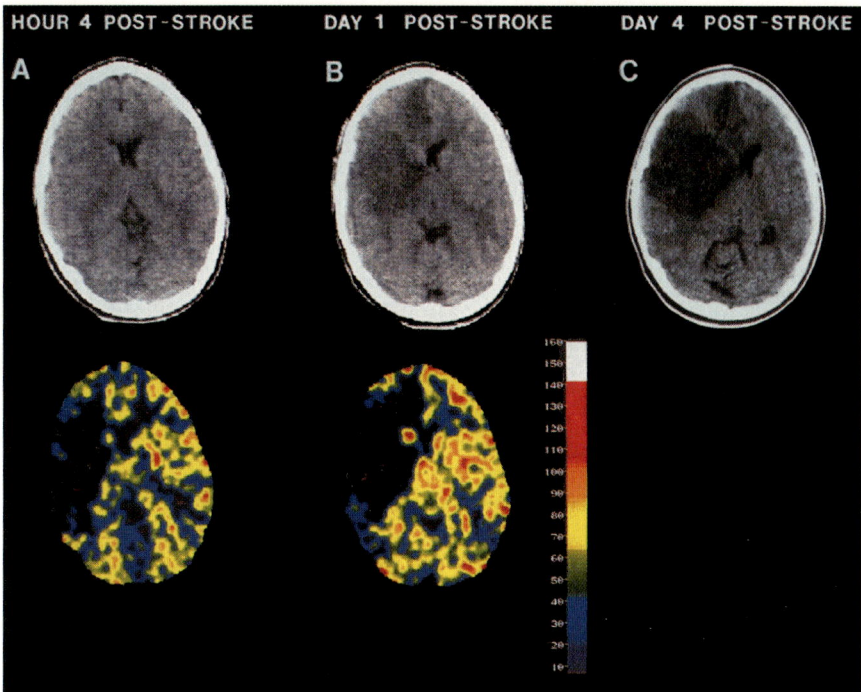

Fig. 2. The first Xe/CT CBF study was obtained within one hour of onset of a right middle cerebral occlusion and an accompanying right hemiplegia. Despite intra-arterial therapy the MCA was not reopened and the patient progressed to a well-defined region of infarction apparent on the CT scan the next day. At that time the area of ischemia was larger than apparent on the CT image. The fixed color scale on the right is in ml/100 g/min

deficit onset. In this setting the emergent use of angioplasty was able to elevate flow levels well above 20 ml/100 g/min and reverse the new clinical deficits [11].

Another independent, validating observation of the importance of 20 ml/100 g/min as a break point between normal function and reversible ischemia was reported by Witt [12] in a series of patients undergoing balloon test occlusion (BTO) of the internal carotid artery (ICA). 160 patients with skull base tumors or intracavernous aneurysms that developed no clinical deficit during a 20 minute ICA BTO underwent a second brief occlusion. A xenon/CT CBF study was obtained prior to and during the second occlusion. In that report no patient that tolerated ICA occlusion had a MCA flow level above 20 ml/100 g/min.

Irreversible Ischemia

While we have learned that CT imaging is capable of defining subtle changes consistent with irreversibly ischemic tissues within 2–3 hours of stroke onset, the changes diagnostic of infarction become more apparent over time. By 5–6 hours

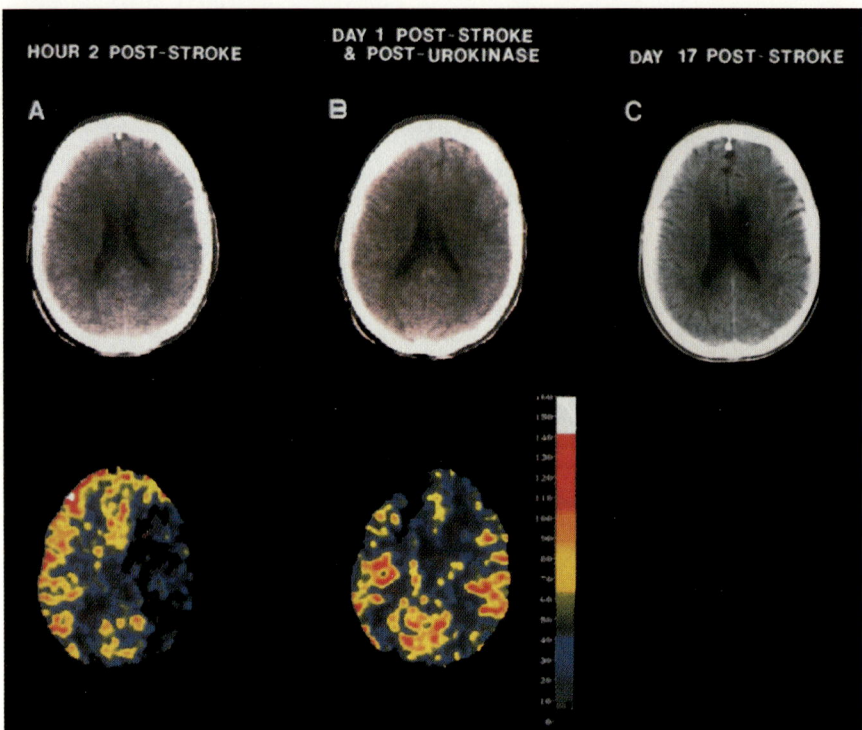

Fig. 3. The first Xe/CT CBF study was obtained four hours after onset of a left middle cerebral artery occlusion. The retention of flow values in the range of 10–20 ml/100 g/min within nearly all of the left MCA territory suggests the possibility of a reversible lesion even though beyond the three hour window for thrombolysis. Intra arterial therapy was successful by hour five post onset and the flow study obtained the next day demonstrated a return to normal flow levels with evidence of infarction on the last CT scan only within a small region of the basal ganglia

even an untrained eye can identify the injury. Because studies have demonstrated that inclusion of patients with large areas of CT defined infarction do suffer an increased risk of bleeding complication presumably with no potential benefit, removal of these patients from thrombolytic trial is obviously important [13]. Unfortunately, even expert panels demonstrate a low accuracy in correctly identifying the earliest CT changes [14]. Thus, there is a role for a physiological study that can accurately define an irreversible injury within the first hours of stroke onset.

The predictive power of a "snap shot" of flow assumes that the flow levels measured were either the same or lowers from the time of onset. While there is little information about sequential alterations of CBF over time during an evolving hemispheric stroke, we have recently examined this question in an animal model of cortical and subcortical stroke. In this model of severe cortical ischemic challenge flow studies performed at hourly intervals for six hours after stroke onset demonstrated that a maximal reduction was achieved with occlusion followed by a gradual tendency toward elevation of flow [15]. Our previously published work with subcortical stroke demonstrated the same stability of very low flows from onset to six hours [2]. Sakoh et al, has recently reported in a pig model of ischemia studies with PET the same stability of very low flow values for regions that initially become severely ischemic [16]. The fact that flow studies obtained in acute stroke victims have been able to distinguish patients that inevitably proceed to CT defined infarctions of a size consistent with the volume of flow <9 ml/100 g/min [17], and when ischemia involved a sufficiently large region was even predictive of herniation [18], lends further support to the power of Xe/CT CBF to measure very low flow levels consistent with irreversible ischemia.

The basis for believing that Xe/CT CBF provides high resolution quantitative CBF information is the series of primate stroke studies performed during the early development of this technology [2, 3]. The initial Xe/CT CBF studies demonstrated the ability of this technology to measure the absence of perfusion in a brain region as small as 100 mm2 located within the basal ganglion [2]. Permanent occlusion of the lateral striate arteries of the baboon consistently produced infarction of the ipsilateral caudate and putamen. CBF studies obtained in the same animal prior to and hourly for six hours following lateral striate occlusion demonstrated the high-resolution capability as well as the stability of the flow information. Opening of the lateral striate vessels after one hour of occlusion resulted in a dramatic hyperemia, accompanied by a hyper acute (<60 minute) development of CT density changes but with irreversible ischemic injury on pathological examination [3]. A more recent study of irreversible MCA cortical ischemia in rhesus monkey has reconfirmed the ability of Xe/CT CBF to define flow levels diagnostic of infarction that are prognostic of cellular change as well as the early appearance of CT defined infarction [19.

Xenon/CT CBF has been shown to be capable of determining the threshold for irreversible ischemia in a number of other clinical disorders. The absence of CBF within all measurable regions has been reported as a useful tool for determining brain death in adults and children [20, 21]. Flow values below 10 ml/100 g/min have predicted areas of infarction in patients following head injury [22]. Following subarachnoid hemorrhage flow values that could not be elevated above 15 ml/100 g/min predicted infarction on subsequent CT scans [23, 24].

Thus, it appears that Xe/CT derived quantitative CBF information would help reduce the fear of primary care and emergency room physicians by making it possible to exclude from thrombolytic therapy those patients who are most likely to be harmed instead of helped by rapid reperfusion.

Ischemic Penumbra-Fact or Fiction?

Although the concept of a significant band of reversibly ischemic tissue around a central core of irreversible ischemia is widely accepted, few studies in man have defined its frequency or significance. While studies have identified a region of incomplete ischemic injury around a core of infarction and many studies have demonstrated the enlargement of an initially smaller central infarction to an eventual larger lesion, the mechanism(s) of this growth are still a matter of speculation [25].

In an effort to examine the clinical significance of tissues with penumbral levels of perfusion (7–20 ml/100 g/min) within the initial hours of ischemic stroke onset, Kaufman et al [17] measured the volume of tissue with flow levels between 7 and 20 ml/100 g/min in 20 acute stroke victims with well defined cortical strokes. Although all patients demonstrated a significant core region with flow values below 7 ml/100 g/min, they observed no significantly greater volume of brain with penumbral levels of flow on the side of the infarction when compared with the normal, opposite side. The transition from the densely ischemic to normally perfused tissue within the cortical mantel was very abrupt measuring, at most, only a few millimeters. Thus a significant volume of reversibly ischemic tissue medial to a core lesion was not a common pattern accompanying cortical infarctions.

A subsequent study by Jovan et al examined the histograms of the hemispheric and MCA territorial flow values of 20 stroke victims selected on the basis of an M1 occlusion. While this study also demonstrated a subgroup with a large core and a small penumbra there was an equal number of patients with a small core and a large penumbra [26]. The latter observation supports the concept of a subgroup with a small irreversibly injured region, most often within the basal ganglia, with the entire cortical mantel surviving in a reversible flow range dependent upon pial collaterals.

Xenon/CT CBF based studies of acute stroke victims have shown that those with proximal vessel occlusion commonly experience cortical flow levels in the mid teens [27]. The fact that the pro-Urokinase stroke trial demonstrated a benefit of reperfusion as late as 6 hours post occlusion onset supports the concept of reversible levels of flow persisting post M1 occlusion. Thus, therapies designed to salvage reversibly ischemic tissues must be focused upon the timely identification and reperfusion of regions with penumbral levels of CBF that are not located medial to core lesions but distal to them.

The concept of a vascular territory developing penumbral levels of perfusion is a well-established mechanism for delayed neurological deficits following subarachnoid hemorrhage. Vasospasm of the Circle of Willis vessels too commonly occurs during the week post SAH causing ischemic levels of perfusion in 10–30% of patients. While delayed neurological deficits may be due to many causes, when flow levels fall below 20 ml/100 g/min deficits occur which can be readily reversed by improving the perfusion pressure [11].

Identification of the Patient That Is No Longer Ischemic

Because thrombolytic therapy must begun as soon as possible after onset to obtain maximal benefit, clinicians are forced to make therapeutic decisions despite the fact that many patients are having TIAs. These are deficits that will resolve over the next few or many hours even without therapy. These patients presumably have already undergone embolus fragmentation, migration and reperfusion. The fact that 40% of the patients in the pro Urokinase trial had no occlusion on angiography despite a stable deficit provides support for the importance of identifying this large subgroup.

Firlik et al [28] examined the flow values of 53 stroke victims studied within eight hours of onset. He reported that 11 patients had no major or minor region with flow values less than 30 ml/100 g/min. Nine of these patients had spontaneous resolution of their deficits within 24 hours without any intervention. The two patients that did not resolve their deficits presumably achieved spontaneously reperfused after they had already suffered irreversible ischemic injuries. The clinical deficit persists presumably due to a functional/perfusion disassociation that can persist for hours.

Because a CBF study does not measure metabolism it has been said that such studies cannot be used effectively to examine acute stroke victims, since without a measure of metabolism it is possible that reperfusion can occur without the return of metabolism. As noted above, in the world of thrombolytic therapy the question of whether an irreversible injury has or has not already occurred is not the key question. In this setting the question is whether a region of reversible or irreversible ischemia is present. If normal or supra normal flow, which is common following reperfusion of a severe ischemic injury, is found throughout the symptomatic hemisphere then the relevant fact is that the patient does not require thrombolytic therapy and its associated risks and expense. Because CT defined densities are altered within minutes of reperfusion of irreversibly ischemic tissues, evidence of the prior ischemic injury is the rule. This was evident in the focal ischemic stroke studies reported by the author in 1990 [3]. Thus, in the acute management of stroke victims quantitative CBF information especially coupled with CT defined anatomy provides exactly the information needed for guiding aggressive therapy.

The Combined Role of Xe/CT CBF and CT/Angiography

Rapid definition of the site or sites of vascular occlusion is important for determining the best course of emergent action. Is the cervical ICA occluded in addition to the MCA or is there no site of major vessel occlusion? Another important question is whether an acute CBF study can identify the patient with an M1 versus a M2 or M3 occlusion? This has become an especially relevant question because intravenous thrombolysis appears to be less effective for opening M1 occlusions [29, 30]. It has been suggested that these patients might, instead, benefit from going directly to intra arterial therapy.

Blood flow information obtained with Xe/CT has shown that patients with M1 occlusion do have a significantly lower territorial flow value (12 vs. 30 ml/100 g/min, $p<.01$, t test). All patients (100%) with CBF in the symptomatic MCA territory <20 ml/100 g/min had M1 occlusions. This association was highly significant ($p<.005$, Fisher exact test) [27]. Although this information is valuable for guiding care toward intra-arterial therapy, the addition of CT angiography provides assessment of the location, degree and extent of vascular occlusion in both extra- and intra-cranial circulations.

If M1 is found to be occluded by CT/A the question is whether there are reversible or irreversible levels of flow within the cortical mantel. If penumbral levels of perfusion are found with only a small percentage of the territory with

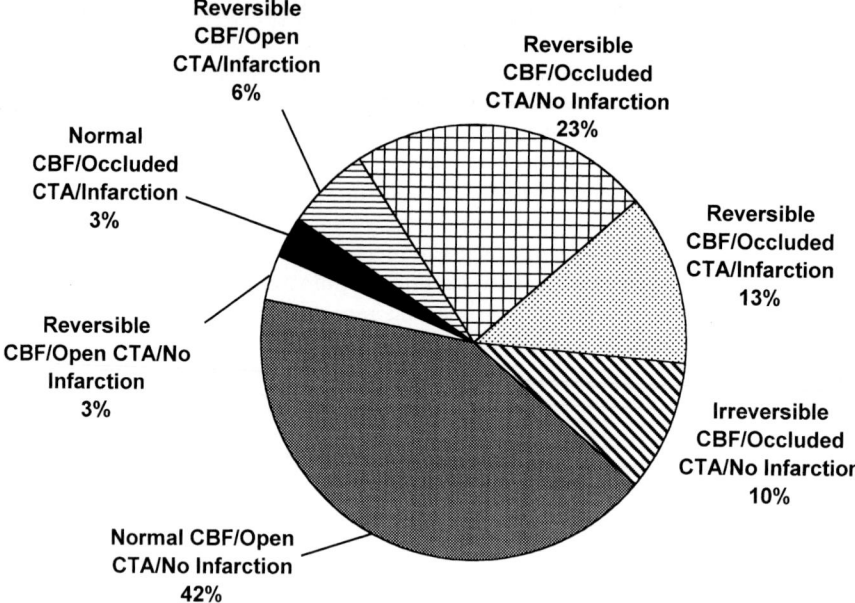

Fig. 4. The "pie chart" was constructed from an analysis of CT, CT angiography and Xenon/CT CBF information obtained in 51 patients with onset of hemispheric ischemic symptoms. Note the large percentage of patients with normal appearing CT scans, normal flow levels and patent vessels. These were patients that also had a benign course with no conversion on late CT scans. Conversely, at all time frames up to 24 hours there remained a subgroup with no evidence of CT defined infarction, flow levels consistent with reversible ischemia and ICA or MCA occlusions. The latter group would be ideal candidates for reperfusion therapy beyond the three-hour window

stagnant (zero) flow aggressive attempts at reperfusion are indicated and we believe that this is the case well past 6 hours of vessel occlusion. If M1 and M2 are open on CTA but islands of low flow are identified distally, then intravenous tPA would be most indicated. If no area is ischemic and all CTA defined vessels are patent then reperfusion therapy and its risks and expenses are not indicated (Fig. 4).

Although the above is a rational approach to the triage of acute stroke victims, a large prospective study is needed to prove the reality of these predictions. In review of 51 acute stroke victims who had CT imaging, Xe/CT CBF and CT angiography performed, both CTA and Xe/CT CBF were highly predictive of later infarction and the disposition to home versus a nursing facility [31]. This review also provided evidence that the level of persistent perfusion was a better predictor of clinical outcome than the time to treatment [10].

Because most stroke patients are emergently studied with CT to rule out a hemorrhagic or other structural cause of new neurological deficit, a xenon/CT CBF study is ideally situated to be rapidly "added on" when no structural cause for the deficit is identified. Because helical scanners are now capable of performing angiography utilizing an intravenous iodine bolus to examine patency of the extra and intra cranial vessels, the combination of Xe/CT CBF and CT angiography has made the CT scanner an ideal tool for functional brain imaging.

References

1. Jones TH, Morawetz RB, Crowell RM, Marcoux FW, FitzGibbon SJ, DeGirolami U, Ojemann, RG. Thresholds of focal cerebral ischemia in awake monkeys. J Neurosurg 1981;54:773–82.
2. Yonas H, Gur D, Claassen D, Wolfson SK, Moossy J. Stable xenon enhanced computed tomography in the study of clinical and pathologic correlates of focal ischemia in baboons. Stroke 1988;19:228–38.
3. Yonas H, Gur D, Claassen D, Wolfson SK, Moossy J. Stable xenon-enhanced CT measurement of cerebral blood flow in reversible focal ischemia in baboons. J Neurosurg 1990;73:266–73.
4. Fisher M, Bogousslavsky J. Further evolution toward effective therapy for acute ischemic stroke. JAMA 1998;279:1298–303.
5. Rubin G, Firlik AD, Pindzola RR, Levy EI, Yonas H. The Effect of Reperfusion Therapy on Cerebral Blood Flow in Acute Stroke. J Stroke Cerebrovasc Dis 1999;8:9–16.
6. Goldstein S, Yonas H, Gebel JM, Kassam A, Jungreis CA, Uzen G, Firlik AD, Rubin G, Wechsler LR. Acute cerebral blood flow as a predictive physiologic marker for symptomatic hemorrhagic conversion and clinical herniation after thrombolytic therapy. Stroke 2000;31:275.
7. Touho H, Karasawa J. Evaluation of Time-Dependent Thresholds of Cerebral Blood Flow and Transit Time During the Acute Stage of Cerebral Embolism: A Retrospective Study. Surg Neurol 1996;46(2):135–146.
8. Goldstein S, Yonas H, Gebel JM, Kassam A, Jungreis CA, Uzen G, Firlik AD, Rubin G, Wechsler LR. Acute cerebral blood flow as a predicative physiologic marker for symptomatic hemorrhagic conversion and clinical herniation after thrombolytic therapy. Stroke 2000;30:275.
9. Brott TG, Haley EC, Levy DE, Barsan W, Broderick J, Sheppard GL, Spilker J, Kongable GL, Massey S, Reed R, et al. Urgent therapy for stroke. Part I. Pilot study of tissue plasminogen activator administered within 90 minutes. Stroke 1992;23:632–40.
10. Kilpatrick MM, Goldstein S, Yonas H, Kassam AB, Gebel J, Wechsler LR, Jungreis CA, Fukui M. Sensitivity and Specificity of Quantitative Cerebral Blood Flow vs. Time from Symptom Onset as a Predictor of Cerebral Infarction. Stroke 2001;32:348a [Abstract].
11. Firlik AD, Kaufmann AM, Jungreis CA, Yonas H: The effect of transluminal angioplasty on cerebral blood flow in the management of symptomatic vasospasm following aneurysmal subarachnoid hemorrhage. J Neurosurg 1997;86:830–839.
12. Witt JP, Yonas H, Jungreis C. Cerebral blood flow response pattern during balloon test occlusion of the internal carotid artery. AJNR 1994;15:847–57.
13. Hacke W, Kaste M, Fieschi C, Toni D, Lesaffre E, von Kummer R, Boysen G, Bluhmki E, Hoxter G, Mahagne MH, et al for the ECASS Study Group. Intravenous thrombolysis with recombinant tissue plasminogen activator for acute hemispheric stroke. The European Cooperative Acute Stroke Study (ECASS). JAMA 1995;274:1017–25.
14. Wardlaw JM, Dorman PJ, Lewis SC, Sandercock PAG. Can stroke physicians and neuroradiologists identify signs of early cerebral infarction on CT? J Neurol, Neurosurg, & Psych 1999;67:651–663.
15. Personal communication with Ed Nemoto, PhD of unpublished data.
16. Sakoh M, Ostergaard L, Rohl L, Smith DF, Simonsen CZ, Sorensen JC, Poulsen PV, Gyldensted C, Sakaki S, Gjedde A. Relationship between residual cerebral blood floe and oxygen metabolism as predicative of ischemic tissue viability: Sequential multitracer positron emission tomography scanning of middle cerebral artery occlusion during the critical first 6 hours after stroke in pigs. J Neurosurg 2000;93:647–57.
17. Kaufmann Am, Firlik AD, Fukui MB, Wechsler LR, Jungreis CA, Yonas H. Ischemic core and penumbra in human stroke. Stroke 1999;30:93–99.

18. Firlik AD, Yonas H, Kaufmann AM, Wechsler LR, Jungreis CA, Fukui MB, Williams RL. Relationship between cerebral blood flow and the development of swelling and life-threatening herniation in acute ischemic stroke. J Neurosurg 1998;89:243–9.
19. Personal communication with Ed Nemoto, PhD of unpublished data.
20. Pistoia F, Johnson DW, Darby JM, Horton JA, Applegate LJ, Yonas H. The role of Xenon CT measurements of cerebral blood flow in the clinical determination of brain death. AJNR 1991;12:97–103..
21. Ashwal S, Schneider S, Thompson J. Xenon computed tomography measuring cerebral blood flow in the determination of brain death in children. Ann Neurol 1989;25:539–546.
22. Astrup J, Bergholt B, Gyldensted C, Bogesvang A, Holdgaard HO, Dahl B. Ischemic Focal Lesions in Acute Head Injury: Correlation to Late Focal Atrophy. Acta Neurol Scand 1996;Suppl 166:118–119.
23. Yonas H, Sekhar L, Johnson DW, Gur D. Determination of irreversible ischemia by xenon-enhanced computed tomographic monitoring of cerebral blood flow in patients with symptomatic vasospasm. Neurosurgery 1989;24:368–72.
24. Fukui MB, Johnson DW, Yon ash, Sekhar L, Latchaw RE, Pentheny S. Xe/CT cerebral blood flow evaluation of delayed symptomatic ischemia after subarachnoid hemorrhage. AJNR 1992;13:265–70.
25. Baron J. Mapping the ischaemic penumbra with PET: Implications for acute stroke treatment. Cerebrovasc Dis 1999;9:193–201.
26. Jovin TG, Goldstein S, Gebel JM, Wechsler LR, Ott MB, Yonas H. Patterns of core and penumbra in acute MI occlusion and their clinical correlates. Stroke 2001;32:348b [Abstract].
27. Firlik AD, Kaufmann AM, Wechsler LR, Firlik KS, Fukui MB, Yonas H. Quantitative cerebral blood flow determinations in acute ischemic stroke: Relationship to computed tomography and angiography. Stroke 1997;28:2208–13.
28. Firlik AD, Rubin G, Yonas H, Wechsler LR. Relation between cerebral blood flow and neurologic deficit resolution in acute ischemic stroke. Neurology 1998;51:177–82.
29. del Zoppo GJ, Poeck K, Pessin MS, Wolpert SM, Furlan AJ, Ferbert A, Alberts MJ, Zivian JA, Wechsler L, Busse O, Greenlee Jr R, Brass L, Mohr JP, Feldmann E, Hacke W, Kase CS, Biller J, Gress D, Otis SM. Recombinant tissue plasminogen activator in acute thrombotic and embolic stroke. Ann Neurol 1992;32:78–86.
30. Mori E, Yoneda Y, Tabuchi M, Yoshida T, Ohkawa S, Ohsumi Y, Kitano K, Tsutsumi A, Yamadori A. Intravenous recombinant tissue plasminogen activator in acute carotid artery territory stroke. Neurology 1992;45:976–982.
31. Kilpatrick MM, Yonas H, Goldstein S, Kassam AB, Gebel JM, Wechsler LR, Jungreis CA, Fukui MB. CT based assessment of acute stroke: CT, CT Angiography and xenon CT cerebral blood flow. (Submitted to Stroke 8–00, pending review.)

Advances in Imaging in Ischemic Stroke

M. Moonis and M. Fisher

Advances in stroke management; acute thrombolytic therapy, trials of neuroprotection are redefining the concepts of stroke management. These have been paralleled by advances in neuroimaging techniques. Rapid improvement in the scanning times and more sensitive methods of defining acute ischemia continue to evolve in CT and MRI. The most significant advances have been in the field of newer MRI techniques; diffusion weighted MRI (DWI) and perfusion imaging (PI) as well as MR Spectroscopy (MRS) [1–5].

Echoplanar DWI is based on the principle of ischemic tissue accumulates intracellular water. This results in a reduction of the apparent diffusion co-efficient (ADC) with a hypointense signal on the ADC maps and a hyperintense signal on the DWI, reflective of cytotoxic edema. This combination is specific to ischemic tissue and is useful in separating other conditions that appear hyperintense on DWI. These include seizure foci, transient global ischemia, migraine, multiple sclerosis and certain tumors [2, 6, 7].

Echoplanar DWI is obtained by applying 2 diffusion-sensitizing gradients placed symmetrically around the 180-degree radiofrequency pulse of a spin echo sequence. Protons that move in the first dephasing sequence change phase randomly as they diffuse in the magnetic field. Areas of restricted diffusion appear hypointense on ADC maps and hyperintense on DWI.

Although most DWI changes reflect irreversible ischemia, several animal and clinical studies suggest that these deficits at least early on in the ischemic process maybe partially reversible. Kidwell et al found that of the 9 patients with transient ischemic attacks and early DWI hyperintensity 45% did not reveal persistent abnormalities on follow-up studies. Similar results have been observed by a few other studies [8].

Current techniques of PI involve either administration of an exogenous bolus of contrast agent that shortens T2 (BT-PI) or arterial spin labeling techniques (ASL-PI). BT-PI utilizes serial multislice T2 weighted images to monitor the signal reduction associated with the passage of the bolus. This is used to generate time curves of signal intensity change that can then be used to estimate the time to peak (TTP), relative mean transit time (MTT), relative cerebral blood flow (CBF) and cerebral blood volume (CBV). Of these, TTP and MTT are utilized to estimate the ischemic area at risk [9–12]. PI abnormalities are a composite of the area of infarction and the area at risk of infarction (penumbra). When used with DWI, PI deficit outside the area of DWI hyperintensity approximates the ischemic penumbra. This is potentially salvageable tissue and typically in untreated patients the area of infarction (DWI) will evolve into the region of the PI deficit [13, 14].

DWI in the Diagnosis of Acute Ischemic Stroke

Evolution of thrombolytic therapy has revolutionized stroke management. Patients with acute ischemic stroke treated with thrombolytics intravenously within 3 hours and intra-arterially within 6 hours have a 33% better relative outcome as compared to patients who did not receive this treatment [15–18]. Patients treated within the first ninety minutes show a better recovery than those treated in the 90–180 minute period [19]. However, the number of patients treated thus far is disappointingly low (10–12%). While part of the process is in delay in arriving at the hospital, we are probably not treating all patients who maybe appropriate for treatment [20]. Accurate selection of appropriate patients based on clinical examination and a CT scan can be misleading [21]. For rational thrombolytic therapy, imaging tools need to be sensitive (identify ischemic infarcts) and specific (exclude other causes of acute neurological deficits and hemorrhage). Furthermore, it should differentiate large vessel and cardioembolic small vessel strokes from lacunar infarcts and other non-embolic stroke.

DWI-PW in Identification of Lesions Suitable for Thrombolysis

Identification of Acute Ischemic Infarcts

DWI is a very sensitive technique in identifying acute ischemic infarcts. DWI changes in ischemic tissue maybe evident within minutes both in experimental and clinical studies. The changes may persist up to a week or even longer in some studies [22–24]. In a study of subacute ischemic strokes, persistent abnormalities on DWI were seen in more patients than on conventional MRI after a period of 6–10 days. Furthermore DWI provided information not evident on conventional MRI in 30% of the patients [25]. In a large prospective study DWI increased the sensitivity of the diagnosis from 48 to 94%. Similar results have been reported by several other studies comparing DWI with CT or conventional T2 weighted MRI imaging. Since DWI usually represents irreversible damage (infarction), it gives valuable information on the size of the stroke at a time when thrombolysis is being considered. DWI hyperintensity greater than one-third the arterial territory would be a contraindication to thrombolytic therapy [26–28]. In patients with pervious strokes DWI is advantageous in differentiating acute from chronic lesions [29–31]. Fitzek reported a sensitivity and specificity approaching 100% in patients with at least one previous imaging abnormality [31]. In our experience, 7 patients imaged within the first 48 hours had a negative CT scan while all patients demonstrated a DWI abnormality (Fig. 1). In 45% of cases DWI changed the original diagnosis to ischemic small vessel stroke which impacted subsequent management.

Fig. 1. Diffusion-weighted image obtained a few hours after stroke onset showing a large left middle cerebral territory stroke not seen on CT

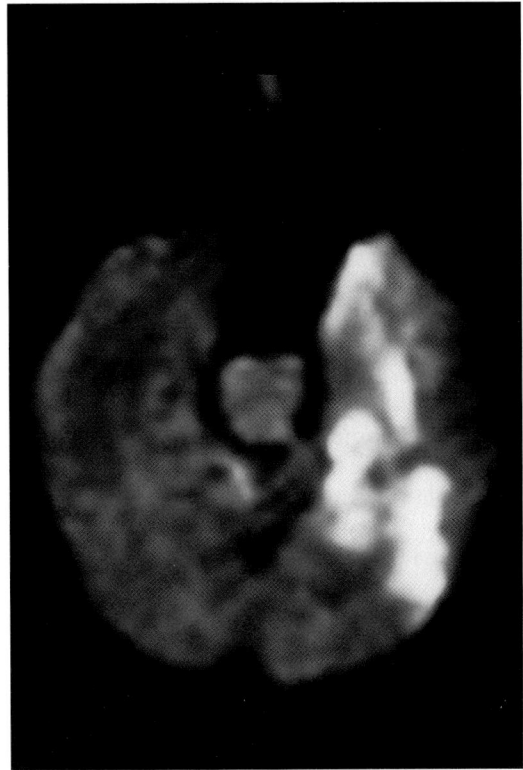

Differentiation of Lacunar Strokes from Thromboembolic Events

Small vessel lacunar strokes are a relative contraindication to thrombolytic therapy in most centers due to their potential of complete recovery and etiopathogenesis other than thromboembolism. Clinical diagnosis of and differentiation of large vessel from small vessel strokes maybe inaccurate in 20–30% of cases. Furthermore, early signs of stroke are often subtle or absent in a large percentage of cases. The sensitivity of the diagnosis is increased with DWI compared to conventional CT and T2 weighted MRI techniques. This is highlighted in several studies that demonstrate that up to 50% of clinically diagnosed small vessel strokes evolved into large cortical strokes [6, 7, 21, 32–34]. Furthermore, location of the DWI hyperintensity is helpful in delineating the extent of the irreversible ischemic lesion and by their location differentiate small vessel from large vessel stroke [25]. In a prospective study of stroke patients presenting with a clinically well defined lacunar syndrome, the authors found multiple DWI abnormalities in nearly 16% suggesting that clinical diagnosis of a lacunar syndrome is not necessarily accurate and 1 of 6 patients who maybe eligible for thrombolytic therapy were wrongly excluded [35].

While perfusion CT scans and CT angiogram (CTA) continue to evolve with faster scan times and more accurate delineation of the area of potential infarction, these techniques have not been widely tested against DWI-PI [36, 37].

Identification of Watershed Infarcts

DWI has been helpful in defining border-zone infarcts that usually result from hypotensive crisis and not thromboembolism. Clinical and early CT diagnosis of watershed infarcts is notoriously inaccurate. DWI on the other hand identifies these lesions and combined with PW helps to differentiate these from similar lesions resulting from thromboembolism or critical carotid artery disease. Matching multiple DWI-PI abnormalities correlated with embolic strokes while abnormal perfusion with normal DWI correlated with transient hypoperfusion. Extensive PW deficits in one or more arterial territories suggested superimposed severe carotid artery disease [9]. Combined DWI-PI imaging correlates well with angiographic lesions during intra-arterial therapy [34].

PI imaging in itself detects early, potentially reversible ischemic changes in stroke and the extent of these deficits suggests whether the main stem or a branch occlusion has occurred. Branch occlusions correlate with a smaller PW deficit. The estimated lesion volumes correlate well with the NIHSS and the RS [38, 39].

Exclusion of Intracerebral Hemorrhage

CT scan has been believed to be a more sensitive tool for detection of intracerebral hemorrhage, which is an absolute contraindication to thrombolytic therapy. However, recent techniques (echoplanar gradient recall echo sequences) have been shown to detect hemorrhage with comparable accuracy [12, 40–42]. In a prospective study of patients with primary intracerebral hemorrhage, Roob et al found MRI evidence of additional microbleeds in 54% of all cases. In the majority of patients microbleeds were located simultaneously in multiple brain regions [40].

DWI-PW in Acute Thrombolytic Therapy

Although not universally accepted because of time limitation and a reported study indicating reversibility of DWI lesions within 24 hours in some cases, DWI-PW offer a powerful combination for rational thrombolytic therapy in acute ischemic stroke. Furthermore it is increasingly becoming possible to image patients within 3–6 hours of onset of their symptoms [43]. Arterial occlusion results in 3 zones in the involved territory. The central core of irreversibly infarcted tissue, the surrounding critically perfused potentially viable and outer zone of normally perfused tissue. This middle zone of critically perfused tissue; the ischemic penumbra is potentially salvageable tissue if re-perfusion occurs in time [2, 44, 45]. There maybe a differential susceptibly of sub-cortical and posterior circulation compared to the large anterior circulation occlusions. Ideally, before attempted re-perfusion, it is important to identify the penumbra i.e. that an area of salvageable tissue is present since there is a substantial iatrogenic risk of causing intra-cerebral hemorrhage. This may be achieved with DWI-PI imaging. Perfusion deficits define the potential area of infarction while to a large extent DWI identifies the area of irreversible infarction. Over time as evident from several large clinical series the DWI deficit expands to match the perfusion deficit [43].

Treatment with thrombolytic therapy should be instituted when there is a PI >DWI volume or an isolated perfusion deficit exists. (DWI-PW mismatch). On the other hand, a DWI-PI match would imply a completed stroke and little role for thrombolysis (Fig. 2).

Even though studies of thrombolytic intervention indicate a definite time window for intervention; up to 3 hours for intravenous and up to 6 hours for intra-arterial thrombolysis there maybe subgroups that may fall outside this range. The second European study ECASS-2 while revealed no overall benefit of rt-PA intravenously at 6 hours demonstrated no significant increase in the risk of hemorrhage as compared to 3 hours. Given this information, patients who fall outside the time frames specified but still demonstrate a DWI-PI mismatch should be candidates for thrombolysis [41, 43, 46].

Role of MRI in Assessment of Re-Perfusion Following Thrombolysis

Thrombolytic therapy can only be useful if there is effective re-perfusion established. Transcranial Doppler (TCD) has been utilized as a non-invasive tool to determine re-perfusion flow. Results of several studies reveal a better outcome in patients with re-established flow and correlates well with the NIHSS as well as

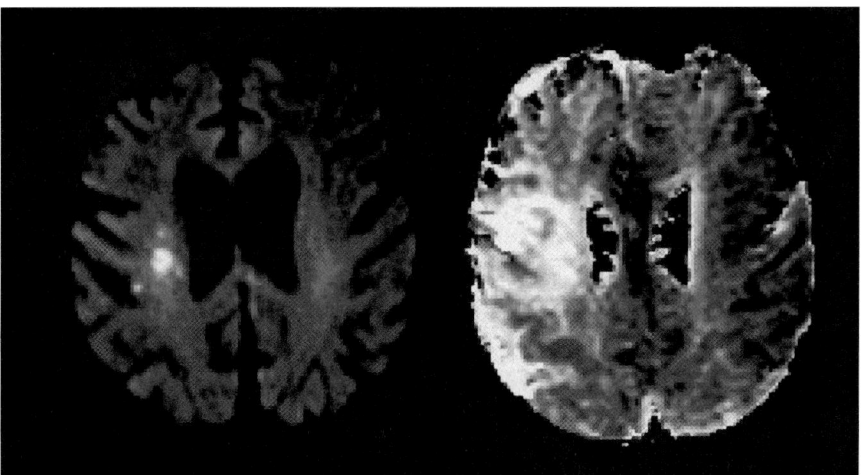

Fig. 2. Perfusion MRI *(on right)* showing a large region of hypoperfusion, while the diffusion-weighted MRI *(on left)* has only a small region of abnormality, confirming a large mismatch

functional scales [47, 48]. More recently, DWI-PI has been shown to be sensitive technique in determining re-perfusion. After successful re-perfusion, the final PI deficits are less than or equal to the initial DWI hyperintensity and correlate with functional outcome [38].

DWI: A Predictor of Stroke Outcome

Hemorrhagic transformation of an embolic stroke is a common phenomenon with some degree of hemorrhagic transformation seen in 50–60% of all embolic strokes. However, clinically significant hemorrhagic transformation is associated with a worse outcome. While studies of contrast extravasation on CT and perfusion deficits on HMPOA-SPECT provide some measure of the possible risk, DWI is beginning to have greater utility in this area [49–51]. In a prospective study Tong et. al assessed the utility of DWI in predicting hemorrhagic conversion. The authors analyzed 17 patients with DWI within 8 hours and at 1 week after the onset of an acute ischemic stroke. ADC for each pixel of the whole ischemic area was calculated. ADC values below 550×10^{-6} correlated well with subsequent hemorrhagic transformation. The authors did not describe the clinical outcome in these cases. Nevertheless, if these results are consistently replicated in other studies, they may provide yet another tool to assess the safety and tailor thrombolytic therapy [52]. Other studies have shown DWI volumes to be predictive of the long term functional outcome and correlate with NIH stroke scale and Rankin Scale [27, 46, 47, 53].

Preoperative Tool in Carotid Endarterectomy (CEA), Alternative to Cerebral Angiography

In patients undergoing CEA it is important to determine both the extent of hemodynamic compromise and the extent of collateral flow. This is one reason for advocating a pre-operative angiogram in this group. However, the morbidity associated with the procedure approaches 1% even in the best of the centers. BT-PI has been utilized to obtain the same information non-invasively. The MTT, TTP, CBF and CBV are compared from side to side. On the side of the critical stenosis, MTT and TTP are increased and CBF and CBV reduced. Along with phase contrast MRA this allows determination of the extent of cross collateral flow. This technique if validated by the larger experience would allow for non-invasive pre-operative assessment [54–56]. TCD monitoring during CEA reveals multiple echogenic signals indicative of multiple upstream emboli during the procedure. It is important to determine if this phenomenon results in cerebral infarction. DWI has been utilized to assess the extent of cerebral microembolism following a CEA. Bath et al evaluated 53 consecutive patients with CEA who had no apparent postoperative neurological deficits. While intraoperative monitoring with TCD detected silent cerebral emboli in 17%, subsequent DWI hyperintensity were found in only 1%, suggesting that most microembolic signals detected on TCD are not associated with cerebral infarction [57].

Future Directions

Other MRI techniques are finding application in the evaluation of acute stroke. Kamran et al describe a hyperintense vessels sign (HSV) on fluid attenuated inversion recovery (FLAIR). The authors correlated these findings with cerebral angiography in selected cases. HSV was an early MRI sign in 10% and indicated the need for reperfusion therapy. There was a correlation with the extent of the HSV sign, NIHSS and functional outcome [58].

MRS is another promising technique in the evaluation of acute stroke and assessment of patients for thrombolytic therapy. MRS is a technique of measuring metabolite peaks in applied pixels on the MRI. The common peaks are lactate, N- acetylaspartate (NAA), creatine and choline. The ratio of the NAA to lactate peaks is important in assessment of acute stroke. NAA peak is reduced with irreversible neuronal damage while lactate increases after ischemic injury and may return to normal with early re-perfusion. Animal studies indicate that a mismatch between NAA and lactate (reduced or normal NAA and elevated lactate) would suggest an incomplete lesion (ischemic penumbra) and maybe another tool to assess patients for re-perfusion therapy [28]. Wild et al prospectively performed MRS in addition to T2 W MRI in 11 patients imaged 24 to 72 hours later. In the center of the T2 lesions, there was a sharp reduction in the NAA peak, the intermediate zone, presumably the penumbra revealed a lesser reduction and the NAA peaks were normal beyond the margins of the lesion. Unfortunately, NAA could not be correlated to DWI in this series [59].

Diffusion Tensor Imaging (DTI) is another MRI technique that allows visualization of the DWI hyperintensity as well as its directionality. DTI has been applied to the visualization of cerebral diaschisis as well as activation of alternative regions after an acute stroke. This may provide useful prognostic information and along with functional MRI promises to be tool in assessment of long term recovery after a stroke [60].

References

1. Beaulieu C, D'Arceuil H, Hedehus M, de Crespigny A, Kastrup A, Moseley ME. Diffusion-weighted magnetic resonance imaging: theory and potential applications to child neurology. Semin Pediatr Neurol 1999;6(2):87–100.
2. Fisher M, Albers GW. Applications of diffusion-perfusion magnetic resonance imaging in acute ischemic stroke [see comments]. Neurology 1999;52(9):1750–6.
3. Hillis AE, Barker PB, Beauchamp NJ, Gordon B, Wityk RJ. MR perfusion imaging reveals regions of hypoperfusion associated with aphasia and neglect [In Process Citation]. Neurology 2000;55(6):782–8.
4. Hoehn-Berlage M. Diffusion-weighted NMR imaging: application to experimental focal cerebral ischemia. NMR Biomed 1995;8(7–8):345–58.
5. Jones SC, Perez-Trepichio AD, Xue M, Furlan AJ, Awad IA. Magnetic resonance diffusion-weighted imaging: sensitivity and apparent diffusion constant in stroke. Acta Neurochir Suppl 1994;60:207–10.
6. Albers GW. Diffusion-weighted MRI for evaluation of acute stroke. Neurology 1998;51(3 Suppl 3):S47–9.
7. Albers GW. Expanding the window for thrombolytic therapy in acute stroke. The potential role of acute MRI for patient selection. Stroke 1999;30(10):2230–7.

8. Kidwell CS, Alger JR, Di Salle F, et al. Diffusion MRI in patients with transient ischemic attacks [see comments]. Stroke 1999;30(6):1174–80.
9. Chaves CJ, Silver B, Schlaug G, Dashe J, Caplan LR, Warach S. Diffusion- and perfusion-weighted MRI patterns in borderzone infarcts. Stroke 2000;31(5):1090–6.
10. Albers GW, Lansberg MG, Norbash AM, et al. Yield of diffusion-weighted MRI for detection of potentially relevant findings in stroke patients [see comments]. Neurology 2000;54(8):1562–7.
11. Jacobs MA, Knight RA, Soltanian-Zadeh H, et al. Unsupervised segmentation of multiparameter MRI in experimental cerebral ischemia with comparison to T2, diffusion, and ADC MRI parameters and histopathological validation. J Magn Reson Imaging 2000;11(4):425–37.
12. Linfante I, Llinas RH, Caplan LR, Warach S. MRI features of intracerebral hemorrhage within 2 hours from symptom onset. Stroke 1999;30(11):2263–7.
13. Neumann-Haefelin T, Moseley ME, Albers GW. New magnetic resonance imaging methods for cerebrovascular disease: emerging clinical applications. Ann Neurol 2000;47(5):559–70.
14. Ozsunar Y, Sorensen AG. Diffusion- and perfusion-weighted magnetic resonance imaging in human acute ischemic stroke: technical considerations.[In Process Citation]. Top Magn Reson Imaging 2000;11(5):259–72.
15. Clark WM, Wissman S, Albers GW, Jhamandas JH, Madden KP, Hamilton S. Recombinant tissue-type plasminogen activator (Alteplase) for ischemic stroke 3 to 5 hours after symptom onset. The ATLANTIS Study: a randomized controlled trial. Alteplase Thrombolysis for Acute Noninterventional Therapy in Ischemic Stroke [see comments]. Jama 1999;282(21):2019–26.
16. Furlan A, Higashida R, Wechsler L, et al. Intra-arterial prourokinase for acute ischemic stroke. The PROACT II study: a randomized controlled trial. Prolyse in Acute Cerebral Thromboembolism [see comments]. Jama 1999;282(21):2003–11.
17. Generalized efficacy of t-PA for acute stroke. Subgroup analysis of the NINDS t-PA Stroke Trial. Stroke 1997;28(11):2119–25.
18. del Zoppo GJ, Higashida RT, Furlan AJ, Pessin MS, Rowley HA, Gent M. PROACT: a phase II randomized trial of recombinant pro-urokinase by direct arterial delivery in acute middle cerebral artery stroke. PROACT Investigators. Prolyse in Acute Cerebral Thromboembolism [see comments]. Stroke 1998;29(1):4–11.
19. Marler JR, Tilley BC, Lu M, et al. Early stroke treatment associated with better outcome: the NINDS rt-PA stroke study [In Process Citation]. Neurology 2000;55(11):1649–55.
20. Lacy CR, Suh DC, Bueno M, Kostis JB. Delay in presentation and evaluation for acute stroke : stroke time registry for outcomes knowledge and epidemiology (S.T.R.O.K.E.) [In Process Citation]. Stroke 2001;32(1):63–9.
21. Lansberg MG, Albers GW, Beaulieu C, Marks MP. Comparison of diffusion-weighted MRI and CT in acute stroke [see comments]. Neurology 2000;54(8):1557–61.
22. Yang Q, Tress BM, Barber PA, et al. Serial study of apparent diffusion coefficient and anisotropy in patients with acute stroke. Stroke 1999;30(11):2382–90.
23. Kohno K, Ohta S, Kumon Y, Sakaki S, Okujima S. Early detection of cerebral ischemic lesion using diffusion-weighted MRI. J Comput Assist Tomogr 1995;19(6):982–6.
24. Yoneda Y, Tokui K, Hanihara T, Kitagaki H, Tabuchi M, Mori E. Diffusion-weighted magnetic resonance imaging: detection of ischemic injury 39 minutes after onset in a stroke patient. Ann Neurol 1999;45(6):794–7.
25. Augustin M, Bammer R, Simbrunner J, Stollberger R, Hartung HP, Fazekas F. Diffusion-weighted imaging of patients with subacute cerebral ischemia: comparison with conventional and contrast-enhanced MR imaging [In Process Citation]. AJNR Am J Neuroradiol 2000;21(9):1596–602.
26. Barber PA, Darby DG, Desmond PM, et al. Identification of major ischemic change. Diffusion-weighted imaging versus computed tomography. Stroke 1999;30(10):2059–65.
27. Warach S, Gaa J, Siewert B, Wielopolski P, Edelman RR. Acute human stroke studied by whole brain echo planar diffusion-weighted magnetic resonance imaging. Ann Neurol 1995;37(2):231–41.
28. Wardlaw JM, Marshall I, Wild J, Dennis MS, Cannon J, Lewis SC. Studies of acute ischemic stroke with proton magnetic resonance spectroscopy: relation between time from onset,

neurological deficit, metabolite abnormalities in the infarct, blood flow, and clinical outcome. Stroke 1998;29(8):1618–24.

29. Geijer B, Brockstedt S, Lindgren A, Stahlberg F, Norrving B, Holtas S. Radiological diagnosis of acute stroke. Comparison of conventional MR imaging, echo-planar diffusion-weighted imaging, and spin-echo diffusion-weighted imaging. Acta Radiol 1999;40(3):255–62.

30. Bartylla K, Hagen T, Globel H, Jost V, Schneider G. [Diffusion-weighted magnetic resonance imaging in the diagnosis of cerebral infarct]. Radiologe 1997;37(11):859–64.

31. Fitzek C, Tintera J, Muller-Forell W, et al. Differentiation of recent and old cerebral infarcts by diffusion- weighted MRI. Neuroradiology 1998;40(12):778–82.

32. Larrue V, von Kummer R, del Zoppo G, Bluhmki E. Hemorrhagic transformation in acute ischemic stroke. Potential contributing factors in the European Cooperative Acute Stroke Study. Stroke 1997;28(5):957–60.

33. Lansberg MG, Norbash AM, Marks MP, Tong DC, Moseley ME, Albers GW. Advantages of adding diffusion-weighted magnetic resonance imaging to conventional magnetic resonance imaging for evaluating acute stroke. Arch Neurol 2000;57(9):1311–6.

34. Lansberg MG, Tong DC, Norbash AM, Yenari MA, Moseley ME. Intra-arterial rtPA treatment of stroke assessed by diffusion- and perfusion-weighted MRI. Stroke 1999;30(3):678–80.

35. Ay H, Oliveira-Filho J, Buonanno FS, et al. Diffusion-weighted imaging identifies a subset of lacunar infarction associated with embolic source. Stroke 1999;30(12):2644–50.

36. Kaufmann AM, Firlik AD, Fukui MB, Wechsler LR, Jungries CA, Yonas H. Ischemic core and penumbra in human stroke [see comments]. Stroke 1999;30(1):93–9.

37. Rother J, Jonetz-Mentzel L, Fiala A, et al. Hemodynamic assessment of acute stroke using dynamic single-slice computed tomographic perfusion imaging. Arch Neurol 2000;57(8): 1161–6.

38. Beaulieu C, de Crespigny A, Tong DC, Moseley ME, Albers GW, Marks MP. Longitudinal magnetic resonance imaging study of perfusion and diffusion in stroke: evolution of lesion volume and correlation with clinical outcome [see comments]. Ann Neurol 1999;46(4):568–78.

39. Thijs VN, Lansberg MG, Beaulieu C, Marks MP, Moseley ME, Albers GW. Is early ischemic lesion volume on diffusion-weighted imaging an independent predictor of stroke Outcome? : A multivariable analysis [In Process Citation]. Stroke 2000;31(11):2597–602.

40. Roob G, Lechner A, Schmidt R, Flooh E, Hartung HP, Fazekas F. Frequency and location of microbleeds in patients with primary intracerebral hemorrhage [In Process Citation]. Stroke 2000;31(11):2665–9.

41. Schellinger PD, Jansen O, Fiebach JB, Hacke W, Sartor K. A standardized MRI stroke protocol: comparison with CT in hyperacute intracerebral hemorrhage [see comments]. Stroke 1999;30(4):765–8.

42. Patel MR, Edelman RR, Warach S. Detection of hyperacute primary intraparenchymal hemorrhage by magnetic resonance imaging. Stroke 1996;27(12):2321–4.

43. Schellinger PD, Jansen O, Fiebach JB, et al. Monitoring intravenous recombinant tissue plasminogen activator thrombolysis for acute ischemic stroke with diffusion and perfusion MRI. Stroke 2000;31(6):1318–28.

44. Flacke S, Urbach H, Folkers PJ, et al. Ultra-fast three-dimensional MR perfusion imaging of the entire brain in acute stroke assessment. J Magn Reson Imaging 2000;11(3):250–9.

45. Heiss WD. Ischemic penumbra: evidence from functional imaging in man. J Cereb Blood Flow Metab 2000;20(9):1276–93.

46. Raha S. ECASS-II: intravenous alteplase in acute ischaemic stroke. European Co- operative Acute Stroke Study-II [letter; comment]. Lancet 1999;353(9146):66; discussion 67–8.

47. Burgin WS, Malkoff M, Felberg RA, et al. Transcranial doppler ultrasound criteria for recanalization after thrombolysis for middle cerebral artery stroke. Stroke 2000;31(5):1128–32.

48. Demchuk AM, Christou I, Wein TH, et al. Specific transcranial Doppler flow findings related to the presence and site of arterial occlusion. Stroke 2000;31(1):140–6.

49. Alexandrov AV, Black SE, Ehrlich LE, Caldwell CB, Norris JW. Predictors of hemorrhagic transformation occurring spontaneously and on anticoagulants in patients with acute ischemic stroke. Stroke 1997;28(6):1198–202.

50. Alexandrov AV, Masdeu JC, Devous MD, Sr., Black SE, Grotta JC. Brain single-photon emission CT with HMPAO and safety of thrombolytic therapy in acute ischemic stroke. Proceedings of the meeting of the SPECT Safe Thrombolysis Study Collaborators and the members of the Brain Imaging Council of the Society of Nuclear Medicine. Stroke 1997;28(9):1830–4.
51. Yokogami K, Nakano S, Ohta H, Goya T, Wakisaka S. Prediction of hemorrhagic complications after thrombolytic therapy for middle cerebral artery occlusion: value of pre- and post-therapeutic computed tomographic findings and angiographic occlusive site. Neurosurgery 1996;39(6):1102–7.
52. Tong DC, Adami A, Moseley ME, Marks MP. Relationship between apparent diffusion coefficient and subsequent hemorrhagic transformation following acute ischemic stroke [In Process Citation]. Stroke 2000;31(10):2378–84.
53. Nighoghossian N, Derex L, Turjman F, et al. Hyperacute diffusion-weighted MRI in basilar occlusion treated with intra-arterial t-PA. Cerebrovasc Dis 1999;9(6):351–4.
54. Maeda M, Yuh WT, Ueda T, et al. Severe occlusive carotid artery disease: hemodynamic assessment by MR perfusion imaging in symptomatic patients [see comments]. AJNR Am J Neuroradiol 1999;20(1):43–51.
55. Rutgers DR, Blankensteijn JD, van Der Grond J. Preoperative MRA flow quantification in CEA patients : flow differences between patients who develop cerebral ischemia and patients who Do not develop cerebral ischemia during cross-clamping of the carotid artery [In Process Citation]. Stroke 2000;31(12):3021–8.
56. Rutgers DR, Klijn CJ, Kappelle LJ, van Huffelen AC, van der Grond J. A longitudinal study of collateral flow patterns in the circle of Willis and the ophthalmic artery in patients with a symptomatic internal carotid artery occlusion. Stroke 2000;31(8):1913–20.
57. Barth A, Remonda L, Lovblad KO, Schroth G, Seiler RW. Silent cerebral ischemia detected by diffusion-weighted MRI after carotid endarterectomy. Stroke 2000;31(8):1824–8.
58. Kamran S, Bates V, Bakshi R, Wright P, Kinkel W, Miletich R. Significance of hyperintense vessels on FLAIR MRI in acute stroke. Neurology 2000;55(2):265–9.
59. Wild JM, Wardlaw JM, Marshall I, Warlow CP. N-Acetylaspartate distribution in proton spectroscopic images of ischemic stroke : relationship to infarct appearance on T2-weighted magnetic resonance imaging [In Process Citation]. Stroke 2000;31(12):3008–14.
60. Conturo TE, Lori NF, Cull TS, et al. Tracking neuronal fiber pathways in the living human brain. Proc Natl Acad Sci U S A 1999;96(18):10422–7.

Assessment of Cerebrovascular Pathophysiology

V. Babikian, J. Gomes, and J. Krejza

Brain embolism and impaired perfusion secondary to severe atherosclerotic disease are considered today the two most common causes of brain ischemia and infarction. In spite of their relative prevalence, the two intravascular processes are not well understood for the lack of technologies that permit to study them. Cerebral angiography, the traditional "gold standard" to assess the intravascular process, is limited by substantial technical shortcomings, associated complications, and exposure to ionizing radiation. In addition, angiography provides only a snapshot of the cerebral circulation at the time of the study rather than a continuous picture of the intravascular process. Other technologies such as positron emission tomography (PET) and magnetic resonance imaging (MRI) are not well suited to monitor the course of intravascular events.

The introduction of ultrasound techniques since the late 1970s has enabled to monitor these phenomena *in vivo* and to provide another glimpse at the intravascular process. In spite of their substantial limitations, these techniques have helped refine previously held notions and have raised new questions. In this chapter, we briefly review the present day understanding of selected aspects of the intravascular process as assessed by transcranial Doppler ultrasonography (TCD).

Intracranial Hemodynamic Changes

Effect of Extracranial Arterial Stenoses on Cerebral Hemodynamics

Middle cerebral artery flow velocities decrease distal to internal carotid artery stenoses, and this finding corresponds to the delayed filling of intracranial branches on angiography. It is quite variable, however, and depends to a large degree on the presence of adequate flow through collateral branches. Anterior and posterior communicating artery collateral flow can be adequately studied with TCD.

In patients with inadequate collateral channels, the middle cerebral artery Doppler waveform changes distal to internal carotid artery stenosis as the perfusion pressure drops. A relative decrease of the peak systolic velocity is coupled with an increase of the end-diastolic velocity, resulting in a drop of the pulsatility index. This reflects the reduction of intracranial vascular resistance secondary to arteriolar autoregulatory vasodilatation. The main corresponding positron emission tomography finding is the increase in the oxygen extraction fraction [1]. The drop in the pulsatility index usually does not occur until the severity of internal carotid stenosis exceeds 85%, and less than 45% of patients with severe stenosis have intracranial hemodynamic changes detectable by TCD.

An impairment in vasomotor reactivity is detected in some patients with extracranial internal carotid artery stenosis or occlusion [2] (Figs. 1 and 2), and it is associated with low-flow rather than thromboembolic infarctions [3]. It is corrected by carotid endarterectomy. Prospective studies suggest that exhausted reactivity is associated with a several fold increased risk for ipsilateral ischemic events in symptomatic and asymptomatic patients [4, 5]. The increased awareness of the role of hemodynamic factors in the cause of symptoms in patients with carotid occlusion [6] has prompted a review of thinking regarding the role of revascularization procedures in this setting.

Thus, extracranial internal carotid artery stenosis causes measurable adaptive changes of the intracranial circulation. These changes are quite variable and are affected by several factors. Although they are associated with future ischemic events, the strength of the association is not known.

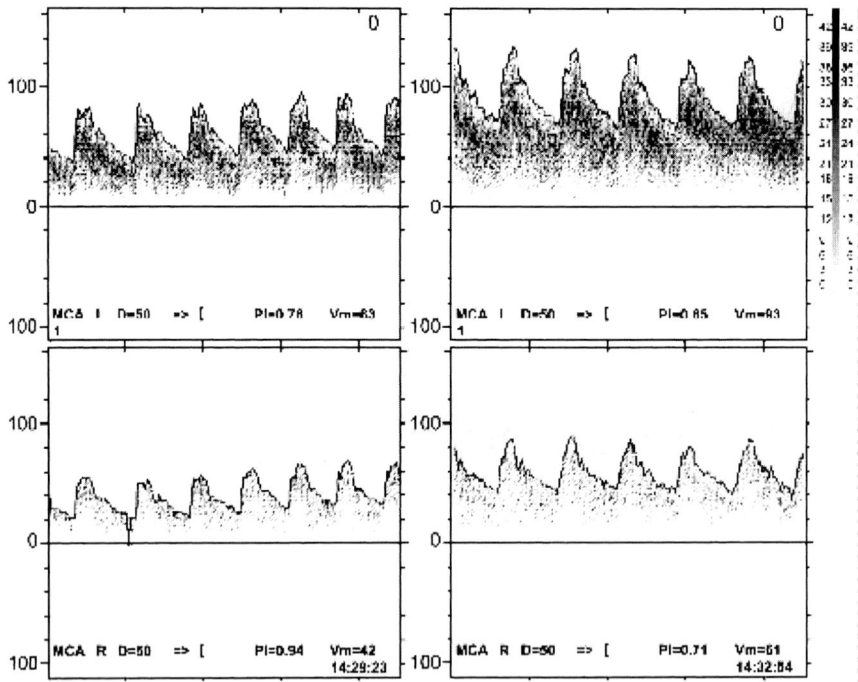

Fig. 1. Preserved vasomotor reactivity. Patient has 90% stenosis at the left internal carotid artery origin and is studied before *(left panel)* and after *(right panel)* hypoventilation. Flow velocities in the left *(MCA L)* and right *(MCA R)* middle cerebral arteries increase by approximately 25%–50%. This suggests adequate collateral flow to the left hemisphere

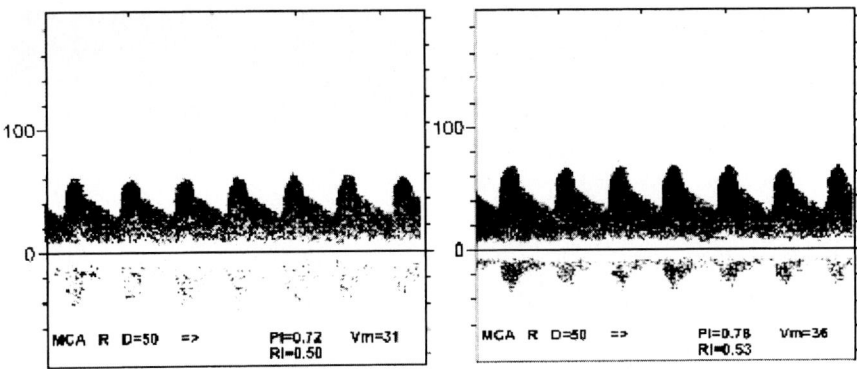

Fig. 2. Impaired vasomotor reactivity in internal carotid artery occlusion. Flow velocities in the middle cerebral artery on the side of the occlusion before an intravenous injection of acetazolamide *(left panel)* are not substantially different from the ones after *(right panel)*

Intracranial Hemodynamic Changes Secondary to Altered Perfusion Pressure

Rapid fluctuations of cerebral blood flow also occur in a variety of other settings. In most patients with internal carotid artery severe stenosis or occlusion who undergo cardiac surgery, there is no substantial and prolonged drop in velocities distal to the occlusive lesion during cardiopulmonary bypass [7], a counter-intuitive and reassuring finding. However, flow velocities fall markedly in patients with intracranial arterial stenosis and transient positional ischemia [8]. The factors that determine this difference between intracranial and extracranial stenosis have not been identified. A key determinant is the severity of the drop in perfusion pressure and whether the lower limit of autoregulation is reached (Fig. 3). TCD studies also confirm that in cough syncope there is a transient cerebral circulatory arrest [9], and a decrease in velocities can be detected in subjects with cardiac rhythm disorders and hypotension [10]. TCD has also been used to monitor brain perfusion during cardiopulmonary resuscitation from cardiac arrest [11].

Cerebral Blood Flow Adjustments in the Elderly

Cerebral blood flow decreases with age, and the corresponding drop in flow velocity is well documented [12]. The mean velocity decreases gradually at a rate of approximately 0.5% per year after the mid-twenties, with slight variations among the different basal cerebral arteries. Flow velocities above age 70 are approximately 20% lower than below age 30. The drop occurs for both men and women, and is partially related to hematocrit and fibrinogen levels. The pulsatility index, an indicator of vascular resistance and stiffness, increases after age 60.

The preceding changes in flow velocity are affected by cerebral, cardiac, and hematological changes secondary to the aging process. They also reflect some of

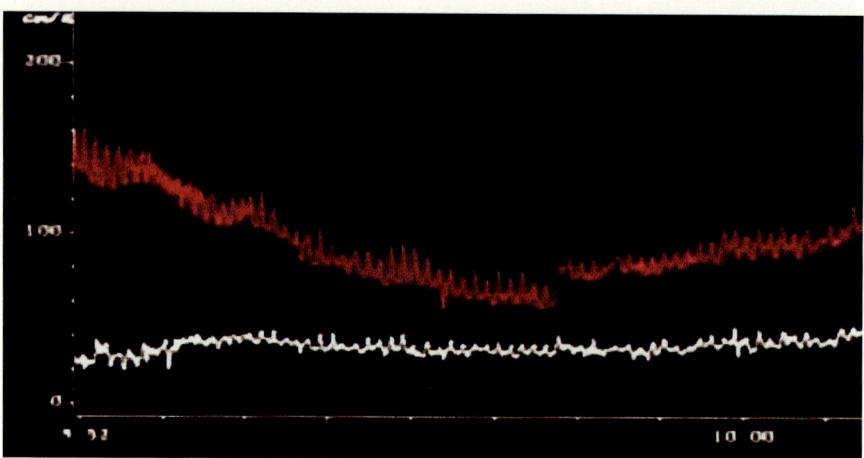

Fig. 3. Effect of hypotension on intracranial hemodynamics. The mean arterial blood pressure *(red line)* drops from approximately 150 mmHg to 70 mmHg. There is no corresponding drop in flow velocities *(white line)*

the structural and physiological alterations in aging brain arteries. Vasomotor reactivity to CO_2 inhalation is impaired in the normotensive elderly, but the autoregulatory response to blood pressure changes is preserved [13, 14]. Because there are only minor fluctuations in the middle cerebral artery M1 segment diameter during hypocapnia [15] or hypoperfusion [16], the impairment in vasoreactivity is thought to be secondary to changes affecting predominantly brain arterioles distal to the M1 segment. The cause(s) of these changes are not well understood. Some may be secondary to alterations in hormonal levels associated with menopause. Hormone replacement therapy appears to enhance reactivity [14].

Periventricular white matter changes detected on MRI testing of healthy elderly persons correspond to astrocytic gliosis, demyelination, and small areas of infarction with thickening of the walls of arterioles less than 150 μm in diameter [17]. They are associated with decreased cerebral blood flow and partially explain the cognitive impairment seen in this population [18]. When measured by TCD, vasomotor reactivity is also decreased. The drop is thought to reflect the severity of the microangiopathy [19], and it may be an independent predictor of lacunar infarction [20].

Thus, in "healthy" elderly patients, the aging process affects the microvasculature and results in measurable physiological changes. The latter are even more marked in hypertensive patients, and can be corrected with successful blood pressure control.

Experience from the Operating Room

Carotid endarterectomy and coronary artery bypass surgery provide unique opportunities to study the brain circulation while it undergoes rapid and occasionally dramatic changes. Endarterectomy is the procedure that has been moni-

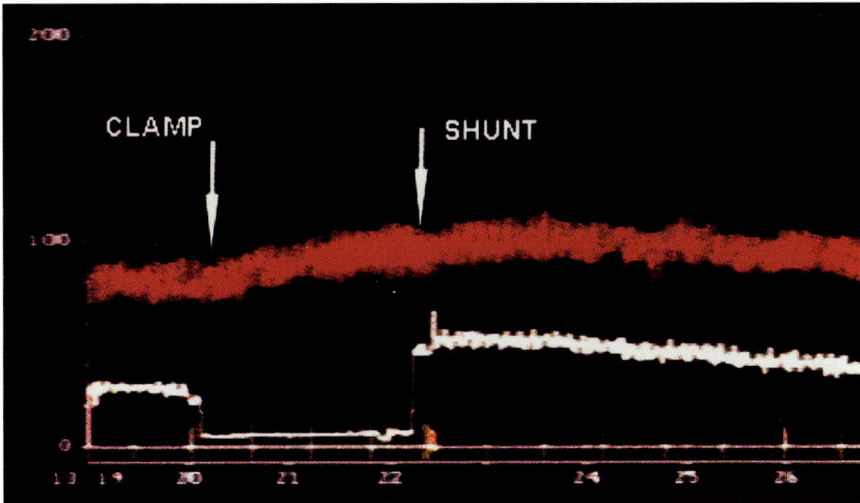

Fig. 4. Effect of cross-clamping on intracranial hemodynamics. During carotid endarterectomy, the flow velocity *(white line)* drops from approximately 30 cm/sec to less than 5 cm/sec as the cross-clamps are placed, and there is a rebound effect when the shunt is opened. No corresponding changes of the mean blood pressure *(red line)* are observed

tored more extensively. Flow velocities in the middle cerebral artery ipsilateral to the side of endarterectomy drop by approximately 20% with the initiation of general anesthesia and the consequent vasodilatation of intracranial arteries. They subsequently remain constant, often in spite of substantial changes in the blood pressure, until cross-clamping, the key hemodynamic "test" of the operation. At cross-clamping, most patients fall into one of two subgroups. Those in the first subgroup have a relatively mild drop in velocities of 15 cm/sec or less. They constitute the majority of patients. The second subgroup is comprised of individuals who have a severe drop in velocity to less than 15% of the pre-clamp values or to post-clamp values ranging between 0 and 20 cm/sec (Fig. 4). When available in this setting, simultaneous electroencephalographic monitoring shows slowing consistent with ischemia in brain regions perfused by the middle cerebral artery. A severe drop identifies patients at an increased risk for perioperative stroke [21]. These patients often have contralateral internal carotid artery stenosis or inadequate collateral channels [22]. They are considered candidates for shunting. The latter restores flow velocities to more than 90% of pre-clamp values (Fig. 4) [23].

Because changes in flow velocity correspond to changes in arterial blood flow, the preceding findings indicate that there is a substantial "reserve" in the volume of blood transiting through the brain at any one time. A threshold effect is present, however, as evidence of tissue ischemia rapidly develops at flow velocity values ranging from 10 to 20 cm/sec in anesthetized patients [24]. Because of the relatively wide margins of this range and in order to err on the safe side, several investigators have recommended shunting when the velocity drops to less than 20 cm/sec or to 30% of the pre-clamp value [25]. There is no consensus in the lit-

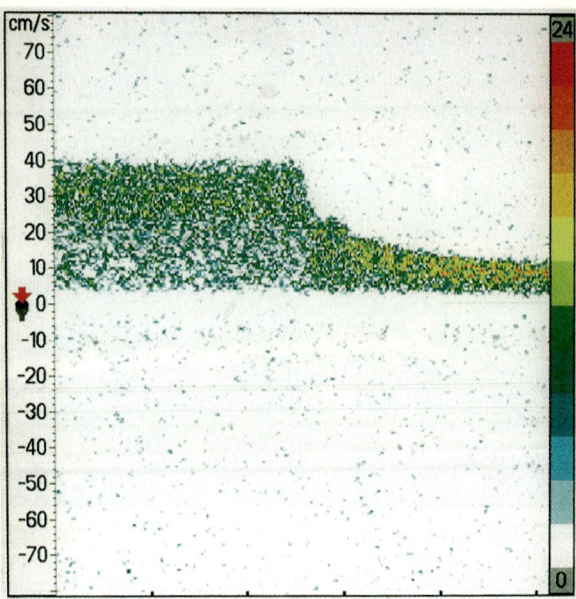

Fig. 5. Monitoring during coronary artery bypass graft surgery. The flow is non-pulsatile during cardiopulmonary bypass and drops from 40 cm/sec to 14 cm/sec secondary to technical difficulties

erature regarding a criterion. It should be noted that transient drops of the flow velocities to even lower levels seem to be tolerated without neurological ill-effects during coronary artery bypass surgery, but the flow is non-pulsatile in that setting as the patients are on cardiopulmonary bypass (Fig. 5).

Carotid endarterectomy also provides an opportunity to monitor collateral flow by simultaneous insonation of the middle and anterior cerebral arteries on both sides. Placement of cross clamps causes an almost immediate drop of the pulsatility index distal to the operated carotid artery, indicating a drop in resistance. Within 2 or 3 heartbeats a rapid increase of collateral flow develops through the anterior communicating artery, reaching a plateau after approximately one minute. It usually persists without substantial change throughout the duration of cross-clamping, returning to baseline after the clamps are released [26]. These findings convincingly demonstrate rapid recruitment of collateral flow, but they do not address more chronic changes.

Vasospasm

Vasospasm is considered a major factor leading to delayed brain ischemia after aneurysmal subarachnoid hemorrhage, and it has been extensively studied by angiography and TCD. Its course and characteristic features are presented elsewhere [27]. Constriction of retinal arteries can be observed during funduscopic examination in some patients who present with amaurosis fugax [28], and symptomatic vasospasm of intracranial arteries is convincingly demonstrated by angiography in patients with hypercalcemia [29] and postpartum angiopathy. Occasionally, vasospasm is also observed during cerebral angiography and angioplasty. Ultrasound studies of vasospasm in these settings are limited.

Vasospasm is not considered a common mechanism of brain ischemia occurring in the context of thromboembolic disease, but its exact role in this setting is not known. Angiographic and TCD studies obtained within hours from the onset of symptoms do not show evidence of vasospasm of the large arteries at the base of the brain [30], and observed "stenoses" are often ascribed to intraluminal emboli or arterial wall atherosclerosis. There is also no substantial evidence to support the occurrence of spasm in more distal arterioles, but these arterial segments are difficult to image, and small changes in diameter can easily be missed.

Both vasoconstriction and dilatation have been reported during the course of migraine attacks [31] and they are also supported by other neuroimaging studies. Although increased velocities confirm the occurrence of vasospasm in migraine [32], a consistent pattern of arterial changes has not emerged from the literature. Constriction of resistance vessels may be common in migraine with aura, particularly during the first 6 hours and specially on the symptomatic side [33]. Dilatation, as evidenced by a drop of flow velocities, can occur during the headache phase of an attack and can be reversed after treatment with sumatriptan [34]. These seemingly contradictory data support the notion of variations in arterial diameter during the course of an attack, and also suggest that the migraine syndrome may have several subtypes. It has been proposed that constriction of resistance arterioles occurs in migraine with aura, and dilatation of the same vessels in migraine without aura [33].

Recreational drugs and pharmacological agents are also associated with vasospasm and occasional cerebral infarction. Chief among them are cocaine, amphetamine, ergotamine, and the triptans. Some drugs, like cocaine and amphetamine, may have synergistic effects. An immediate and transient increase in flow velocities is detected following the intravenous administration of cocaine [35], and a milder and more prolonged effect is seen after intranasal administration [36]. Although the amplitude of the increase was mild to moderate in these experimental settings, and patients remained asymptomatic, more substantial elevations may occur when larger doses of the drug are injected and when several, potentially synergistic drugs are administered. These findings are consistent with the development of vasospasm in the large arteries at the base of the brain and support the notion of vasospasm as a cause of cerebral ischemia following cocaine use.

Brain Embolism

High intensity transient signals corresponding to microemboli coursing in intracranial arteries were first detected by TCD in the context of carotid endarterectomy [37]. They have since been reported in other conditions associated with brain ischemia such as myocardial infarction and internal carotid artery stenosis. These signals can correspond to gaseous microbubbles as well as particles composed of cholesterol, platelets and fibrin [38]. Several studies suggest it might be feasible to differentiate between gaseous and particulate microemboli based on an analysis of corresponding signal characteristics, but a considerable degree of overlap between these characteristics has been a limiting factor. Gaseous microbubbles are associated with signals of higher intensity and longer duration than particulate microemboli of the same size (Figs. 6–8). The

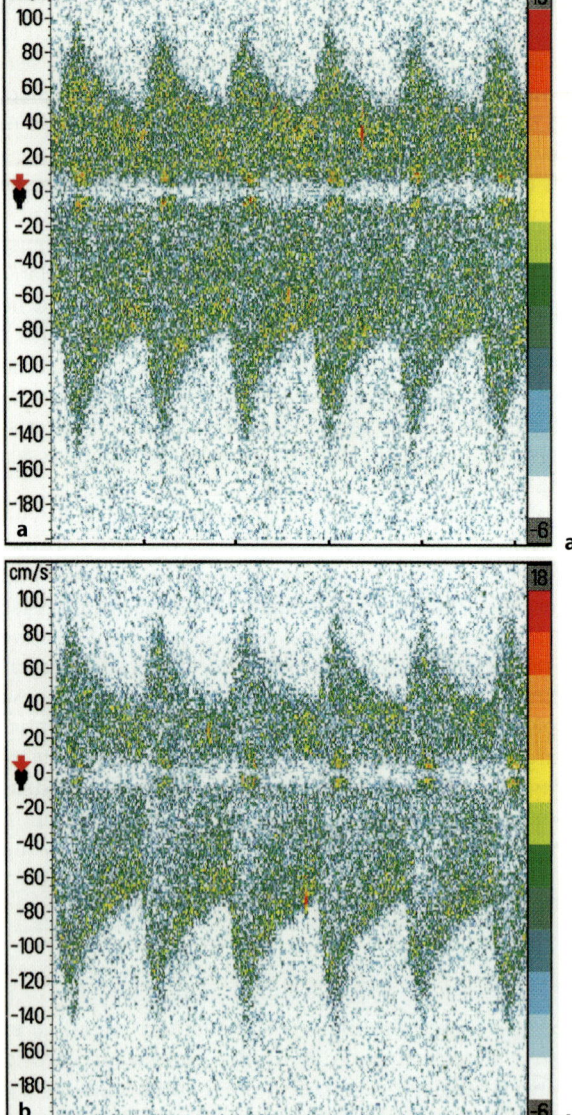

Fig. 6a,b. Microembolism distal to extracranial internal carotid artery stenosis. Microembolic signals (red dots that appear within the Doppler spectrum) are detected in the ipsilateral middle **a** and anterior **b** cerebral arteries. When compared to gaseous microbubbles (Figs. 7 and 8), these signals have lower intensities and shorter durations

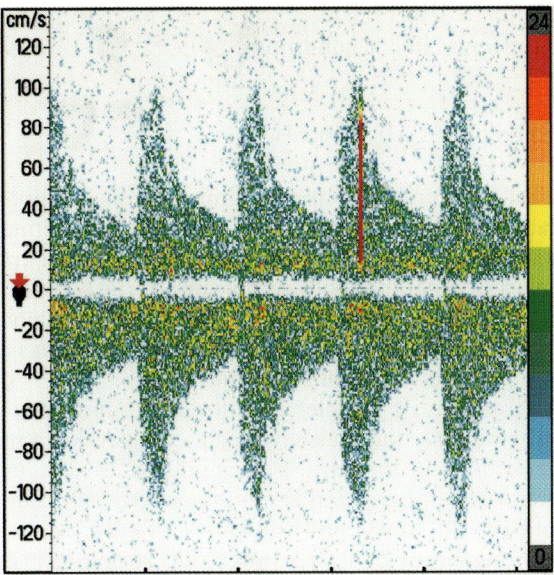

Fig. 7. Gaseous microembolism in a patient with a prosthetic cardiac valve. The (suspected) microbubble appears as a red line in the fourth cardiac cycle

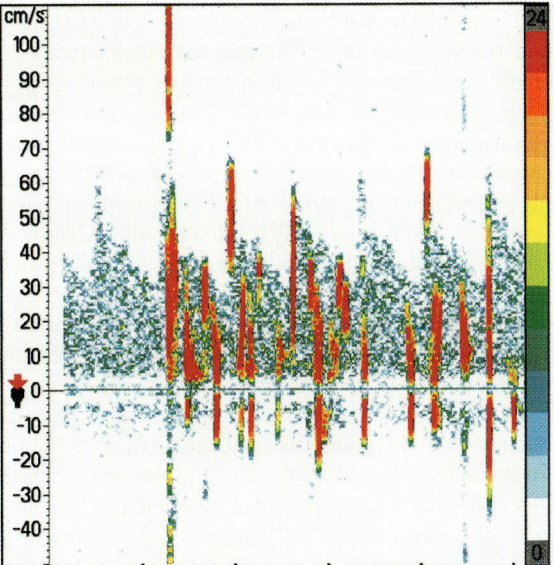

Fig. 8. Gaseous microembolism in a patient with patent foramen ovale. Air microbubbles appeared in the middle cerebral artery approximately 8 seconds after injection in a brachial vein. Transesophageal echocardiographic monitoring showed their passage from the right side of the heart to the left through a patent foramen ovale

ability to detect microemboli *in vivo* has permitted the study of brain embolism in various clinical conditions.

Embolism As a Dynamic Process

That brain embolism is a dynamic process is supported by extensive clinical and laboratory experience. The finding of mobile retinal emboli during funduscopic examination [39], the observation of recurrent transient ischemic attacks and infarcts in patients with cardiac or arterial sources of emboli, and the finding of multiple arteriolar occlusions during neuropathological examination of the brains of patients who die from the complications of stroke are just examples of the dynamic nature of brain embolism.

Transcranial Doppler monitoring studies have refined and expanded these observations, and they have enabled to develop a new, and hopefully more accurate, image of the intravascular process. In symptomatic internal carotid artery stenosis monitored for 30 minutes, microembolism can be detected in 20 to 30% of patients [40, 41], and these rates are even higher when patients are monitored for longer periods of time (Fig. 6). Microembolism fluctuates during the course of the 24 hour day, being most prominent during early morning hours. It is also detected in more than 20% of patients with acute myocardial infarction and reduced ejection fraction [42], and it is ubiquitous during certain surgical procedures such as carotid endarterectomy [21, 43]. Thus, these studies lend strong support to the notion of embolism as a recurrent and frequent phenomenon.

The doubt raised regarding the preceding observations concerns their validity and clinical relevance. The majority of particles detected by TCD are relatively small with diameters of 50 to 100 µm. When the collateral flow is adequate, these particles are presumably washed out without causing brain ischemia. Laboratory studies suggest that particles 200 to 500 µm particles in diameter consistently cause a scattered pattern of neuronal cell death [44]. Larger particles are even more likely to cause brain ischemia, and those 2 to 3 mm in size can occlude the middle cerebral artery M1 segment. Emboli less than 200 µm in diameter are not harmless, but the pattern of damage is less clear. The composition of emboli is also relevant with regards to their potential to occlude brain arteries. The finding of intra-arteriolar platelet-fibrin aggregates without associated tissue necrosis on pathological examination suggests that not all emboli necessarily cause ischemia, and that some platelet clumps can perhaps disaggregate spontaneously.

Differences between the characteristics of symptomatic and asymptomatic microembolism remain to be determined. Data supporting the association between microembolic signals and recent symptoms of brain ischemia are strong [21, 40, 41], and both the percentage of patients and the rate of microembolism is lower in asymptomatic patients [40]. Evidence of brain ischemia is often preceded by a sudden and substantial surge of the rate of embolism, and monitoring in the operating room reveals that patients who develop cerebral ischemia in the context of carotid endarterectomy have a relatively high microembolic count, usually exceeding 50 over a 60 minute period [45]. In addition, microemboli are less frequently detected when patients are evaluated more than a week after onset of symptoms.

In patients with symptoms of brain ischemia, the detection of microembolism denotes an increased risk for recurrent brain ischemic events [41]. This has led researchers to consider it a surrogate end-point for therapy. Several investigations have addressed the impact of pharmacological interventions, but published conclusive studies are limited. In patients with prosthetic cardiac valves, the intensity of warfarin anticoagulation has no substantial effect on the microembolic signal rate, an observation explained by the recent finding that microemboli in this setting are gaseous and not particulate. The rapid decline of microemboli of arterial origin after the intravenous administration of salicylic acid confirms the promise of the technique [46]. In patients with extracranial internal carotid artery stenosis, microembolism resolves after endarterectomy.

Distribution of Microemboli in Brain Arteries

Epidemiological studies consistently show that middle cerebral artery territory infarcts are 15 to 20 times more common than those in the area supplied by the anterior cerebral artery. This has raised questions regarding the distribution of emboli in intracranial arteries and the factors that affect it. TCD detected microemboli that reach the terminal bifurcation of the internal carotid artery preferably enter the middle, rather than the anterior, cerebral artery, and this uneven distribution is more marked in patients with ipsilateral internal carotid artery stenosis than those with cardiac embolism (Figs. 6, 7) [47]. It partially explains the difference in the frequency of brain infarction in the territories of the 2 arteries.

In laboratory animals, emboli introduced into the cardiac circulation are equally distributed throughout the brain [48]. This seems to be also the case in patients with a cardiac lesion such as a patent foramen ovale (Fig. 8) [49]. However, within an arterial segment streamlining does occur, causing emboli to preferentially choose one branch rather than another. For example, emboli originating in one vertebral artery may predominantly enter one, rather than the other, posterior cerebral artery [50], and particles originating at a lesion of the internal carotid artery origin may cross the anterior communicating artery to enter the contralateral middle cerebral artery. Additional factors that seem to affect distribution include the relative size of an embolus to the arterial diameter, the composition of emboli, and the anatomical features of an arterial bifurcation [51].

Fat Embolism Syndrome

Most often diagnosed a complication skeletal trauma, the fat embolism syndrome can be encountered in other conditions as well. Its exact pathogenesis remains unknown, but there is consensus that at least some of its manifestations are secondary to massive embolism to the lungs, brain and other organs. Pathological examination of the brains of patients who die from complications of the condition shows extensive petechial hemorrhages, specially in the white matter, and anemic lesions 1 to 4 mm in diameter [52].

Transcranial Doppler evidence of fat embolism remains limited. Available data support the notion of extensive microembolism to the brain during the days following injury, and signals suggestive of larger microemboli are present when a patent foramen ovale is present [53]. The frequency of microembolic signals drops rapidly after the fifth day following the traumatic event, but intramedullary nail insertion during hip surgery, a procedure known to cause paradoxical embolism across a patent foramen ovale, causes a transient relapse.

Experience from Carotid Endarterectomy

Brain infarction is a frequent complication of carotid endarterectomy, and is a major reason why the procedure is not recommended more frequently. It is clinically detected in 3 to 10% of surgeries, and in an additional 5 to 10% of cases "silent" infarcts are detected by CT or MRI studies [54]. More than 70% of these infarcts are thought to be secondary to brain embolism. The topography and distribution of the silent infarcts is of particular interest. Most are less than 10 mm in diameter and tend to involve subcortical regions. Their relatively small size suggests that intraoperative small emboli are potentially damaging to brain tissue even when a "stroke" is not diagnosed by the clinician.

Intraoperative microembolism ipsilateral to the side of endarterectomy is detected by TCD monitoring in 50 to 80% of patients. Occasionally, microemboli are large enough to transiently occlude the middle cerebral artery M1 segment on the side of surgery. Microembolism can occur throughout the course of the operation, and it tends to cluster around specific surgical stages [43]. It is particularly common during the dissection phase of surgery, at shunt insertion and removal, at clamp release, and during the immediate postoperative period [43] (Fig. 9). Microembolism during dissection occurs in 20% of patients and has been associated with internal carotid artery ulcerated plaque formation. It can also be secondary to the usual pushing and pulling of the exposed carotid artery that occurs during that phase of surgery. Microembolism also occurs in more than 70% of patients during the 6 to 12 hours immediately following surgery, and it is particularly relevant when it is early and persistent. Thrombus formation at the endarterectomy site acts as a source for microemboli during this period. When detected during dissection and the immediate postoperative period, microembolism is associated with perioperative brain infarction [45, 55].

Intraoperative microembolism tends to be most dramatic at clamp release and shunt insertion, but it has been difficult to characterize and has not been associated with ischemic brain damage. The main reason for this lack of association is the composition of the mixture of microembolic particles, as air microbubbles occur in conjunction with particulate microemboli, and they are less prone to cause brain ischemia. Signals detected during dissection and the immediate postoperative period tend to have characteristics similar to those of particulate emboli. Although reliable and tested TCD criteria predictive of cerebral ischemic complications have not been established at the time of this writing, available data suggest cerebral ischemia occurs when the microembolus count is high. In one

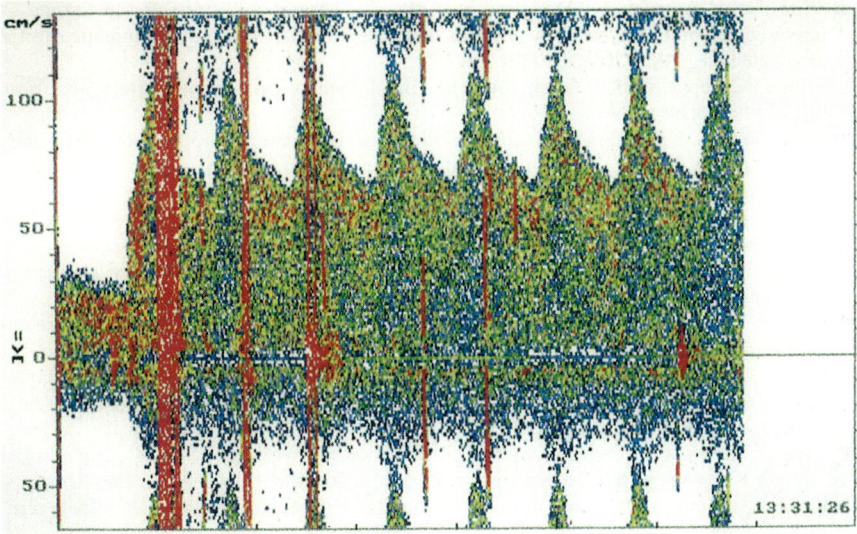

Fig. 9. Microembolism at clamp release during internal carotid endarterectomy. Microembolic signals *(in red)* are seen with the restoration of flow in the middle cerebral artery on the side of endarterectomy

study, a rate of more than 50 microemboli/hour during the first postoperative hour was observed in most patients who developed symptoms of perioperative brain ischemia, and it had a positive predictive value of 0.71 [45].

Thus, microembolism is ubiquitous during carotid endarterectomy, and the large majority of brain microemboli remains asymptomatic. It has a predictable pattern and is often the result of specific actions taken by the surgeon. This information has been used to improve the outcome of the procedure. During the dissection phase of surgery, the availability of immediate feedback information allows the surgeon to introduce specific changes as needed. In addition, in selected patients, postoperative embolism has been treated with antithrombotic agents, such as dextran-40 or a platelet glycoprotein IIB/IIIA receptor antagonist, with a reduction of its frequency and of the postoperative complication rate [56].

References

1. Derdeyn CP, Grubb RL, Powers WJ. Cerebral hemodynamic impairment. Neurology 1999; 53:251–259.
2. Furst H, Hartl W, Janssen I. Patterns of cerebrovascular reactivity in patients with unilateral asymptomatic carotid artery stenosis. Stroke 1994;25:1193–1200.
3. Ringelstein EB, Weiller C, Weckesser M, Weckesser S. Cerebral vasomotor reactivity is significantly reduced in low-flow as compared to thromboembolic infarctions: The key role of the circle of Willis. J Neurol Sci 1994;121:103–109.
4. Kleiser B, Widder B. Course of carotid artery occlusions with impaired cerebrovascular reactivity. Stroke 1992;23:171–174.

5. Silvestrini M, Vernieri F, Pasqualetti P, Matteis M, Passarelli F, Troisi E, Caltagirone C. Impaired cerebral vasoreactivity and risk of stroke in patients with asymptomatic carotid artery stenosis. JAMA 2000;283:2122–2127.
6. Klijn CJN, Kappelle LJ, Tulleken CAF, van Gijn J. Symptomatic carotid artery occlusion. Stroke 1997;28:2084–2093.
7. von Reutern GM, Hetzel A, Birnbaum D, Schlosser V. Transcranial Doppler ultrasonography during cardiopulmonary bypass in patients with severe carotid stenosis or occlusion. Stroke 1988;19:674–680.
8. Marti-Fabregas J, Cocho D, Lleo A, Marti-Vilalta JL. Transcranial Doppler recording in a patient with transient positional cerebral ischemia. Neurology 2000;55:731–732.
9. Mattle HP, Nirkko AC, Baumgartner RW, Sturzenegger M. Transient cerebral circulatory arrest coincides with fainting in cough syncope. Neurology 1995;45:498–501.
10. Carey BJ, Eames PJ, Panerai RB, Potter JF. A case of arrhythmia induced transient cerebral hyperaemia. Cerebrovasc Dis 2000;10:330–333.
11. Gomez CR, Lewis LM, Gomez SM, Ruoff BE, Gasirowski B, Hall IS. Transcranial Doppler assessment of the cerebral hemodynamic effetc of cardiopulmonary ressucitation in fatal cardiac arrest. J Neuroimaging 1992;2:8–11.
12. Tong DC, Albers GW. Normal values. In, Babikian VL, Wechsler LR (eds), Transcranial Doppler Ultrasonography. Second edition. Boston: Butterworth Heinemann, 1999;33–46.
13. Lipsitz LA, Mukai S, Hamner J, Gagnon M, Babikian V. Dynamic regulation of middle cerebral artery blood flow velocity in aging and hypertension. Stroke 2000;31:1897–1903.
14. Kastrup A, Dichgans J, Niemeier M, Schabet M. Changes of cerebrovascular CO_2 reactivity during normal aging. Stroke 1998;29:1311–1314.
15. Kleiser B, Scholl D, Widder B. Doppler CO_2 and diamox test: Decreased reliability by changes of the vessel diameter? Cerebrovasc Dis 1995;5:397–402.
16. Giller CA, Bowman G, Dyer H, Mootz L, Krippner W. Cerebral arterial diameters during changes in blood pressure and carbon dioxide during craniotomy. Neurosurgery 1993; 32:737–742.
17. Van Swieten JC, Van Den Hout JHW, Van Ketel BA, Hijdra A, Wokke JHJ, Van Gijn J. Periventricular lesions in the white matter on magnetic resonance imaging in the elderly. Brain 1991;114:761–774.
18. Ylikoski R, Ylikoski A, Erkinjuntti T, Sulkava R, Raininko R, Tilvis R. White matter changes in healthy elderly persons correlate with attention and speed of mental processing. Arch Neurol 1993;50:818–824.
19. Terborg C, Gora F, Weiller C, Rother J. Reduced vasomotor reactivity in cerebral microangiopathy. Stroke 2000;31:924–929.
20. Molina C, Sabin JA, Montaner J, Rovira A, Abilleira S, Codina A. Impaired cerebrovascular reactivity as a risk marker for first-ever lacunar infarction. Stroke 1999;30:2296–2301.
21. Ackerstaff RGA, Moons KGM, van de Vlasakker CJW, Moll FL, Vermeulen FEE, Algra A, Spencer MP. Association of intraoperative transcranial Doppler monitoring variables with stroke from carotid endarterectomy. Stroke 2000;31:1817–1823.
22. Schwartz RB, Jones KM, LeClercq G, Ahn SS, Chabot R, Whittemore A, Mannick JA, Donaldson MC, Gugino LD. The value of cerebral angiography in predicting cerebral ischemia during carotid endarterectomy. AJR 1992;159:1057–1061.
23. Hayes PD, Vainas T, Hartley S, Thompson MM, London NJM, Bell PRF, Naylor AR. The Pruitt-Inahara shunt maintains mean middle cerebral artery velocities within 10% of preoperative values during carotid endarterectomy. J Vasc Surg 2000;32:299–306.
24. Halsey JH, McDowell HA, Gelmon S, Morawetz RB. Blood velocity in the middle cerebral artery and regional cerebral blood flow during carotid endarterectomy. Stroke 1989;20:53–58.
25. Spencer MP. Transcranial Doppler monitoring and causes of stroke for carotid endarterectomy. Stroke 1997;28:685–691.
26. Babikian VL, Schwarze JJ, Cantelmo NL, Pochay V, Winter M. Collateral flow changes through the anterior communicating artery during carotid endarterectomy. J Neurol Sci 1996; 138:53–59.

27. Sloan MA, Wozniak MA, Macko RF. Monitoring vasospasm after subarachnoid hemorrhage. In, Babikian VL, Wechsler LR (eds), Transcranial Doppler Ultrasonography. Second edition. Boston: Butterworth Heinemann, 1999;109–127.

28. Winterkorn JMS, Kupersmith MJ, Wirtschafter JD, Forman S. Treatment of vasospastic amaurosis fugax with calcium channel blockers. N Engl J Med 1993;329:396–398.

29. Walker GL, Williamson PM, Ravich RB, Roche J. Hypercalcemia associated with cerebral vasospasm causing infarction. J Neurol Neurosurg Psychiatry 1980; 43:464–467.

30. Alexandrov AV, Demchuk AM, Felberg RA, Christou I, Barber PA, Burgin WS, Malkoff M, Wojner AW, Grotta JC. High rate of complete recanalization and dramatic clinical recovery during tPA infusion when continuously monitored with 2 MHz transcranial Doppler monitoring. Stroke 2000;31:610–614.

31. Solomon S, Lipton RB, Harris PY. Arterial stenosis in migraine: spasm or arteriopathy?. Headache 1990;30:52–61.

32. Thie A, Spitzer K, Lachenmayer L, Kunze K. Prolonged vasospasm in migraine detected by noninvasive transcranial Doppler ultrasound. Headache 1988;28:183–186.

33. Zanette EM, Agnoli A, Roberti C, Chiarotti F, Cerbo R, Fieschi C. Transcranial Doppler in spontaneous attacks of migraine. Stroke 1992;23:680–685.

34. Friberg L, Olesen J, Iversen HK, Sperling B. Migraine pain associated with middle cerebral artery dilatation: Reversal by sumatriptan. Lancet 1991;338:13–17.

35. Herning RI, Better W, Nelson R, Gorelick D, Cadet JL. The regulation of cerebral blood flow during intravenous cocaine administration in cocaine abusers. Ann N Y Acad Sci 1999; 890:489–494

36. Fayad P, Price LH, McDougle CJ, Pavalkis FJ, Brass LM. Acute hemodynamic effects of intranasal cocaine on the cerebral and cardiovascular systems. Abstract. Stroke 1992;23:159.

37. Padayachee TS, Gosling RG, Bishop CC, Burnand K, Browse NL. Monitoring middle cerebral artery blood flow velocity during carotid endarterectomy. Br J Surg 1986;73:98–100.

38. Markus HS, Brown MM. Differentiation between pathological cerebral embolic materials using transcranial Doppler in an in vitro model. Stroke 1993;24:1–5.

39. Wijman C, Babikian V, Matjucha I. Monocular visual loss and platelet fibrin embolism to the retina. J Neurol Neurosurg Psychiatry 2000;68:386–387.

40. Babikian VL, Hyde C, Pochay V, Winter MR. Clinical correlates of high-intensity signals detected on transcranial Doppler sonography in patients with cerebrovascular disease. Stroke 1994;25:1570–1573.

41. Valton L, Larrue V, Pavy le Traon A, Massabuau P, Geraud G. Microembolic signal and risk of early recurrence in patients with stroke or transient ischemic attack. Stroke 1998;29:2125–2128.

42. Nadareishvili ZG, Choudary Z, Joyner C, Brodie D, Norris JW. Cerebral microembolism in acute myocardial infarction. Stroke 1999;30:2679–2682.

43. Gavrilescu T, Babikian VL, Cantelmo N, Rosales R, Pochay V, Winter M. Cerebral microembolism during carotid endarterectomy. Am J Surg 1995;170:159–164.

44. Rapp JH, Pan XM, Sharp FR, Shah DM, Wille GA, Velez PM, Troyer A, Higashida RT, Saloner D. Atheroemboli to the brain: Size threshold for causing acute neuronal cell death. J Vasc Surg 2000;32:68–76.

45. Levi CR, O'Malley H, Fell G, Roberts AK, Hoare MC, Ryle JP, Chan A, Beiles BC, Chambers BR, Bladin CF, Donnan GA. Transcranial Doppler detected cerebral microembolism following carotid endarterectomy. Brain 1997;120:621–629.

46. Goertler M, Baeumer M, Kross R, Blaser T, Lutze G, Jost S, Wallesch CW. Rapid decline of cerebral microembolism of arterial origin after intravenous acetylsalicylic acid. Stroke 1999;30:66–69.

47. Wijman CAC, Babikian VL, Winter MR, Pochay VE. Distribution of cerebral microembolism in the anterior and middle cerebral arteries. Acta Neurol Scand 2000;101:122–127.

48. Svensson LG, Robinson MF, Esser J, Fritz VU, Levien LJ. Influence of anatomic origin on intracranial distribution of microemboli in the baboon. Stroke 1986;17:1198–1202.

49. Venketasubramanian N, Sacco RL, Di Tullio M, Sherman D, Homma S, Mohr JP. Vascular distribution of paradoxical emboli by transcranial Doppler. Neurology 1993;43:1533–1535.

50. Diehl RR, Sliwka U, Rautenberg W, Schwartz A. Evidence for embolization from a posterior cerebral artery thrombus by transcranial Doppler monitoring. Stroke 1993;24:606–608.
51. Liebeskind DS, Saver JL, Lim SR, Villablanca JP. CT angiography of the middle cerebral artery elucidates the association of Wernicke's aphasia with cardioembolic stroke. Abstract. Stroke 2000;31:294.
52. Kamenar E, Burger PC. Cerebral fat embolism: A neuropathological study of a microembolic state. Stroke 1980;11:477–484.
53. Forteza AM, Koch S, Romano JG, Zych G, Bustillo IC, Duncan RC, Babikian VL. Transcranial Doppler detection of fat emboli. Stroke 1999;30:2687–2691.
54. Cantelmo NL, Babikian VL, Samaraweera RN, Gordon JK, Pochay VE, Winter MR. Cerebral microembolism and ischemic changes associated with carotid endarterectomy. J Vasc Surg 1998;27:1024–1031.
55. Jansen C, Ramos LMP, van Heesewijk JPM, Moll FL, van Gijn J, Ackerstaff RGA. Impact of microembolism and hemodynamic changes in the brain during carotid endarterectomy. Stroke 1994;25:992–997.
56. Lennard N, Smith J, Dumville J, Abbott R, Evans DH, London NJ, Bell PR, Naylor AR. Prevention of postoperative thrombotic stroke after carotid endarterectomy: The role of transcranial Doppler ultrasound. J Vasc Surg 1997;26:579–584.

Cerebral Blood Flow Measurement with Positron Emission Tomography

W.J. Powers

This research was supported by USPHS grants NS39529, NS35966, NS28947, NS06833 and The Lillian Strauss Fund of the Jewish Hospital of St. Louis

Measurement of cerebral blood flow (CBF) has provided much valuable information about normal physiology and disease-induced pathophysiology. A variety of techniques currently are available to measure quantitative regional CBF in the living human brain. Among these, positron emission tomography (PET) has both distinct advantages and disadvantages. PET can provide accurate quantitative regional measurements of CBF with excellent reproducibility, but spatial resolution is somewhat limited. The real advantage of PET over other techniques, however, stems from its capacity to provide measurements of metabolism as well. This combination has been especially useful for the study of ischemia, providing new insights into the role of ischemia in various disease states.

Positron Emission Tomography

Certain radionuclides decay by emission of a positron, a small particle with the same mass as an electron but the opposite charge. After traveling a few millimeters through tissue, the positron interacts with an electron, resulting in the destruction of both. This annihilation creates two photons (gamma rays) that travel away from the annihilation site in opposite directions. A pair of external radiation detectors positioned on either side of a positron-emitting source will register these photons at almost the same time. (The difference in time is equivalent to the difference in the distance the two photons travel divided by the speed of light.) If this detector pair is connected by an electronic circuit that records a signal only when two photons arrive within this short time interval, then only photons arising from positron annihilations occurring between the detector pair will be recorded. A positron emission tomograph consists of a large number of detector pairs connected by coincidence circuits. The information obtained from each of these detector pairs is used to construct a series of projections, each representing the distribution of regional radioactivity as viewed from a different angle. These projections are then combined to produce a two-dimensional reconstruction of the regional radioactivity within the combined field of view of all the detectors. Multiple rings of detectors generate multiple reconstructed slices simultaneously, each depicting a different level of the brain and together providing a true three-dimensional image [1–4].

A particular advantage of PET over other radiotracer imaging methodologies such as single photon emission computed tomography (SPECT) is that the fraction of radioactivity lost due to absorption by surrounding tissue can be measured accurately and then corrected for. For an individual photon, this attention fraction depends on the tissue composition and the distance the photon travels through the tissue. For a pair of annihilation photons, the tissue composition and total distance traveled by *both* gamma photons will be the same regardless of where between the detector pair the annihilation occurs. The attenuation fraction for a given path through an object will, therefore, be the same whether the annihilation occurs internally or externally to the object. The attenuation fraction for any pair of coincidence detectors relative to a specific object can be measured accurately prior to the internal administration of any radiotracers. First, a positron emitting source is placed between the detector pair and the total number of coincidences per unit time is recorded. The head (or other part of the body to be studied) is then also placed between the detector pair and the number of coincidences per unit time is again measured. The fractional reduction in the initial radioactivity represents the annihilation photons absorbed by the head for the tissue path between the detector pair. When a radiotracer is administered, this individually measured attenuation fraction is used to correct the number of coincidence events recorded by the detector pair to yield the actual number of positron annihilations that took place with its field of view [1–4].

The accuracy of the reconstructed PET image as a quantitative measure of regional radioactivity depends on a variety of technical factors beyond the scope of this article. There is one technical concept, however, that is crucial for the proper interpretation of any PET measurement. This is the effect of image resolution on the accuracy of the measurement of regional radioactivity. In the PET image, radioactivity from a given region in the object is redistributed or smeared over a larger area. For a point source of radioactivity, this redistribution approximates the form of a Gaussian (bell-shaped) curve with the maximum value occurring at the original point. As a consequence of this redistribution of radioactivity, a given region in the reconstructed image, regardless of its size, contains only a portion of the radioactivity actually within that region in the original structure. The remainder has been redistributed into surrounding regions of the image. Similarly, some radioactivity originally in these surrounding regions has been redistributed into the region of interest. Thus, the regional radioactivity measurement made with PET represents some portion of the radioactivity actually within that region plus a contribution from radioactivity in surrounding regions. This is known as the partial volume effect [5, 6]. Thus, PET will always demonstrate a gradual transition of values between two structures even when there is an abrupt change, such as at the edge of a cerebral infarct or hemorrhage. Under certain conditions, this partial volume effect can be corrected for to provide truly accurate measurement of regional CBF at the edge of pathological structures [7].

Most positron-emitting radionuclides have half-lives of minutes to a few hours. This allows relatively large amounts of radioactivity to be administered while keeping the radiation dose to the subject at a safe level. Since the radioactivity often decays rapidly, sequential studies may be easily performed. The disadvantage to these short-lived radionuclides is obvious. In most cases, they must be prepared on site or shipped only short distances. Since production of the more commonly used positron emitters (^{11}C, [15]O and ^{18}F) requires a cyclotron or linear accelerator, their availability depends on proximity to one of these facilities. Synthesis of molecules incorporating short-lived radionuclides is a specialized field requiring great expertise. The synthesis must be performed rapidly and, at the same time, yield substances that are of sufficient purity to be safe for administration to human subjects [3–4].

PET measurements of physiology employ a mathematical model that quantitatively relates tissue concentration of the positron-emitting radiotracer (as measured by PET) to the physiologic variable under study. This model must take into account a variety of factors including delivery of the tracer to the tissue, distribution and metabolism of the tracer within the tissue, egress of tracer and labeled metabolites from the tissue, recirculation of metabolized and unmetabolized tracer, and the amount of tracer and labeled metabolites remaining in the blood. Furthermore, the model must be practically applicable given the constraints imposed by PET designs and the amount of radioactivity that can be safely administered to human subjects. Finally, the validity of the underlying assumptions and possible sources of error for each model when applied to the study of both normal physiology and disease states must be clearly understood. Ideally, each PET technique should be validated by pair-wise comparison to a "gold standard" under the conditions for which it will be used.

PET Measurement of CBF

A wide variety of methods for measuring cerebral blood flow with PET are available. These use different radiotracers and different mathematical models [8–14]. The most commonly used radiotracer is ^{15}O-H$_2$O. ^{15}O-H$_2$O is easy to synthesize and the 122 s half-life of oxygen-15 permits multiple studies in rapid sequence. This short half-life also necessitates an on site cyclotron or linear accelerator for production. A problem with the use of ^{15}O-H$_2$O arises because the blood-brain barrier is incompletely permeable to water [15]. As a result, ^{15}O-H$_2$O is incompletely extracted at high rates of flow causing underestimation of CBF. This inaccuracy at high flow rates can be overcome with the use of a freely permeable tracer such as ^{15}O-butanol. ^{15}O-butanol is, however, much more difficult to synthesize and has not seen widespread use [14]. Nevertheless, since measurements of CBF made with ^{15}O-H$_2$O are accurate at low flow rates (within the limitations of partial volume averaging), they have proven to be valuable for the study of cerebral ischemia [4–16].

The method for measuring CBF with ^{15}O-H$_2$O that we have extensively employed at Washington University is based on the tissue autoradiographic technique of Kety and coworkers [17, 18]. This method utilizes a bolus intravenous injection of ^{15}O-H$_2$O followed by a 40 second PET scan. During this period, sequential samples of arterial blood are collected to determine the time-activity curve for ^{15}O-H_2O [13]. Because of the almost linear relationship between region-al radioactivity and CBF with this model, the measured regional CBF closely approximates the weighted mean for tissues within the region [12]. The major disadvantage of this technique is its dependence on the arterial time-activity curve. This curve, obtained by sampling from a peripheral artery, is assumed to be the same as that for the cerebral circulation. Any difference between the peripheral curve and the cerebral curve will lead to errors in calculated CBF, the worst errors occurring when the radiotracer bolus arrives in the brain at a differ-ent time than it arrives in the peripheral artery. This problem can largely be over-come by timing the arrival of the radiotracer bolus in the brain by the sudden increase in PET counts and shifting the peripheral curve to match [12, 13]. This technique has been validated by comparison to the intracarotid height/area method and shown to be accurate at CBF below 60 ml $100g^{-1}$ min^{-1} [13].

This technique provides excellent within session reproducibility and thus is well suited to look at the short term acute physiologic and pharmacological manipulations. We have recently studied the effects of moderate hyperventilation on hemispheric CBF in 9 subjects within 8–14 hours following severe traumatic brain injury (Glasgow coma score 5.6 ± 1.8). Baseline $PaCO_2$ was 38 ± 4 mmHg and dropped to 30 ± 2 mmHg during hyperventilation. Baseline hemispheric CBF of 38 ± 14 ml $100g^{-1}$ min^{-1} decreased to 26 ± 9 ml $100g^{-1}$ min^{-1} during hyperventilation ($p<.001$) [19]. We have also investigated the effect of pharmacological blood pres-sure reduction on the regional CBF around the clot in patients with acute intrac-erebral hemorrhage (ICH) . Twelve hypertensive patients with supratentorial ICH within 24 hours after onset had measurements of CBF and then received nicardip-ine($n=5$) or labetalol ($n=7$) to produce a 15% reduction in mean arterial pressure (MAP). Global CBF was computed from slice averages above the pineal gland identified on a high resolution co-registered CT. Peri-clot CBF was measured in a 1 cm wide region around the hyperdense clot drawn on the CT. All PET images were masked to exclude non-cerebral structures and corrected for partial volume effects due to clot, CSF spaces and skull. MAP was reduced from 142 ± 9 to 120 ± 8 mmHg. Global CBF was 40 ± 12 at baseline and 37 ± 8 ml $100g^{-1}$ min^{-1} after MAP reduction (95% CI of the difference = $+2$ to -6). Peri-clot CBF was 21 ± 8 at baseline and 21 ± 8 ml $100g^{-1}$ min^{-1} after blood pressure reduction (95% CI of the difference = $+0$ to -2) [20]. Due to the excellent reproducibility of this technique, the 95% confidence intervals for the differences in CBF produced by MAP reduc-tion are small, allowing us to conclude with a high degree of certainty that MAP reduction of this degree does not lead to a reduction in CBF in the area sur-rounding acute intracerebral hemorrhage.

Measurement of Cerebral Oxygen Metabolism

The unique value of PET for investigating cerebral physiology and pathophysiol-ogy stems from its capability to provide physiologic data other than CBF. In stud-ies of ischemia, combined measurements of CBF and cerebral oxygen metabolism ($CMRO_2$) have proven to be particularly valuable [4, 16]. Measurements of CBF alone cannot determine whether low CBF is due to a primary reduction in supply (ischemia) or simply a reflection of the reduced metabolic demand of injured tissue. Measurements of the relationship between CBF and $CMRO_2$ can often help make this distinction. This relationship is often expressed in terms of the oxygen extraction fraction (OEF) = $CMRO_2/(CBF \times CaO_2)$ where CaO_2 is the arterial oxygen content. OEF is normally 0.3 –0.5 and is uniform throughout the brain. When CBF is primarily reduced due to ischemia, OEF will initially increase to maintain $CMRO_2$. If CBF is reduced due to low metabolic demand, OEF will remain normal. With severe and prolonged ischemia, cerebral infarction occurs. $CMRO_2$ will eventually decrease and OEF will return to normal [4, 21].

The original method described for measuring $CMRO_2$ involves the continuous inhalation of ^{15}O-CO_2 followed by the continuous inhalation of ^{15}O-O_2. In the pulmonary vessels, ^{15}O-CO_2 is rapidly converted to ^{15}O-H_2O by carbonic anhydrase in red blood cells. The resultant ^{15}O-H_2O circulates throughout the body. After five to ten minutes, a steady state is reached in the brain such that the amount of radioactivity entering as ^{15}O-H_2O is equal to the amount lost via radioactive decay and venous outflow. During this equilibrium, the relationship between regional CBF and regional radioactivity can be expressed by a simple, non-linear equation. Calculation of quantitative values for CBF requires, in addition to the regional radioactivity data obtained by PET, measurement of the arterial concentration of ^{15}O-H_2O is and knowledge of the specific volume of distribution of water (often called the partition coefficient). The latter is derived from previous experimental data. Following the ^{15}O-CO_2 scan, a second continuous inhalation of ^{15}O-O_2 is performed. ^{15}O-O_2 binds to hemoglobin and circulates throughout the body. A fraction of the ^{15}O-O_2 in the blood is extracted by the brain and locally metabolized to water. This ^{15}O-H_2O exits the brain and a portion then recirculates back to the brain where it is distributed in proportion to regional CBF. The OEF can be calculated and is, in fact, proportional to the ratio of the regional radioactivities measured by the two scans: ^{15}O-$O_2/^{15}O$-CO_2. Regional $CMRO_2$ can then be calculated by multiplying OEF $\times$ CBF $\times$ CaO_2 where CaO_2 is measured from a peripheral arterial sample [8]. As originally described and implemented, this method failed to correct for radioactivity from intravascular ^{15}O-O_2 still bound to hemoglobin. As a result, OEF and $CMRO_2$ were overestimated. This overestimation of OEF depends upon the local intravascular volume and is greatest at low values of OEF and CBF. Correction for the effect of intravascular ^{15}O-O_2 hemoglobin using data from a separately performed cerebral blood volume (CBV) measurement using ^{15}O – CO to label red blood cells is now routinely used [22, 23].

At Washington University, we have used a different method for measuring OEF and $CMRO_2$ employing a brief inhalation of air containing ^{15} O-O_2 [24]. Following inhalation, a 40 second PET scan is performed and arterial blood samples are collected. Data from separately performed ^{15}O-H_2O CBF and ^{15}O-CO CBV studies is also required. A two-compartment model describing the production and egress of water of metabolism in cerebral tissue, recirculating water of metabolism in the brain, and the arterial, venous, and capillary contents of ^{15}O-hemoglobin is used to calculate OEF. This accuracy of method has been extensively validated under conditions of both low and high CBF, OEF and $CMRO_2$ [24, 25].

Other methods for measuring $CMRO_2$ using dynamic multiple scan sequences and more complex mathematical models have also been described [26].

PET Studies of Cerebral Ischemia with CBF and $CMRO_2$ at Washington University

We used combined measurements of CBF, OEF and $CMRO_2$ to investigate the low CBF that occurs following aneurysmal subarachnoid hemorrhage [27]. Global CBF, OEF and $CMRO_2$ in 8 patients with subarachnoid hemorrhage (SAH) prior to the onset of vasospasm were compared to 20 controls. In the patients CBF (SAH 38 ± 8 ml $100g^{-1}$ min^{-1} vs control 48 ± 9 ml $100g^{-1}$ min^{-1}) and $CMRO_2$ (SAH 2.0 ± 0.2 ml $100g^{-1}$ min^{-1} vs control 2.6 ± 0.5 ml $100g^{-1}$ min^{-1}) were reduced (p<.02), whereas there was no difference in OEF (SAH 0.34 ± 0.04 vs control 0.35 ± 0.07). We interpreted this to mean that the reduction in CBF occurring prior to the onset of vasospasm was caused by a primary reduction in metabolic demand, perhaps from an effect of blood or blood products on the brain. We then compared regions with no, mild or severe angiographic vasospasm which did not go on to infarction in the patients with SAH. Angiographic vasospasm was associated with a progressive reduction in CBF combined with an increase in OEF (p<.02) with no changes in $CMRO_2$ (p=.2). We interpreted this to mean that vasospasm is a primary problem with blood vessels that causes cerebral ischemia rather that a secondary decrease in vessel caliber in response to reduced metabolic demand for oxygen.

In a recent study of 16 patients with acute intracerebral hemorrhage, we compared CBF, OEF and $CMRO_2$ in the region around the clot to a mirror region on the contralateral side. In the peri-clot region CBF and $CMRO_2$ were reduced (CBF: 21 ± 8 ml $100g^{-1}$ min^{-1} vs contralateral 37 ± 14 ml $100g^{-1}$ min^{-1}, p <.001; $CMRO_2$: 1.4 ± 0.5 ml $100g^{-1}$ min^{-1} vs contralateral 2.9 ± 1.0 ml $100g^{-1}$ min^{-1}, p<.0001). OEF was reduced, not elevated, in the peri-clot area as compared to the opposite side (0.44 ± 0.18 vs contralateral 0.51 ± 0.13, p=.05) indicating that there was no ischemia in the peri-clot region when these scans were performed a median of 16(range 5–22) hours after onset [28].

We have also investigated whether the reduction in CBF produced by hyperventilation (HV) in patients with traumatic brain injury is severe enough to reduce cerebral oxygen supply below that needed to meet metabolic needs. We measured CBF, OEF and $CMRO_2$ with PET before ($PaCO_2=38\pm4$ mmHg) and during HV ($PaCO_2=29\pm1$ mmHg) in 8 subjects with severe TBI (Glasgow Coma Score 3–7) 13 ± 6 hours after injury. Whole brain data for these patients showed significant reductions in CBF (see above, one patient had CBF measurements only), increase in OEF (p <0.01) and no change in CMRO2 [19]. To study regional effects of HV, an automated search routine was used to identify 5 ml spherical regions with the lowest CBF during each patient's HV study. Regional $CMRO_2$ before and during HV were compared for these regions. There were no significant changes in $CMRO_2$ for those regions with CBF <20 during HV (before $1.2\pm.3$ vs during $1.2\pm.3$, p=.86), CBF <15 during HV ($1.0\pm.2$ vs $1.0\pm.3$, p=.75) or CBF <10 during HV ($0.8\pm.3$ vs $0.9\pm.4$, p=.70). We concluded that moderate HV to $PaCO_2$ 29 ± 1 mmHg in patients with severe TBI did not produce regional deterioration in $CMRO_2$ in areas where CBF dropped to the lowest levels. This was due to low pre-HV $CMRO_2$ in these areas and adequate compensatory increases in OEF during HV. We, therefore, found no evidence of regional ischemia under these conditions [29].

In 1987, we proposed a three stage classification for the hemodynamic status of the cerebral circulation based upon the compensatory responses made by the brain to progressive reductions in cerebral perfusion pressure (CPP) [30]. When CPP is normal (Stage 0), CBF is closely matched to the resting metabolic rate of the tissue. As a consequence of this resting balance between flow and metabolism, the oxygen extraction fraction (OEF) shows little regional variation. With moderate reductions in CPP, vasodilation of arterioles reduces cerebrovascular resistance, thus maintaining a constant CBF (Stage I). This phenomenon is known as cerebrovascular autoregulation. As a consequence, the intravascular cerebral blood volume (CBV) is elevated and the capacity of the vessels to respond to further vasodilatory stimuli is impaired. With more severe reductions in CPP, the capacity for compensatory vasodilation is exceeded and autoregulation fails. CBF begins to decline. A progressive increase in OEF now maintains cerebral oxygen metabolism and brain function (Stage II).

In a previous study using historical controls, we failed to demonstrate a relationship between Stage I autoregulatory vasodilation and the subsequent risk of stroke [31]. To test the hypothesis that Stage II cerebral hemodynamic failure (increased oxygen extraction measured by positron emission tomography) distal to symptomatic carotid artery occlusion is an independent risk factor for subsequent stroke in medically treated patients, we carried out a prospective, blinded, longitudinal cohort study of patients referred from a group of regional hospitals between 1992 and 1996 [32]. From 419 subjects referred, 81 with previous stroke or transient ischemic attack in the territory of an occluded carotid artery were enrolled. All were followed to completion of the study with average follow-up of 31.5 months. Every six month telephone contact recorded the subsequent occurrence of all stroke, ipsilateral ischemic stroke and death. Stroke occurred in 12/39 with Stage II hemodynamic failure and in 3/42 without [p=.005]. Ipsilateral stroke occurred in 11/39 with Stage II hemodynamic failure and in 2/42 without [p=.004]. Six deaths occurred in each group. After adjustment for 17 baseline patient characteristics and interval medical treatment, the relative risk conferred by Stage II hemodynamic failure was 6.0 (95% CI 1.7–21.6) for all stroke and 7.3 (95% CI 1.6–33.4) for ipsilateral stroke. We concluded that Stage II hemodynamic failure defines a subgroup of patients with symptomatic carotid occlusion who are at high risk for subsequent stroke when treated medically.

Conclusions

Within the limits of tracer methodology and spatial resolution, PET can provide accurate quantitative regional measurements of regional CBF. PET CBF measurements can be used to investigate a variety of physiological, pathophysiological and pharmacological phenomena in the human brain. The unique value of PET in investigating cerebral ischemia stems from its capability to provide measurements of $CMRO_2$ as well. By combining measurements of CBF with $CMRO_2$ it is possible to determine whether low CBF is due to ischemia or reduced metabolic demand. Studies using this combined methodology has lead to increased understanding of the role of ischemia in aneurysmal subarachnoid hemorrhage, intracerebral hemorrhage, traumatic brain injury and the long term prognosis of carotid artery occlusion.

References

1. Ter-Pogossian MM: Positron emission tomography instrumentation In: Reivich M, Alavi A eds.Positron Emission Tomography. New York: Alan R. Liss, Inc.; 1985:43–61.
2. Hoffman EJ, Phelps ME: Positron emission tomography: Principles and quantitation In: Phelps M, Mazziotta J, Schelbert H; eds. Positron Emission Tomography and Autoradiography: Principles and Applications for the Brain and Heart. New York: Raven Press; 1986:237–286.
3. Lammertsma AA, Frackowiak RSJ: Positron emission tomography. CRC Crit Rev Biomed Eng 1985;13:125–169.
4. Powers WJ, Raichle ME: Positron emission tomography and its application to the study of cerebrovascular disease in man. Stroke 1985;16:361–376
5. Hoffman EJ, Huang SC, Phelps ME: Quantitation in positron emission computed tomograph: 1. Effect of object size. J Comput Assist Tomogr 1979;3:299–308.
6. Budinger TF, Derenzo SE, Gullberg GT, Greenberg WL, Huesman RH: Emission computer assisted tomography with single-photon and positron annihilation photon emitters. J Comput Assist Tomogr 1977;l:131–145.
7. Videen TO, Dunford-Shore JE, Diringer MN, Powers WJ: Correction for partial volume effects in regional blood flow measurements adjacent to hematomas in humans with intracerebral hemorrhage: Implementation and validation. J Comput Assist Tomogr 1999;23:248–256
8. Frackowiak RSJ, Lenzi GL, Jones T, Heather JD: Quantitative measurement of regional cerebral blood flow and oxygen metabolism in man using ^{15}O and positron emission tomography: Theory, procedure and normal values. J Comput Assist Tomogr 1980;4:727–736.
9. Ohta S, Meyer E, Fujita H, Reutens DC, Evans A, Gjedde A: Cerebral [^{15}O] water clearance in humans determined byPET: I. Theory and normal values. J Cereb Blood Flow Metab 1996 ; 16: 765–780
10. Carson RE, Huang S, Green MV: Weighted integration method for local cerebral blood flow measurements with Positron emission tomography. J Cereb Blood Flpw Metab 1986
11. Holden JE, Gatley SJ, Hichwa RD, Ip WR, Shaughnessy WJ, Nickles RJ, Polcyn RE: Cerbral blood flow using PET measurements of fluoromethane kinetics J Nucl Med 1981 22:1084–1088
12. Herscovitch P, Markham J, Raichle ME: Brain blood flow measured with intravenous $H_2^{15}O.I.$ Theory and error analysis. J Nucl Med 1983;24:782–789.
13. Raichle ME, Martin WRW, Herscovitch P, Mintun MA, Markham J: Brain blood flow measured with intravenous $H_2^{15}O$. II. Implementation and validation. J Nucl Med 1983;24:790–798.
14. Berridge MS, Adler BL, Nelson AD, Cassidy EH, Muzic RF, Bednarczyk EM, Miraldi F: Measurement of human cerebral blood flow with [^{15}O]butanol positron emission tomography. J Cereb Blood Flow Metab 1991;ll:707–715.
15. Eichling JO, Raichle ME, Grubb RL Jr, Ter-Pogossian M: Evidence of the limitations of water as a freely diffusible tracer in brain of the rhesus monkey. Circ Res 1974;35:358–364.
16. Baron J, Frackowiak RSJ, Herholz K, Jones T, Lammertsma AA, Mazoyer B, Wienhard K: Use of PET methods for measurement of cerebral energy metabolism and hemodynamics in cerebrovascular disease. J Cereb Blood Flow Metab 1989;9:723–742.
17. Landau WM, Freygang WH Jr, Rowland LP, Sokoloff L, Kety SS: The local circulation of the living brain: Values in the unanesthetized and anesthetized cat. Trans Am Neurol Assoc 1955 ;80:l25–129.
18. Kety SS: Measurement of local blood flow by the exchange of an inert diffusible substance. Methods Med Res 1960;8:228–236.
19. Diringer MN, Yundt K, Videen TO, Adams RE, Zazulia AR, Deibert E, Aiyagari V, Dacey RGJr, Grubb RLJr, Powers WJ: No reduction in cerebral metqbolism as a result of early moderat hyperventilation following severe traumatic brain injury. J Neurosurg 2000; 92: 7–13

20. Powers WJ, Zazulia AZ, Videen TO, Diringer MN: Effect of Phamacologic Blood Pressure Reduction on CBF in Patients with Acute Intracerebral Hemorrhage. Society of Nuclear Medicine Abstracts, May 2000

21. Powers WJ: Cerebral hemodynamics in ischemic cerebrovascular disease. Ann Neurol 1991;29:231–240.

22. Lammertsma AA, Jones T: Correction for the presence of intravascular oxygen-is in the steady state technique for measuring regional oxygen extraction ratio in the brain: 1. Description of the method. J Cereb Blood Flow Metab1983; 13:416–424.

23. Pantano P, Baron J-C, Crouzel C, Collard P, Sirou P, Samson Y: The 150 continuous-inhalat$_1$_on method: Correction for intravascular signal using C 0. Eur J Nuci Med 1985;l0:387–391.

24. Mintun MA, Raichle ME, Martin WRW, Herscovitch P: Brain oxygen utilization measured with 0-15 radiotracers and positron emission tomography. J Nucl Med 1984;25:177–187

25. Altman DI, Lich LL, Powers WJ: Brief inhalation method to measure cerebral oxygen extraction with PET: Accuracy determination under pathological conditions. J Nucl Med 1991; 32:1738–1741.

26. Ohta S, Meyer E, Thompson CJ, Gjedde A: Oxygen consumption of the living human brain measured after a single inhalation of positron emitting oxygen. J Cereb Blood Flow Metab 1992 ; 12: 179–192.

27. Carpenter DA, Grubb RL Jr, Tempel LW, Powers WJ: Cerebral oxygen metabolism after aneurysmal subarachnoid hemorrhage. J Cereb Blood Flow and Metab 1991;ll:837–844.

28. Zazulia AR, Diringer MN, Videen TO, Aiyagari V, Deibert EM, Powers WJ: Acute intracerebral hemorrhage does not produce peri-clot cerebral ischemia. Neurology 2000; 54(Suppl 3): A261

29. Powers WJ, Zazulia AZ, Videen TO, Dacey RJJr, Grubb RLJr, Diringer MN: Effect of hyperventilation on regional cerebral oxygen metabolism following severe traumatic brain injury. Society of Nuclear Medicine Abstracts, May 2000

30. Powers WJ, Press GA, Grubb RL, Jr., Gado M, Raichle ME. The effect of hemodynamically significant carotid artery disease on the hemodynamic status of the cerebral circulation. Ann Int Med 1987; 106:27–35.

31. Powers WJ, Tempel LW, Grubb RL, Jr. Influence of cerebral hemodynamics on stroke risk: One–year follow–up of 30 medically treated patients. Ann Neurol 1989; 25:325–330.

32. Grubb RLJr, Derdeyn CP, Fritsch SM, Carpenter DA, Yundt KD, Videen TO, Spitznagel EL, Powers WJ: The importance of hemodynamic factors in the prognosis of symptomatic carotid occlusion. JAMA 1998; 280:1055–1060.

Section IV:
Current Status of Clinical Trials
in Acute Stroke

Thrombolysis for Acute Stroke

L.R. Wechsler

Introduction

Trials of intravenous thrombolytic agents in acute stroke date back to the early 1960s. At that time, several trials of streptokinase, fibrinolysin and urokinase were performed and demonstrated either no effect or higher mortality in patients treated with thrombolysis [1–3]. Because these studies preceded CT scanning, patients with hemorrhage were not necessarily excluded. The discouraging results inhibited further acute stroke trials until the 1980 s when several reports appeared showing favorable outcomes with local intra-arterial thrombolytic therapy within a few hours of stroke onset [4, 5]. These reports renewed interest in thrombolysis and led to several feasibility studies and small randomized trials of intravenous thrombolysis [6, 7]. In 1995 the results of the National Institute of Neurological Disorders and Stroke (NINDS) intravenous tPA study, a multicenter, randomized, controlled trial of intravenous tPA for acute ischemic stroke, were published, demonstrating for the first time a beneficial effect of acute stroke treatment when given within three hours of onset [8] (Table 1).

Intravenous Thrombolysis

The NINDS acute stroke study included over 600 patients with acute ischemic stroke within 3 hours of onset [8]. Half of the patients were treated within 90 minutes. Patients were randomly assigned to receive either intravenous tPA at a dose of 0.9 mg/kg up to a maximum of 90 mg, or intravenous placebo. Primary outcome measures consisted of favorable outcomes at 90 days measured by a combination of the NIH stroke scale, Barthel Index, Glasgow outcome scale, and Rankin Scale. By all four measures, significantly more patients had a favorable outcome at 90 days in the tPA group when compared with the placebo group. Intracerebral hemorrhage (ICH) with clinical deterioration occurred in 6.4% of tPA-treated patients, but in only 0.6% of placebo patients. Despite the increase in hemorrhages, there was no significant increase in mortality or severe disability in the tPA group when compared with the placebo group. When strokes were classified according to initial impression of stroke subtype, all types had more favorable outcomes with tPA. There were no clear factors that predicted response to tPA [9], but those patients with large strokes (NIHSS >20) and evi-

Table 1. Clinical trials of thrombolytic therapy for stroke

Study	Design	Dose	Time to Rx	Results
ASK	SK v. Pl	1.5 MU	4 hr	No benefit
MAST-I	SK v. Pl	1.5 MU	6 hr	No benefit
MAST-E	SK v. Pl	1.5 MU	6 hr	No benefit
NINDS	IV tPA v. Pl	0.9 mg/kg	3 hr	TPA
ECASS I	IV tPA v. Pl	1.1 mg/kg	6 hr	No benefit
ECASS II	IV tPA v. Pl	0.9 mg/kg	6 hr	No benefit
ATLANTIS A	IV tPA v. Pl	0.9 mg/kg	0–6 hr	No benefit
ATLANTIS B	IV tPA v. Pl	0.9 mg/kg	3–5 hr	No benefit
PROACT	IA r-proUK v. Hep	9 mg	6 hr	r-proUK

dence of early low density or edema on CT had a higher rate of hemorrhage after tPA [10].

The European Cooperative Acute Stroke Study (ECASS) I, was also a blinded, randomized, controlled trial including 620 patients treated with intravenous tPA within 6 hours of stroke onset [11]. This trial differed from the NINDS trial in several important ways. In addition to the longer time window for treatment, ECASS I used a higher tPA dose of 1.1 mg/kg. Patients with early signs of infarction on initial CT, including extensive low density, mass effect, or sulcal effacement, were intended to be excluded. However, many protocol violations occurred, particularly the inclusion of patients with early CT changes. The primary analysis was based upon intent to treat, but a target population was prospectively identified, including only those patients without protocol violations. The primary endpoints were improvement on the Rankin and Barthel Index at 90 days. In the intent-to-treat group, there was no significant difference between the tPA-treated patients and those receiving placebo on either of the primary endpoints. However, in the target population, there was a significant benefit in favor of tPA as evidenced by improvement in the Rankin scale. Mortality was greater in tPA-treated patients, but the difference did not reach statistical significance (17.9% v 12.7%, p=0.08). Intracerebral hemorrhage occurred in 19.8% of those treated with tPA and in 6.5% of patients given placebo (p<0.001). The inclusion of patients with early CT abnormalities contributed to this increased risk.

ECASS II, similar to ECASS I, randomized patients with stroke less than 6 hours from onset to receive either IV tPA at the same dose used in the NINDS trial (0.9 mg/kg) or placebo [12]. A concerted effort was made to avoid the pitfalls of ECASS I by instructing each center on acute interpretation of CT and identification of extensive early low density. Patients with low density areas exceeding one-third of the MCA territory were excluded. Despite these additional efforts, no significant benefit from tPA was found in this study, although there was a trend favoring tPA treatment (Rankin = 1–40% tPA, 37% control). The placebo group had fewer events and a better outcome than in the NINDS study. The lower event rate in the placebo group made demonstration of a benefit from tPA more difficult. If the results were analyzed using Rankin of ≤ 2, the study showed a significant benefit in favor of tPA.

However, the prespecified primary outcome was Rankin ≤ 1, and by this measure the difference between groups did not reach statistical significance.

The ATLANTIS trial started as a randomized trial of IV tPA *v* placebo between 0 and 6 hours from stroke onset. Following FDA approval of tPA for treatment of stroke under 3 hours, the entry criteria were modified to include only patients beyond 3 hours, and later 3–5 hours, from stroke onset [13, 14]. No significant difference was found in either the 0–6 hour or 3–5 hour groups between those treated with IV tPA v. placebo in outcome at 30 days or 90 days. Despite the lack of clinical benefit, symptomatic hemorrhages were more frequent in the patients treated with tPA (7% tPA *v* 1% placebo). Overall, these results do not support the use of intravenous tPA beyond 3 hours from stroke onset.

Although only one study clearly demonstrated a benefit, in June 1996, the FDA approved intravenous tPA for treatment of stroke within 3 hours of onset. Since then reports of patients treated with IV tPA both in a community setting and at university centers suggest similar efficacy and safety results as long as the NINDS protocol is used for patient selection [15, 16]. Unfortunately, only a minority of stroke patients arrive at the hospital within the 3-hour time window for intravenous tPA treatment. Hopefully, additional patient and professional education will increase this percentage.

Intra-Arterial Thrombolysis

Intravenous tPA was the first treatment shown to improve outcome from stroke when given within 3 hours of stroke onset. tPA presumably causes lysis of arterial thrombus resulting in reperfusion of ischemic brain. However, the effectiveness of tPA in recanalizing arterial occlusions is not known from intravenous thrombolytic studies since in most cases no angiographic information was obtained. Angiographically-based studies of IV tPA demonstrate recanalization rates of approximately 30% [17, 18]. The probability of recanalization decreases with more proximal location of the occlusion in the arterial circulation [17].

Tomsick et al reported that intravenous tPA was not effective in patients with NIHSS score greater than 10 and a hyperdense middle cerebral artery (MCA) sign when treated within 3 hours of stroke onset [19]. Intra-arterial thrombolysis is an alternative approach that might be more effective for thrombosis of larger intracranial arteries such as the MCA.

Intra-arterial infusion of thrombolytic agents through a catheter placed within a thrombus should allow more direct delivery to the site of occlusion and require less lytic agent with less activation of systemic thrombolytic activity. Unlike the intravenous route in which a fixed weight-based dose is given, intra-arterial therapy allows the amount of lytic agent given to be titrated to the response. When the thrombus is lysed, no additional infusion is needed. In addition, if no thrombus is found at angiography, no lytic agent is administered. This approach also provides documentation of the effectiveness of treatment in terms of angiographic evidence of recanalization.

The major drawback of intra-arterial therapy is the additional time necessary to perform angiography and place a microcatheter into the intracranial circulation.

This requires specialized skills and equipment usually only available at tertiary care hospitals. Patients may need to be transferred from community hospitals, further delaying treatment. Intravenous tPA can be given at many community hospitals without delays for transfer or angiography, thereby greatly reducing the time from stroke onset to start of treatment. However, time to start of treatment is probably not as important as time to arterial recanalization and brain reperfusion. Whether the benefits of direct infusion and visualization of results outweigh the additional time needed for the intra-arterial approach remain to be determined.

The results of previously reported series of patients treated with either local or selective infusion of thrombolytics for the carotid territory demonstrated favorable outcomes in 30 –70% of patients, and, in most studies, recanalization was associated with a greater probability of clinical improvement [4, 20–23]. Similar results were found with infusion in the vertebral-basilar circulation [5]. These anecdotal series suggest a benefit from intra-arterial therapy, but, without appropriate controls, conclusions are limited. However, outcomes in both circulations were improved when compared to previous reports of patients with similar disease, suggesting that a randomized controlled trial was warranted.

The long-term outcome of patients treated with intra-arterial thrombolysis has not been examined in most previous studies that limited follow up to 30 –90 days. We recently studied the longer term outcome of 49 patients treated with intra-arterial urokinase with at least one year of follow-up [24]. Duration of follow-up ranged from 1 to 7 years with a mean of 34 months. Outcome was classified based upon a Barthel index of minimal or no disability (MND) (Barthel 90–100), moderate disability (MD) (Barthel <90, >50), severe disability (SD) (Barthel <50), or dead. At the time of follow up, 22 patients had MND (45%), 4 MD (8%), 4 SD (8%) and 19 died (39%). In those patients with recanalization (n=33), 48% had MND, whereas in those without recanalization (n=16), only 36% had MND. Mortality was greater in the group without recanalization (50% v. 33%), but the small numbers preclude any meaningful statistical analysis.

The Prolyse in Acute Cerebral Thromboembolism study (PROACT) was the first randomized, controlled trial of intra-arterial therapy for acute stroke. Prourokinase (r-proUK) is a single-chain proenzyme that preferentially activates fibrin-bound plasminogen and is converted to two-chain urokinase by locally produced fibrin. These properties provide greater clot specificity than urokinase, as well as local amplification at the site of the thrombus. The PROACT I study randomized patients within 6 hours of stroke onset due to occlusion in the M1 or M2 segment of the MCA to either 6 mg of r-proUK infused directly into the clot or infusion of saline in a similar manner [25]. All patients were also treated with intravenous heparin, although the dose of heparin was reduced during the study because of hemorrhagic complications in the r-proUK group. A total of 26 patients received r-proUK and 14 received placebo infusions. Recanalization occurred in 58% of those treated with r-proUK and in only 14% of patients given placebo. In the group given higher doses of heparin in addition to r-proUK (n=11), the recanalization rate was 82% v. 40% with lower doses of heparin. This suggests a significant augmentation of r-proUK activity by heparin, although hemorrhagic complications were also increased. There was a trend toward greater neurological improvement and more good outcomes with r-proUK, but in this small group of patients the difference did not reach statistical significance. Mortality was lower in the r-proUK group, but again the difference between groups was not statistically significant.

Based on these encouraging data, PROACT II randomized 180 patients with occlusion of the M1 or M2 segment of the MCA within 6 hours of stroke onset to treatment either with 9 mg of r-proUK and low-dose intravenous heparin (2000u bolus followed by 500u/hr for 4 hours) or low-dose heparin alone [18]. After 90 days, 40% of patients treated with r-proUK reached the primary endpoint of modified Rankin scale $\leq$ 2 compared with 25% of the control group (p=.04). There was a 15% absolute increase in good outcomes with r-proUK. Partial or complete recanalization after 2 hours occurred in 66% of the r-proUK group and in only 18% of the control patients (p<.001). Symptomatic ICH was more common in those treated with r-proUK (10% v. 2% at 24 hours), but there was no significant difference in mortality (25% v 27%). The median time from stroke onset to randomization was 4.7 hours for patients treated with r-proUK. These results indicate that treatment with intra-arterial r-proUK up to 6 hours after stroke onset improves outcome and extends the window for acute stroke therapy from 3 to 6 hours. In addition, the median NIHSS for both the r-proUK and control groups was 17, significantly greater than in any previous thrombolytic trial. Thus intra-arterial therapy appears to be effective not only in a longer time window, but also for patients with more severe clinical deficits due to MCA occlusion.

Combined Intravenous/Intra-Arterial Thrombolysis

A third approach to thrombolysis combines the intravenous and intra-arterial methods. This combination allows immediate initiation of thrombolysis, thereby avoiding the delay of 1 hour or more that is typically necessary for administration of intra-arterial therapy. For patients at centers without interventional capabilities, it also provides a means of starting therapy while transfer to an interventional center is in progress. In these cases, intravenous therapy continues while transport and cerebral arteriography occur. If an arterial thrombosis persists despite intravenous treatment, further thrombolysis can be performed intra-arterially until the thrombus is completely dissolved.

Lewandowski et al reported a small double-blind trial of 35 patients randomized to IV tPA or placebo followed by arteriography and intra-arterial tPA [26]. The intravenous dose of tPA was reduced to 0.6 mg/kg over 30 minutes, and up to 20 mg of tPA was given intra-arterially at a rate of 10 mg/hr. Eleven of 17 patients initially treated with IV tPA had residual thrombus at the time of arteriography. Recanalization was greater in the IV/IA group (partial or complete recanalization 81% IV/IA v 50% placebo/IA). Symptomatic hemorrhage occurred in only 1 placebo/IA patient at 24 hours, but in 2 IV/IA patients after 24 hours. Asymptomatic ICH was also more common in the IV/IA group. Life-threatening systemic bleeding occurred only in the IV/IA group (2 patients). There was no difference between the groups in the primary clinical outcome measure, the proportion of patients improving 7 or more points on the NIHSS, or NIHSS of 0 or 1 at 7 days (24% v 24%). Whether improved recanalization and clinical outcome with combined treatment will be offset by increased bleeding complications is an important issue. A multicenter NIH funded study of combined IV/IA treatment is planned and should provide additional information regarding the efficacy and safety of this promising approach to thrombolytic therapy.

Future Considerations

The technique of intra-arterial therapy is rapidly evolving, but the r-proUK administration in PROACT II probably does not represent the optimal method. This agent was infused over a long time interval (2 hours), and mechanical disruption of the clot was not permitted. In practice, intra-arterial infusion of thrombolytic agents can be given much more quickly, and manipulation of the clot may help establish recanalization. The optimal agent for intra-arterial thrombolysis and the most effective dose are unknown. Since urokinase was removed from the market and prourokinase is not available, most centers use intra-arterial tPA for thrombolysis. Doses of 20–30 mg are commonly used, but much lower doses may be equally effective. Finally, devices using laser, ultrasound, or high speed saline jets to agitate and lyse intracranial clots have now been developed and are undergoing initial clinical testing. The PROACT study is a beginning for intra-arterial therapy, and we hope that improvements in technique and the addition of devices will further improve recanalization rates, as well as excellent clinical outcomes.

References

1. Meyer JS, Gilroy J, Barnhart MI, al. e. Anticoagulants plus streptokinase therapy in progressive stroke. JAMA 1963;189:373.
2. Meyer JS, Gilroy J, Barnhart MI, Johnson JF. Therapeutic thrombolysis in cerebral thromboembolism. Neurology 1963;13:927–937.
3. Fletcher AP, Alkjaersig N, Lewis M, Tulevski V, Davies A, Brooks JE, Hardin WB, Landau WM, Raichle ME. A pilot study of urokinase therapy in cerebral infarction. Stroke 1976;7:135–42.
4. del Zoppo GJ, Ferbert A, Otis S, Bruckmann H, Hacke W, Zyroff J, Harker LA, Zeumer H. Local intra-arterial fibrinolytic therapy in acute carotid territory stroke. A pilot study. Stroke 1988;19:307–13.
5. Hacke W, Zeumer H, Ferbert A, Bruckmann H, del Zoppo GJ. Intra-arterial thrombolytic therapy improves outcome in patients with acute vertebrobasilar occlusive disease. Stroke 1988;19:1216–22.
6. Mori E, Yoneda Y, Tabuchi M, Yoshida T, Ohkawa S, Ohsumi Y, Kitano K, Tsutsumi A, Yamadori A. Intravenous recombinant tissue plasminogen activator in acute carotid artery territory stroke [see comments]. Neurology 1992;42:976–82.
7. Haley EC, Jr., Brott TG, Sheppard GL, Barsan W, Broderick J, Marler JR, Kongable GL, Spilker J, Massey S, Hansen CA, et al. Pilot randomized trial of tissue plasminogen activator in acute ischemic stroke. The TPA Bridging Study Group. Stroke 1993;24:1000–4.
8. Tissue plasminogen activator for acute ischemic stroke. The National Institute of Neurological Disorders and Stroke rt-PA Stroke Study Group. N Engl J Med 1995;333:1581–7.
9. Generalized efficacy of t-PA for acute stroke. Subgroup analysis of the NINDS t-PA Stroke Trial. Stroke 1997;28:2119–25.
10. Intracerebral hemorrhage after intravenous t-PA therapy for ischemic stroke. The NINDS t-PA Stroke Study Group. Stroke 1997;28:2109–18.
11. Hacke W, Kaste M, Fieschi C, Toni D, Lesaffre E, von Kummer R, Boysen G, Bluhmki E, Hoxter G, Mahagne MH, et al. Intravenous thrombolysis with recombinant tissue plasminogen

activator for acute hemispheric stroke. The European Cooperative Acute Stroke Study (ECASS) [see comments]. Jama 1995;274:1017–25.

12. Hacke W, Kaste M, Fieschi C, von Kummer R, Davalos A, Meier D, Larrue V, Bluhmki E, Davis S, Donnan G, Schneider D, Diez-Tejedor E, Trouillas P. Randomised double-blind placebo-controlled trial of thrombolytic therapy with intravenous alteplase in acute ischaemic stroke (ECASS II). Second European-Australasian Acute Stroke Study Investigators [see comments]. Lancet 1998;352:1245–51.

13. Clark WM, Wissman S, Albers GW, Jhamandas JH, Madden KP, Hamilton S. Recombinant tissue-type plasminogen activator (Alteplase) for ischemic stroke 3 to 5 hours after symptom onset. The ATLANTIS Study: a randomized controlled trial. Alteplase Thrombolysis for Acute Noninterventional Therapy in Ischemic Stroke [see comments]. Jama 1999;282:2019–26.

14. Clark WM, Albers GW, Madden KP, Hamilton S. The rtPA (alteplase) 0- to 6-hour acute stroke trial, part A (A0276 g) : results of a double-blind, placebo-controlled, multicenter study. Thromblytic therapy in acute ischemic stroke study investigators. Stroke 2000;31:811–6.

15. Chiu D, Krieger D, Villar-Cordova C, Kasner SE, Morgenstern LB, Bratina PL, Yatsu FM, Grotta JC. Intravenous tissue plasminogen activator for acute ischemic stroke: feasibility, safety, and efficacy in the first year of clinical practice [see comments]. Stroke 1998;29:18–22.

16. Albers GW, Bates VE, Clark WM, Bell R, Verro P, Hamilton SA. Intravenous tissue-type plasminogen activator for treatment of acute stroke: the Standard Treatment with Alteplase to Reverse Stroke (STARS) study [see comments]. Jama 2000;283:1145–50.

17. Wolpert SM, Bruckmann H, Greenlee R, Wechsler L, Pessin MS, del Zoppo GJ. Neuroradiologic evaluation of patients with acute stroke treated with recombinant tissue plasminogen activator. The rt-PA Acute Stroke Study Group [see comments]. AJNR Am J Neuroradiol 1993;14:3–13.

18. Furlan A, Higashida R, Wechsler L, Gent M, Rowley H, Kase C, Pessin M, Ahuja A, Callahan F, Clark WM, Silver F, Rivera F. Intra-arterial prourokinase for acute ischemic stroke. The PROACT II study: a randomized controlled trial. Prolyse in Acute Cerebral Thromboembolism [see comment]. Jama 1999;282:2003–11.

19. Tomsick T, Brott T, Barsan W, Broderick J, Haley EC, Spilker J, Khoury J. Prognostic value of the hyperdense middle cerebral artery sign and stroke scale score before ultraearly thrombolytic therapy. AJNR Am J Neuroradiol 1996;17:79–85.

20. Zeumer H, Freitag HJ, Zanella F, Thie A, Arning C. Local intra-arterial fibrinolytic therapy in patients with stroke: urokinase versus recombinant tissue plasminogen activator (r-TPA). Neuroradiology 1993;35:159–62.

21. Sasaki O, Takeuchi S, Koike T, Koizumi T, Tanaka R. Fibrinolytic therapy for acute embolic stroke: intravenous, intracarotid, and intra-arterial local approaches. Neurosurgery 1995;36:246–52; discussion 252–3.

22. Mori E, Tabuchi M, Yoshida T, Yamadori A. Intracarotid urokinase with thromboembolic occlusion of the middle cerebral artery. Stroke 1988;19:802–12.

23. Barnwell SL, Clark WM, Nguyen TT, O'Neill OR, Wynn ML, Coull BM. Safety and efficacy of delayed intraarterial urokinase therapy with mechanical clot disruption for thromboembolic stroke. AJNR Am J Neuroradiol 1994;15:1817–22.

24. Wechsler LR, Junreis CA, Massaro LM, Wehner JJ, Knepper LE, Yonas H, Kaufman AM, Barch CA, Johnson DW. Long term followup of patients treated with intaarterial urokinase for acute stroke. Stroke 1998;29:303.

25. del Zoppo GJ, Higashida RT, Furlan AJ, Pessin MS, Rowley HA, Gent M. PROACT: a phase II randomized trial of recombinant pro-urokinase by direct arterial delivery in acute middle cerebral artery stroke. PROACT Investigators. Prolyse in Acute Cerebral Thromboembolism [see comments]. Stroke 1998;29:4–11.

26. Lewandowski CA, Frankel M, Tomsick TA, Broderick J, Frey J, Clark W, Starkman S, Grotta J, Spilker J, Khoury J, Brott T. Combined intravenous and intra-arterial r-TPA versus intra-arterial therapy of acute ischemic stroke: Emergency Management of Stroke (EMS) Bridging Trial. Stroke 1999;30:2598–605.

Neuroprotective Stroke Trials: A Ten Year Dry Season

A.M. Buchan

Introduction

For stroke patients presenting within 3 hours of a significant hemispheric ischemic stroke, thrombolysis induced by the administration of exogenous tPA will reduce death and disability [1]. For every thousand stroke patients treated, an additional 160 will recover to an independent status within three months. The data for patients treated between three and six hours suggests there may be a signal of efficacy but neither the clinical trials [2] nor the meta-analysis has yet to give us a robust answer [3]. The fact that patients benefit within three hours, but not between three and six, is not because of an excess of hemorrhages in the three to six hour group [3], but because of a lack of cell recovery following brain resuscitation with delayed reperfusion. Simply stated the reperfusion is too late. While the best neuroprotectant will always be the rapid return of oxygen and glucose, the fact that attempts to restore circulation within the first three hours are highly effective confirms the concept that reperfusion will salvage brain tissue. A successful neuroprotectant must either increase the time window to allow more patients to be effectively reperfused, perhaps up to six hours, or reduce the injury sustained during ischemia. In the event that reperfusion is injurious, it must reduce not only the initial reperfusion injury but also sustain cells which are left ailing in the hours and days that follow successful reperfusion.

Neuroprotective evidence is sought first in models of cell culture exposed to either anoxia or glutamate insults and then developed in rodent models of both global and focal ischemia. The evidence that neuroprotection works is based on *in vivo* models of focal stroke, largely using mice and rats. This paper will review the background of the models, will overview the theory of neuroprotection and the experimental and clinical data that can be drawn for the various agents which have gone to Phase III clinical trials.

A recurrent theme will be that, in the animal models, a lack of physiological control may have led to spurious results [4]. In the clinical trials there have also been physiological perturbations which may have resulted in deleterious side effects either leading to excess toxicity or causing futility in terms of improving outcome.

A second major problem has been the difficulty of achieving drug levels in humans comparable to those that were equated with neuroprotection in animal models. A third difficulty is that in the animal models a slow maturation of injury following the first few days may account for observed "neuroprotection" which in reality is only a postponement of injury [5]. In humans where three month outcomes are the gold standard, any early neuroprotection may have evaporated as the injury slowly matures.

Neuroprotection in Animal Models

Agents demonstrated to protect cells drawn from cell lines or primary cell culture have been taken forward into models of both global and focal ischemia. Two models of global or severe forebrain ischemia are used in the rat: the 4-VO transient severe forebrain ischemia model [6, 7] and the 2-VO plus hypotension model [8]. Both have been used to examine selective CA_1 death.

These models, when properly used, create a transient oligaemia (no blood flow) to the hippocampus, cortex and striatum during ischemia and are then followed by a prompt recovery of both flow and energy (ATP) after 5, 10, 15 or even 30 minutes of transient forebrain ischemia [9]. The ischemic insult although brief is very severe, and drugs, if given following reperfusion, cannot influence the degree of blood flow during the ischemic insult. The use of hypothermia even 6 to 24 hours after reperfusion allows for long-term recovery of cells [10]. There appears to be a fairly prolonged interval of depressed energy in the hippocampal neurons prior to cell death. Given the extraordinary sensitivity of CA_1 cells *vis a ` vis* CA_3 cells, any agent that reverses this selective vulnerability can be defined as a neuroprotectant. *Drugs which prevent CA_1 cell death (cytoprotective) are logically taken forward, to see if they attenuate cortical and striatal injury (brain protection) following either permanent or transient focal ischemia.*

Models of focal ischemia generally use either a suture, which induces severe ischemia in the striatum and relatively milder ischemia in the cortex, or a more distal clip, which spares the striatum but results in more severe cortical ischemia [11]. These vascular occlusions can be either permanent or transient [12]. The striatum undergoes fairly rapid necrosis and then there is a gradual recruitment of the cortex to the infarct, the speed of which depends on the duration of the ischemic insult [13]. Much of the cortex will receive at least partial recovery of cerebral blood flow from collaterals. Transient models are less severe as are the models which employ either a clip or a ligation of the artery in the rhinal fissure, and result in a different pattern of injury. Distal models can be engineered to produce cortical injury only [13]. With permanent ischemia, a fairly generous infarct evolves over 24 hours. In reperfusion models transient ischemia results in less injury, if a critical ischemic threshold is exceeded then the infarct volume in the cortex will mature over time, ultimately achieving the same volume of infarction as that seen with a permanent occlusion [14]. The infarction in the cortex is associated with a breakdown in the blood brain barrier, an inflammatory response and edema causing swelling. The process of necrosis, components of apoptosis and a neuro inflammatory reaction all work in parallel, resulting in the full evolution of the infarct.

It is worth pointing out that in lissencephalic species such as mice and rats there is very little white matter, the striatum is very hard to protect, and while 50% infarct volume reductions are often seen, this reduction in injury may not be static. In the same way that brief ischemia results in less infarction, if a longer interval is allowed to elapse this small infarct will recruit the penumbral zones. It remains to be proven, in many instances, when infarct volume reductions are seen at 24 or 48 hours, whether this protection can be maintained out to 7–28 days or even three months, which is the standard follow-up period to assess recovery in patients in neuroprotective trials.

Neuroprotection in the rat ideally should involve cytoprotection of CA_1 cells following transient forebrain ischemia. It should result in lasting cortical protection, which should be translated to reductions in focal infarction, which must also be lasting. While it is very difficult to protect the striatum, a lasting cortical infarct volume reduction would be enough to warrant development of clinical trials, assuming comparable drug levels needed to protect the rat can be achieved in the clinic.

The Biology of Cell Death

Much has been written about ischemia in terms of the critical reductions in cerebral blood flow and levels which result in the inhibition of protein synthesis, the loss of membrane potential, the loss of high energy ATP and terminal anoxic depolarization. Energy failure is clearly a prerequisite to cell loss. In humans, using PET metabolic imaging, it is possible to examine regions where there may be increased oxygen utilization (CMRO2) suggesting potentially critical hypoperfusion (misery perfusion). Much of the data from the animal kingdom with respect to neuroprotectants is derived from severely ischemic tissue where there is a loss of all electric potential, a loss of energy and a loss of protein synthesis. A penumbra must be defined as an area in which there is still residual energy but protein synthesis is inhibited (see Hossman in this volume). The recruitment of the penumbra to the infarct relates to a secondary failure of energy with a secondary loss of ion homeostasis followed by activation of either apoptotic or inflammatory pathways.

From the global models it is clear that both the loss of energy and the loss of ion homeostasis is recoverable [9]. The reasons for a secondary decline in energy and ion homeostasis are not fully understood. The acute insult is associated with a massive release of glutamate. Calcium entering the N-type calcium channels promotes the synaptic release of glutamate, which in turn will have action on the post-synaptic glutamate receptors namely the NMDA, AMPA and the metabotropic receptor [15]. The NMDA receptor has been much studied and drugs have been developed which act on the glutamate site, the ion channel, and the polyamine and glycine modulatory sites. During depolarization there is a release of the magnesium block of the channel and glutamate in conjunction with glycine and polyamine will stimulate calcium entry into post-synaptic neurons through the NMDA channel. The AMPA channel was initially thought to be less significant, as it gates sodium rather than calcium, but evidence from the sub-unit examination of the heteromeric channel receptor complex suggests that following ischemia, there is a loss of GluR2, making the post-ischemic AMPA channel highly conductive of calcium [16]. The metabotropic receptor, by stimulating second messengers, may activate events in a similar way to calcium entry, resulting in endogenous release of high levels of intracellular calcium.

The corollary is that inhibitory receptors such as serotonin and the GABA A receptors when stimulated will abrogate the levels of calcium seen in the intracellular compartment.

High levels of calcium, which can injure mitochondria releasing cytochrome C [17] which initiates apoptotic pathways [14], can also stimulate enzymes resulting in lipolysis, proteolysis and endonuclease activation, which will also result in apoptosis. Calcium, which is said to hold "centre stage" [15], activates death processes, and so the hope was that by preventing calcium influx the multitude of downstream events could be arrested prior to the initiation of a multitude of injurious parallel pathways. If one pathway is inhibited it may have resulted in increased activity of another, so caution must be exercised.

Most of the clinical trials have tested the hypothesis that NMDA antagonism, either non-competitively or by blocking the glycine or polyamine sites, would reduce clinical injury and result in better neurological outcomes at three months.

Neuro-Protective Trials

The trials of antagonists to the excitotoxicity pathway (mainly NMDA antagonists) will be reviewed in terms of the specific mechanism of action of the compound, the pre-clinical data as it reflects CA_1 protection, focal infarct reduction, and, in particular, the dose of the drug required to produce a 30–50% infarct volume. The therapeutic temporal thresholds are important, in terms of how quickly following ischemia the drug has to be infused to achieve the effect. Toxicity will be discussed as it pertains to the animal models, as well as the known human toxicity in Phase I and II trials. In those trials that went to Phase III, discussion will be made about the reason for failure of the pivotal trial as it has currently been reported. Trials which block downstream events will similarly be discussed. These include drugs which stabilize membranes, reduce free radicals, promote recovery through cytokine action, and work as inhibitors of inflammatory secondary injury.

MK-801 (Dizoclopine)

MK-801 is the prototypic neuroprotectant. It is a powerful non-competitive NMDA antagonist which, in early studies, appeared to dramatically prevent CA_1 injury [18] and to reduce volumes of focal infarction provided that it was given either as a pre-treatment or during ischemia [19]. Further experiments demonstrated its cytoprotective abilities hinged on the co-concurrent hypothermia seen in the comatose period following transient forebrain ischemia [4, 20], and in its ability to enhance cerebral blood flow through vasodilatory mechanisms [21]. The drug had side effects in the animals and one early concern was its ability to induce psychotomimetic effects in animals associated with a tachycardia and hyperglycemia. The observation that there were neuronal vacuoles in both ischemic treated and naïve animals raised serious concern within the regulatory agencies [22]. Nevertheless, clinical trails were initiated, although the development was discontinued at the Phase II level, largely because the psychotomimetic side effects and the need to give Labetalol to control heart rate and blood pressure as it induced vascular instability [23].

CGS-19755 (Selfotil)

The competitive NMDA antagonist CGS-19755 was never clearly shown to prevent CA_1 cell death. It appeared to produce focal protection in cortex but never striatum (as with MK-801), but only if it was given during ischemia in transient models and early (within an hour of occlusion) in permanent models [24]. Once again there was data to suggest that changes in blood flow may well have accounted for reductions in focal infarct volume [25].

The drug had poor blood brain barrier penetration [25] but enough of the drug clearly got into the nervous system to account for the agitation and delirium seen in not only Phase II, but also Phase III trials [26, 27].

The clinical trials were suspended because of the psychotic behavior of the treated patients, but despite demonstrating brain penetration of the agent, no effect was demonstrable in the treated patients compared to controls regardless of a reasonable sample size [26]. One of the reasons for this may be that in the rat the drug dose to achieve a 30%–50% reduction in infarct size (the IC50) was 10 mg/kg, while the maximal tolerated dose achieved in the human was 2 mg/kg, ie. a TI of 0.2. *Despite reaching high levels in a head injury trial, CGS-19755 failed to improve outcome following trauma* [28].

Table 1. Clinical trials for acute stroke treatment

Drugs to Improve Blood Flow
  Anti-thrombotic
    Heparin
    Nadroparin (Low molecular weight heparin)
    Tinzaparin (Low molecular weight heparin)
    Danaparoid (Low molecular weight heparinoid, Org 10172)
  Anti-platelet
    Aspirin
    Abciximab
  Fibrinogen depleting
    Ancrod
  Improve capillary flow
    Pentoxuylline
  Thrombolytics
    Pro-urokinase
    Tissue plasminogen activator
    Streptokinase
    Urokinase
Drugs to Protect Brain Tissue (neuroprotective agents)
  Glutamate agonists
    AMPA antagonists
    GYKI 52466
    NBQX
    YM90K
    YM872
    ZK-200775 (MPQX)
  Kainate antagonist
    SYM 2081

Table 1. *Continued*

NMDA antagonists
  Competitive NMDA antagonists
    CGS 19755 (Selfotel)
  NMDA channel blockers
    Aptiganel (Cerestat)
    Dextrorphan
    Dextromethorphan
    Magnesium
    Memantine
    MK-801
    NPS 1506
    Remacemide
    AR-R15896AR
    HU-211
  Glycine site antagonists
    ACEA 1021
    GV150526
  Polyamine site antagonists
    Eliprodil
    Ifenprodil
Free radical scavengers – Antioxidants
  Ebselen
  Tirilazad
  NXY-059
Growth factors
  Fibroblast growth factor (bFGF)
Leukocyte adhesion inhibitor
  Anti-ICAM antibody (Enlimomab)
  Hu23F2G
Nitric Oxide Inhibitor
  Lubeluzole
Opioid antagonists
  Naloxene
  Nalmefene
Phosphatidylcholine precursor
  Citicholine (CDP-choline)
Serotonin agonists
  Bay X 3072
Sodium channel blockers
  Fosphenytoin
  Lubeluzole
  619C89
Calcium channel blockers
  Nimodipine
  Flunarizine
GABA agonists
  Clomethiazole
Potassium channel opener
  BMS-204352

CNS1102 (Cerostat)

The non-competitive NMDA antagonist CNS1102 again demonstrated no CA_1 protection, but with a dose of 0.25 mg/kg achieved a 50% infarct volume reduction, provided it was given during early ischemia [29]. There were problems at Phase II with side effects and elevations of blood pressure. The dose settled on in the Phase III study was limited to 0.03 mg/kg, giving it a TI of 0.125. Six hundred and twenty-eight patients were randomized in the Phase III trial before it was suspended; no efficacy was demonstrated [30]. The traumatic brain injury trial went on longer because it was possible to give a much higher dose ($16\times0.03=0.48$ mg/kg) to ventilated ICU patients who were far more physiologically easy to stabilize and would not have noticed the psychotomimetic side effects. This trial was also negative [31].

Eliprodil

Eliprodil was a non-competitive NMDA antagonist acting on the polyamine side which, while demonstrating no CA_1 protection in forebrain ischemia, did result in infarct volume reduction in the wide range of species climbing the phylogenetic tree: from mouse to rat to cat to primate. In the rat, doses of 1 mg/kg, achieved a 30–40% infarct volume reduction [32]. Because of cardiovascular side effects, including a prolonged QT interval, the maximum dose achieved in humans was 0.1 mg/kg, giving it a TI of 0.1 [32].

Clinical trials were discontinued because of lack of effects through futility analysis and because of the risk of prolongation of the QT interval [33].

Lubeluzole – Prosynap

Janssen, while initially purporting Lubeluzole to be an NMDA antagonist, concluded at the time of the clinical trials that Lubeluzole inhibited glutamate mediated nitric oxide, or NO, toxicity. CA_1 protection was never disclosed, but robust focal infarct volume reductions were achieved and at Phase II this compound was felt to have a good safety profile. The drug had to be given early during ischemia and, although rat doses to achieve infarct volume reductions were 5 mg/kg, the maximum human dose was 0.1 mg/kg, giving it the lowest TI of any of the neuroprotectants tested at Phase IIII, at 0.02 [34].

LUB-INT 9, which was performed in the U.S., showed a non-significant reduction in mortality from 26% to 21% [34]. The European study, LUB-INT 5, was entirely negative [35], but a meta-analysis of the "target group" suggested that mortality was reduced from 20% to 14%, so LUB-INT 13 was launched to study whether or not, in moderate to severe stroke, mortality could be reduced [34,35]. Despite early attempts to obtain licensing for this compound through the FDA, the program was discontinued in June 1998. More recently, studies in which Lubeluzole was combined with tPA, with tPA being given within 3 hours and Lubeluzole shortly after, also demonstrated no efficacy in what is the first clinical thrombolysis plus neuroprotectant clinical trial [36].

GV150256 – GAIN Trials

The Glaxo Wellcome GAIN trials were performed with a glycine antagonist, GV150256 [37]. This compound antagonized the allosteric site of the NMDA receptor [38]. These extremely well conducted trials were performed in both Europe and America in the so-called GAIN trials (GAIN and GAIN-Americas) [37, 39]. Initial concerns about cholestasis were overcome [37]. The in-house dose required to produce a 30–40% infarct volume reduction of 10 mg/kg [38] was actually matched in the human, giving it a therapeutic index, at least, by dose of 1 (achieving unity for the first time). Unfortunately, despite achieving doses comparable to that seen with neuroprotection in the rat, the ability of this compound to reduce infarct volume in extramural laboratories was not demonstrated. The trials were completely neutral on both sides of the Atlantic [37, 39]. It is sad that, in the instance of the first drug to achieve levels that might have translated neuroprotection into humans (in well done trials), the neuroprotection in the animal models was not substantiated by an independent laboratory.

Problems with NMDA Antagonists

NMDA antagonists have been the prototypic neuroprotectants. Despite this, they do not protect the white matter (there are no NMDA receptors in white matter) and they have never protected the striatum in experimental focal ischemia. They have never been effective if given late, ie. during reperfusion. In normothermically controlled animals there has never been any cytoprotective effect for CA_1 cells. The focal infarct reductions may in part have related to changes in vasoactivity (increased rCBF), and increases in tachycardia and blood pressure (also resulting in a relative change of cerebral blood flow). The side effects have included cardiotoxicity, psychotomimetic reactions and, of concern to the neuropathologists, the appearance of vacuolations in the limbic cortex in, not only post-ischemic, but also naïve, brain.

AMPA Antagonists

While AMPA antagonists have yet to make it to Phase III clinical trials, they are potent neuroprotectants, which have been demonstrated to both protect CA_1 [40, 41] and to reduce infarct volumes, even when given quite late during reperfusion following transient ischemia or late in the process of permanent focal ischemia [42]. These compounds block either the AMPA channel or the AMPA receptor and, because post-ischemic receptors may be permissive to calcium, they have a good rationale [43]. Of importance, these agents have been given very late, up to 12–24 hours after global ischemia [44] and in the first hour or two after reperfusion following focal ischemia and have still resulted in protection [43]. This protection has not been demonstrated to be indefatigable [5] and although recurrent administration of the drug might result in this, because of the toxicity (mainly nephrotoxicity) [44], these compounds have been stuck in development. The Yamanouchi compound YM-90K now seems poised for clinical development [45].

Given the putative mechanism of action, for these drugs to produce permanent salvage [10] would require the cells to recover their ability to make edited GluR2 [46]. Although this may be possible with hypothermia [10], it has not been demonstrated with neuroprotectants [5]. Continuous administration of the drugs will require a soluble compound; there is hope that soluble AMPA antagonists, which reduce infarct volume, and protect CA_1 cells, are in development [45].

Glutamate Release Blockers

Drugs which block N-type calcium channels, namely derivatives of the conus snail peptide toxins, prevent calcium entering the pre-synaptic bouton and prevent the release of glutamate. Unfortunately, these compounds, although they can protect CA_1 cells [47, 48], many hours, perhaps 24 hours, after global ischemia and during reperfusion following focal ischemia, have side effects resulting from their lack of selectivity. By blocking adrenergic synapses, profound hypotension results [48], which is what ultimately limited the development of L-type calcium channel blockers such as nimodipine in acute stroke. Many stroke patients are hypertensive and drops in blood pressure have precluded the use of this class of drug following cardiac arrest, focal stroke, or in high-risk vascular procedures such as carotid endarterectomy or coronary artery bypass surgery. N-type calcium channel blockade, which can be separated from hypotensive side effects, are an extremely promising approach [49]. An approach which blocks both AMPA and voltage dependent channels might be the most promising avenue [50]. By preventing the excito-toxic cascade at its source, lasting benefit might result. That these drugs can be given late, however, suggests that the initial release of glutamate results in an acquired increased susceptibility to glutamate and, of course, to achieve lasting or "indefatigable" protection, this acquired susceptibility would have to be reversed [46]. If cells become so sensitive to glutamate then, unless the sensitivity reverses, normal neural processing needed for behavioral recovery may not be achieved in either animals or in humans.

Inhibitory Mechanisms

The corollary to blocking excito-toxicity is to agonize inhibitory pathways. The most studied site of action is the GABA A receptor.

Chlomethiazole

GABA A receptors may be up-regulated following ischemia and the drug clomethiazole is a GABA A agonist derived from thiamine. Pre-clinically, although there were initial claims of CA_1 protection [51], this was not confirmed. Early administration of the agent in focal ischemia, be it permanent or transient, resulted in modest infarct volume reductions [52]. The drug is in clinical practice in the U.K.

and is used as an anti-convulsant and as a sedative during alcohol withdrawal. It has a long history of safety. The problem, though, is that it is sedative and while doses of 100 mg/kg were needed to achieve maximal infarct volume reduction, levels of 75 mg/kg have been somewhat toxic in the form of sedation in humans. The largest clinical trial to date with clomethiazole, the CLASS study [53], demonstrated no overall efficacy but there was a promising reduction in death and disability in those presenting with a large stroke ie total anterior cerebral syndrome [54]. Accordingly, a confirmatory study is underway, the CLASS I study, in which patients with total anterior cerebral ischemia only are randomized to cytoprotective doses of clomethiazole. Concurrent studies in which clomethiazole was given to patients with hemorrhage (CLASS H) [55] and to patients getting thrombolysis (CLASS T for tPA) [56] have been negative. The results of the main ischemic stroke study (CLASS I) are expected by December 2000.

Note added in proof: and as predicted from the animal Studies the trial was negative.

Bayer-X3702: Brains

Bayer X3702 which was studied in the Brain Study Phase II study also examined safety. This 5HT agonist acts on the 5HT 1 A receptor. Preclinically, although no CA_1 protection was seen, infarct volume reductions were demonstrated. In terms of development the biggest problem has been its interaction with a myriad of compounds used in stroke patients for blood pressure control, depression, [57] etc. The BRAINS study examined 200 patients and showed reasonable safety at drug levels which approximated those given to rats to achieve infarct volume reduction. A Phase III study is now planned for the fourth quarter of 2000, but one of the problems has been a need to perform bedside monitoring of the "drug levels" to see which patients metabolize the compound and which do not. For those patients who do not, the drug has to be withdrawn. There has been no evidence of sedation or increased broncho-pulmonary secretions which might have been predicted from the serotonergic mechanism of action.

BMS – The Post Study

Bristol Myers Squibb are currently testing a potassium channel agonist which is in a Phase III clinical trial, the "POST" study. Although there is no evidence for CA_1 protection, there is evidence of focal infarct volume reduction and levels have been achieved in the absence of toxicity. The drug is being studied in cortical infarction and is distinctly different from many of the studies which included lacunar stroke and patients with sub-cortical ischemia. The rationale for this, of course, is that in the animal models protection was seen in the cortex and not the striatum.

In patients co-concurrently receiving tPA there has been no excess risk of hemorrhage in those randomized to receive the potassium channel agonist, compared with placebo.

Results reported in the second quarter of 2001, were negative.

Downstream Events

Following the loss of energy in the form of ATP, the depolarization and the transient acidosis, recovery is associated with a variety of putative mechanisms of maturation of the injury. These include parallel pathways: a stimulation of apoptotic pathways, free radical mediated injury, a loss of membrane stability, and a loss of cytokine activity. During or following cell death there is evidence (causal or secondary) for a deleterious neuro-inflammatory response. Agents have therefore been developed which test most of these putative mechanisms.

U74006F – (Tirilazad)

This 21 amino steroid is a lipid peroxidation inhibitor and thereby acts as a free radical scavenger [58]. Pre-clinically, early claims of CA_1 protection were not confirmed [59], but focal infarction was reduced in transient focal ischemia, but not permanent ischemia [60]. That it would be more effective in transient or reperfusion ischemia is logical, given that it was blocking lipid peroxidation and the exposure to oxygen-derived free radicals.

Extensive clinical trials have been done despite the fact that this drug is somewhat insoluble and certainly in a sub-arachnoid hemorrhage trial there was evidence for protection in men, but not women [58]. A series of trials were performed but the most recent trial, Ranitas, was negative, and the subsequent Ranitas II was canceled because of lack of efficacy [58].

There is hope that the spin trap nitrone derivative from PBN [61], NXY-059, which appears to protect after really quite prolonged delays, one to two hours after transient focal ischemia, may proceed to Phase III clinical trials [62, 63]. Interestingly, the dose given at Phase II has far exceeded that which was needed to reduce infarct volume in the rat.

Cytokines – Fiblast

The Fiblast cytokine b-FGF, failed to protect CA_1 cells, but did reduce infarct volume. Pre-clinically there were suggestions of vasodilation, which were confirmed in humans, and the drug was suspended after the randomization of approximately 1800 patients with a six hour window [64]. The vasodilatory effects caused side effects in patients and, through a similar mechanism of action, that could have accounted for the focal infarct volume reduction in the rodents.

ICAM-1 – Enlimomab

The use of the first monoclonal antibody against ICAMs was studied in a trial known as the Enlimomab study. This human ICAM receptor antibody was, in fact, a murine antibody that was developed and shown to be neuroprotective [65]. The Phase III study of 625 patients, treated in under six hours, resulted in only half the number recovering with treatment as those recovered after placebo. There was also an excess rate of death in the treatment group. There was serious concern that this murine-derived antibody aggravated inflammatory responses [65]. There appeared to be fever, but analysis of those patients with a fever suggested that, in those patients, but not afebrile patients, there was some benefit. It is possible that relevant quantities of the antibody were associated with fever. The sequel to this trial, the ICOS trial, has also been discontinued for reasons which are as yet not apparent. The ICOS trial used a humanized ICAM antibody and was discontinued prematurely some months ago.

Citicholine

Citicholine is essentially phosphatidyl choline, used as a membrane stabilizer. It affords some evidence of focal infarct volume reduction. One of the problems was that the high doses needed to reduce infarction in the rat, induced human side effects which included dizziness, hypotension and the risk of falls. Nevertheless, trials went ahead; initial studies of 500 mg doses looked like they were optimal but, on close analysis of the early trials, it appears that the 500 mg group (with the most benefit) had the lowest glucose concentrations compared with those in the 1,000 or 1,500 mg groups [66]. The Phase III trial has now been completed with 2,000 mg doses, but the trial failed to achieve significant benefit. Of great importance is that in both the Phase II and Phase III trials there was evidence for cytoprotection in an MRI sub-study. In patients studied with MR, using diffusion (DWI) and perfusion (PWI) weighted imaging and analyzed for a mismatch, those treated with Citicholine had less progression of their predicted infarct than those treated with placebo [67]. Not only were the groups different, but patients, using their own baseline scans (and mismatch) as their own controls, clearly benefited by the drug treatment, while placebo treatment had no effect. The failure to translate this surrogate effect to a clinical effect raises many questions for the conduct of future trials.

For the first time it looks as though the rodent effect was translated to a human effect, ie. "the rat experiment done in man" [67], which raises the question as to why this did not predict or correlate with a positive clinical trial outcome. It would be important to know if those patients who had smaller infarcts as a result of treatment also had behavioral benefit, given that the clinically relevant outcome has to be one of recovery to either independence or improvements in activities of daily living. It suggests a great deal of concern regarding the validity of the outcome of trials as they are now conducted.

Summary

In summary, for a drug to be effective, the *in vitro* protection must be translated to studies of both global, cellular neuroprotection (cytoprotection) and focal ischemia parenchymal neuroprotection(infarct reduction or brain protection). Drug levels that suggest that the mechanism is active, in vitro, must result in infarct volume reductions, in vivo, which are sustained (indefatigable) and initiation of therapy should be delayed in order to be clinically relevant. Most importantly, the "effective dose" plasma level reached in rodents to achieve the neuroprotective effect must be matched in humans in the absence of toxicity.

There are a number of problems with "cytoprotective drugs" to date – in rats, in particular, their inability to protect white matter and striatum. The dose in rats is rarely achieved in humans.

In humans, the study design appears to be inadequate but one of the things which is recurrently apparent is that, although toxicity has stopped much of the development in those trials which have been completed, there have been difficulties with fever, glucose, changes in blood pressure, changes in blood flow, and above all, an inability to get concentrations of drug into patients that approximate those needed to reduce infarct volume in the rat. The ability to reduce injury as measured by a surrogate MRI market while failing to achieve a functional result has raised many questions about the conduct of future trials.

References

1. National Institute of Neurological Disorders and Stroke rt-PA Stroke Study Group. Tissue plasminogen activator for acute ischemic stroke. New England Journal of Medicine 1995; 333:1581–1587.
2. Hacke W, Kaste M, Fieschi C, et al. Randomised double blind placebo-controlled trial of thrombolytic therapy with intravenous alteplase in acute stroke (ECASS II). Lancet 1998; 352:1245–1251.
3. Wardlaw JM, Yamaguchi T, del Zoppo G. Thrombolytic therapy versus control in acute ischaemic stroke. Stroke module of the Cochrane Database of Systematic Reviews. Available in the Cochrane Library (database on disk and CDROM). Oxford: Update software, 1999.
4. Buchan AM, Pulsinelli WA. Hypothermia but not the N-methyl-D-aspartate antagonist, MK-801, attenuates neuronal damage in gerbils subjected to transient global ischemia. J Neurosci 1990;10:311–316.
5. Colbourne F, Li H, Buchan AM. Continuing post-ischemic neuronal death in CA1: Influence of ischemia duration, and cytoprotective doses of NBQX and SNX-111. Stroke 1999;30:662–668.
6. Pulsinelli WA, Brierly JB. A new model of bilateral hemispheric ischemia in the unanesthetized rat. Stroke 1979;10:267–272.
7. Pulsinelli WA, Buchan AM. The four-vessel occlusion rat model: method for complete occlusion of vertebral arteries and control of collateral circulation. Stroke 1988;19:913–914.
8. Smith ML, Bendek G, Dahlgren N, Rosen I, Wieloch T, Siesjo BK. Models for studying long-term recovery following forebrain ischemia in the rat. 2. A 2-vessel occlusion model. Acta Neurol Scand 1984;69;385–401.
9. Pulsinelli WA, Duffy TE. Regional energy balance in rat brain after transient forebrain ischemia. J Neurochem 1983;40:1500–1503.
10. Colbourne F, Li H, Buchan AM. Indefatigable CA1 sector neuroprotection with mild hypothermia induced 6 hours after severe forebrain ischemia in rats. J Cereb Blood Flow Metab 1999;19:742–749.
11. Buchan AM, Xue D, Slivka A. A new model of temporary focal neocortical ischemia in the rat. Stroke 1992;23:273–279.
12. Kaplan B, Brint S, Tanabe J, Jacewicz M, Wang XJ, Pulsinelli W. Temporal thresholds for neocortical infarction in rats subjected to reversible focal cerebral ischemia. Stroke 1991; 22:1032–1039.

13. Li H, Sun P, Buchan AM. Maturation of ischemic neuronal death following focal cerebral ischemia. Stroke 2000;31:275

14. Li H, Colbourne F, Sun P, Zhao Z, Buchan AM. Caspase inhibitors reduce neuronal injury after focal but not global cerebral ischemia in rats. Stroke 2000:31:176–182.

15. Choi DW. Calcium-mediated neurotoxicity: relationship to specific channel types and role in ischemic damage. Trends Neurosci 1988;11:465–469.

16. Pellegrini-Giampietro DE, Zukin RS, Bennett MVL, Cho S, Pulsinelli WA. Switch in glutamate receptor subunit gene expression in CA_1 subfield of hippocampus following global ischemia in rats. Proc Natl Acad Sci USA 1992;89:10499–10503.

17. Sugawara T, Fujimura M, Morita-Fujimura Y, Kawase M, Chan PH. Mitochondrial release of cytochrome c corresponds to the selective vulnerability of hippocampal CA1 neurons in rats after transient global cerebral ischemia. J Neurosci 1999:19:39

18. Gill R, Foster AC, Woodruff GN. Systematic administration of MK-801 protects against ischemia-induced hippocampal neurodegeneration in the gerbil. J Neurosci 1987;7:3343–3349.

19. Park CK, Nehls DG, Graham DI, Teasdale GM, McCulloch J. Focal cerebral ischemia in the cat: treatment with the glutamate antagonist MK-801 after induction of ischaemia. J Cereb Blood Flow Metab 1988;8:757–762.

20. Buchan AM, Li H, Pulsinelli WA. The N-methyl-D-aspartate antagonist, MK-801, fails to protect against neuronal damage caused by transient severe forebrain ischemia in adult rats. J Neurosci 1991;11:1049–1056.

21. Buchan AM, Slivka A, Xue D. The effect of the NMDA receptor antagonist MK-801 on cerebral blood flow and infarct volume in experimental focal stroke. Brain Res 1992;574:171–177.

22. Olney JW, Labruyere J, Price MT. Pathological changes induced in cerebrocortical neurons by phencyclidine and related drugs. Science 1990;244:1360–1362.

23. Buchan AM. Do NMDA antagonists protect against cerebral ischemia: are clinical trials warranted? Cerebrovas Brain Metab Rev 1990;2:1–26.

24. Simon R, Shiraishi K. N-methyl-D-aspartate antagonist reduces stroke size and regional glucose metabolism. Ann Neurol 1990;27:606–611.

25. Takizawa S, Hogan M, Hakim AM. The effects of a competitive NMDA receptor antagonist (CGS 19755) on cerebral blood flow and pH in focal ischemia. J Cereb Blood Flow Metab 1991;11:786–793.

26. Davis SM, Lees KR, Albers GW, Diener HC, Markabi S, Karlsson G, et al. for the ASSIST Investigators. Selfotel in acute ischemic stroke: possible neurotoxic effects of an NMDA antagonist. Stroke 2000;31:347–354.

27. Davis SM, Albers GW, Diener HC, Lees KR, Norris J. Termination of acute studies involving selfotel treatment. ASSIST Steering Committee. Lancet 1997;349:32.

28. Morris GF, Bullock R, Marshall SB, Marmarou A, Maas A, Marshall LF. Failure of the competitive N-methyl-D-aspartate antagonist Selfotel (CGS 19755) in the treatment of severe head injury: results of phase III clinical trials. The Selfotel Investigators. J Neurosurg 1999;91:737–743.

29. Meadows M-E, Fisher M, Minematsu K. Delayed treatment with a noncompetitive NMDA antagonist, CNS-1102, reduces infarct size in rats. Cerebrovasc Dis 1994;4:26–31.

30. Gamzu ER. CERESTAT® in the treatment of acute cerebral ischemia and TBI. In: Grotta J, Miller LP, Buchan AM, eds. Ischemic Stroke: Recent Advances in Understanding and Therapy. International Business Communications. 1995:86–110.

31. Gamzu ER, for the CNS 1102–002 Study Group. CERESTAT™ (CNS-1102), an NMDA antagonist in severe traumatic brain injury (TBI) patients: a safety study. American Neurology Association 1994 Oct.

32. Scatton B, Giroux C, Thenot JP, et al. Eliprodil hydrochloride. Drugs Future 1994;19:905–909.

33. Carter C, Avenet P, Benavides J, et al. Ifenprodil and eliprodil: neuroprotective NMDA receptor antagonists and calcium channel blockers. In: Herrling PL, ed. Excitatory Amino Acids – Clinical results with Antagonists. San Diego, CA: Academic Press; 1997:57–80.

34. US and Canadian Lubeluzole Ischemic Stroke Study Group. Lubeluzole treatment of acute ischemic stroke. Stroke 1997;28:2338–2346.

35. Diener HC, Hacke W, Hennerici M, Radberg J, Hantson L, DeKeyser J, for the Lubeluzole International Study Group. Lubeluzole in acute ischemic stroke. A double-blind placebo-controlled phase II trial. Stroke 1996;27:76–81.

36. Grotta J. Acute stroke therapy at the millennium: consummating the marriage between the laboratory and bedside. The Feinberg lecture. Stroke 1999;30:1722–1728.

37. Dyker AG, Lees KR. Safety and tolerability of GV150526 (a glycine site antagonist at the N-methyl-D-aspartate receptor) in patients with acute stroke. Stroke 1999;30:986–992.

38. Warner D, Martin D, Ludwig P, McAllister A, Keana J, Weber E. In vivo models of cerebral ischemia: effects of parenterally administered NMDA receptor glycine site antagonists. J Cereb Blood Flow Metab 1995;15:188–196.

39. The North American Glycine Antagonist in Neuroprotection (GAIN) Investigators. Phase II studies of the glycine antagonist GV150526 in acute stroke. The North American experience. Stroke 2000;31:358–365.

40. Sheardown MJ, Nielson EØ, Hansen AJ, Jacobsen P, Honre T. 2,3-dihydroxy-6-nitro-7-sulfamoyl-benzo(F)quinoxaline: a neuroprotectant for cerebral ischemia. Science 1990;247:571–574.

41. Buchan AM, Li H, Cho SH, Pulsinelli WA. Blockade of the AMPA receptor prevents CA_1 hippocampal injury following severe but transient forebrain ischemia in adult rats. Neurosci Let 1991;132:255–258.

42. Buchan AM, Xue D, Huang ZG, Smith KE, Lesiuk H. Delayed AMPA receptor blockade reduces cerebral infarction induced by focal ischemia. NeuroReport 1991;2:473–476.

43. Xue D, Huang ZG, Barnes K, Lesiuk HJ, Smith KE, Buchan AM. Delayed treatment with AMPA, but not NMDA, antagonists reduces neocortical infarction. J Cereb Blood Flow Metab 1994;14:251–261.

44. Li H, Buchan AM. Treatment with an AMPA antagonist 12 hours following severe normothermic forebrain ischemia prevents CA1 neuronal injury. J Cereb Blood Flow Metab 1993;13:933–939.

45. Yao H, Ibayashi S, Nakane H, Cai H, Uchimura H, Fujishima M. AMPA receptor antagonist, YM90 K, reduces infarct volume in thrombotic distal middle cerebral artery (MCA) occlusion in spontaneously hypertensive rats (SHR). J Cereb Blood Flow Metab 1997;17, Suppl 1.

46. Grooms SY, Colbourne F, Zukin RS, Bucham AM, Bennett MVL. Delayed postischemic hypothermia attenuates downregulation of the AMPA receptor Subunit GluR2 and promotes its recovery. Society for Neuroscience annual meeting, November 2000. P 909 Vol. 2000

47. Valentino K, Newcomb R, Gadbois T, et al. A selective N-type calcium channel antagonist protects against neuronal loss after global cerebral ischemia. Proc Natl Acad Sci USA 1993;90:7894–7897.

48. Buchan AM, Gertler SZ, Li H, et al. A selective N-type CA^{++} channel blocker prevents CA1 injury 24 h following severe forebrain ischemia and reduces infarction following focal ischemia. J Cereb Blood Flow Metab 1994;14:903–910.

49. Carter AJ, Grauert M, Pschorn U, et al. Potent blockade of sodium channels and protection of brain tissue from ischemia by BIII 890 CL. Proc Natl Acad Sci USA 2000;97:4944–4949.

50. Weiser T, Brenner M, Palluk R, et al. BIIR 561 CL: A novel combined antagonist of α–amino-3-hydroxy-5-methyl-4-isoxazolepropionic acid receptors and voltage-dependent sodium channels with anticonvulsive and neuroprotective properties. J Pharmacol Exper Therap 1999;289:1343–1349.

51. Cross AJ, Jones JA, Baldwin MA, Green AR. Neuroprotective activity of clomethiazole following transient forebrain ischemia in the gerbil. Br J Pharmacol 1991;104:406–411.

52. Sydserff SG, Cross AJ, West KJ, Green AR. The effect of chlomethiazole on ischaemic neuronal damage in a model of transient focal ischaemia. Br J Pharmacol 1995;114:1631–1635.

53. Wahlgren NG, Ranasinha KW, Rosolacci T, et al. for the CLASS Study Group. Clomethiazole Acute Stroke Study (CLASS): results of a randomized controlled trial of clomethiazole versus placebo in 1360 acute stroke patients. Stroke 1999;30:21–28.

54. Wahlgren NG, Bornhov S, Sharma A, et al. for the CLASS Study Group. The Clomethizaole Acute Stroke Study (CLASS): efficacy results in 545 patients classified as total anterior circulation syndrome (TACS). J Stroke Cerebrovasc Dis 1999;8:231–239.

55. Shuaib A. Safety of chlomethiazole for acute stroke – hemorrhages (CLASS-H): final results. Neurology 2000;54(suppl 3):A64.

56. Lyden PD. Safety and efficacy of combined chlomethiazole and tPA for acute stroke – CLASS-T: a pilot study. Neurology 2000;54(suppl 3):A88.

57. Teal P, on behalf of the BRAIN study group. BRAINS, a phase II study of the neuroprotectant BAY x3702 in patients with ischemic stroke. Cerebrovasc Dis 1998;8:51–103.

58. Hall ED. Free radicals in stoke. In: Miller LP, ed. Stroke Therapy: Basic, Preclinical and Clinical Directions. New York, NY: John Wiley & Sons, Inc; 1999:245–270.

59. Buchan AM, Bruederlin B, Heinicke E, Li H. Failure of the lipid peroxidation inhibitor, U74006F, to prevent post-ischemic selective neuronal injury. J Cereb Blood Flow Metab 1992;12:250–256.

60. Xue D, Slivka A, Buchan AM. Trilazad reduces cortical infarction after transient but not permanent focal cerebral ischemia in rats. Stroke 1992;23:894–899.

61. Cao X, Phillis J. α-phenyl-tert-butyl-nitrone reduced cortical infarct and edema in rats subjected to focal ischemia. Brain Res 1994;644:267–272.

62. Kuroda S, Tsuchidate R, Smith M-L, Maples KR, Siesjo BK. Neuroprotective effects of a novel nitrone, NXY-059, after transient focal cerebral ischemia in the rat. J Cereb Blood Flow Metab 1999;19:778–787.

63. Zhao Z, Cheng M, Maples KR, Ma SY, Buchan AM. NXY-059, a novel free radical trapping compound, reduces cortical infarction after permanent focal cerebral ischemia in the rat. Brain Research 2001; in press.

64. Cramer SC, Finkelstein SP. Reparative approaches: growth factors and other pharmacological treatments. In: Miller LP, ed. Stroke Therapy: Basic, Preclinical and Clinical Directions. New York, NY: John Wiley & Sons, Inc; 1999:321–336.

65. The Enlimomab Acute Stroke Trial Investigators. The Enlimomab acute stroke trial: final results. Neurology 1997;48:A270.

66. Clark WM, Warach SJ, Pettigrew LC, Gammans RE, Sabounjian LA, for the Citicoline Stroke Study Group. A randomized dose-response trial of citicoline in acute ischemic stroke patients. Neurology 1999;49:671–678.

67. Chaves CJ, Silver B, Schlaug G, Dashe J, Caplan LR, Warach S. Diffusion- and perfusion-weighted MRI patterns in borderzone infarcts. Stroke 2000;31:1090–6.

Interventional Neuroradiology in Acute Ischemic Stroke: Extracranial and Intracranial Angioplasty and Stenting

R.T. Higashida, A.M. Malek, C.C. Phatouros,
C.F. Dowd, and Van V. Halbach

Introduction

Atherosclerotic disease as a cause for stroke represents a major source of mortality in North America and is associated with high medical and social cost. Currently there are more than 700,000 cases of new or recurrent strokes per year [1], of which 20%–30% is attributed to atherosclerosis of the carotid bifurcation and proximal internal carotid artery. Recent advances in neurointerventional catheter-based techniques and microballoon and stent design have occurred in the past decade which have enabled the treatment of complex vascular lesions, previously deemed unapproachable using catheter-based techniques [2]. The endovascular approach is providing greater therapeutic options for patients with increased surgical risk and who are symptomatic despite maximal medical therapy. Such lesions include severe atherosclerosis in patients with significant co-morbidity such as tandem intracranial stenosis, contralateral carotid occlusion and recurrent stenosis of vessels having previously undergone surgical carotid endarterectomy. Percutaneous balloon angioplasty alone or when combined with stent placement (stent-assisted angioplasty) is also providing alternatives to treatment of carotid dissection, intracranial atherosclerosis, or recalcitrant acute thrombosis refractory to intraluminal thrombolysis, wide-necked aneurysms, and intracranial vasospasm resulting from subarachnoid hemorrhage. The technique of angioplasty and stent deployment and their current role in the management of cerebrovascular ischemic disease are presented.

Balloon Angioplasty of the Extracranial Vessels

Percutaneous balloon angioplasty was first reported by Dotter and Judkins [3], and subsequent innovation led to the first report of coronary artery angioplasty 15 years later [4] resulting in a subsequent revolution in coronary intervention. Percutaneous angioplasty of the extracranial carotid artery was initially tempered by fears of distal intracranial embolization from plaque rupture during this procedure [5]. A review by Kachel summarizing the cumulative experience of balloon angioplasty of the carotid, vertebral, subclavian, and innominate artery reported in 1995, described 1,971 cases with a technical success rate of 94.6% [6] (Table 3). The mortality varied by territory from 0 to 2.1% with overall morbidity of 0.9%

Table 1. Location of reported arterial and venous sites where a stent has been deployed either primarily or following percutaneous balloon angioplasty

Arterial	
Anterior Circulation	Posterior Circulation
Innominate Artery	Subclavian Artery
Common Carotid Artery	Vertebral Artery
Carotid Artery Bifurcation	Origin stenosis
Internal Carotid	Cervical vertebral artery
Cervical	Intracranial vertebral artery[a]
Petrous[a]	Basilar artery[a]
Cavernous[a]	Midbasilar trunk[a]
Supraclinoid[a]	
Venous	
Internal Jugular Vein	
Transverse Sinus[a]	
Occipital Sinus[a]	

[a]Intracranial location.

Table 2. Various indications for which a stent has been deployed intravascularly

Arterial
  Atherosclerotic Stenosis (>70% NASCET criteria)
  Restenosis following carotid endarterectomy
  Tandem stenotic lesions
  Intimal Dissection (Spontaneous, iatrogenic, chronic)
  Pseudoaneurysm without coiling (spontaneous thrombosis)
  Scaffold for coiling of wide-necked intracerebral aneurysm
  Scaffold for coiling of pseudoaneurysm
Venous
  Maintain patency
  Recanalization of occluded sinus

and minor technical complications of 0–6.3%. The author's experience included percutaneous angioplasty of 74 symptomatic carotid lesions with a technical success of 93%, 1 major stroke (1.4%), 2 minor complications (2.7%) and no reported restenosis at 70-month follow-up. Higashida and Tsai reported angioplasty of 256 extracranial vessels with greater than 70% stenosis with 1 major stroke (0.4%), 5 transient ischemic events (2%), no mortality, and 15 cases (6%) of restenosis at 6–12 months of follow-up [7].

In the posterior circulation, Higashida reported percutaneous angioplasty in 42 patients of the vertebral artery (34 proximal, 5 distal, 3 basilar) with stroke in 2 cases and vessel rupture in 1 (7.1% permanent complications), 2 cases of spasm, and 2 cases of cerebral ischemia lasting less than 30 minutes (9.5% transient complications). Clinical improvement was noted in 92.9% of patients at follow-up, with 3 cases of restenosis (7.1%) of the proximal vertebral artery, two of which underwent successful repeat percutaneous angioplasty [8].

Table 3. Summary of technical success, complications, and morbidity in reported studies in the literature

Author	Number of Patients	Technical Success	Major Complications or Stroke	Minor Complications or TIAs	Mortality Rate	Restenosis Rate
Angioplasty						
Kachel [6] (review)	1971	94.6%	0.9%	4.2%	0%	–
Kachel [6] (series)	74	93.2%	1.4%	1.4%	0%	0%
Higashida []2	325	100%	2.4%	5.5%	0%	7.4%
Iyer [17]	100	97%	7%	3%	3%	1%
Mathias [82]	79	100%	0%	2.5%	2.5%	0%
Théron [35]	482	100%	2%	2%	0.6%	16%
Stent-Assisted Angioplasty						
Diethrich [83]	110	99%	6.4%	4.5%	1.8%	4%
Vitek [21]	404	98%	0.7%	5.8%	1.9%	0%
GSCAS [15]	2048	98.6%	1.32%	3.1%	1.37%	4.8%
Vozzi [84]	22	96%	4%	4%	0%	–
Henry [85]	163	99.4%	1.8%	3%	0%	2.3%

GSCAS Global status of carotid artery stent placement. *TIA* Transient ischemic attack.

Measurements of middle cerebral artery velocity using transcranial Doppler insonation has also enabled the assessment of intracranial hemodynamics, prior to and after angioplasty. Although restenosis is one of the reported concerns following angioplasty, there is evidence for a delayed and persistent improvement in cerebral reactivity and hemodynamics beyond the immediate post-angioplasty period, to 1 and 6 months [9]. Quantitative angiographic measurement of stenotic lesions (mean of 87%), treated with percutaneous angioplasty, showed an improvement from 47% immediately post-dilatation, to 28%, and a 1-year follow-up suggested an active expansile structural remodeling process that was ongoing [10].

Recent experience in the percutaneous angioplasty of subclavian artery for aortoarteritis (32 vessels) and atherosclerosis (23 vessels) has been performed by Tyagi et al., with a 92.8% success in stenotic lesions, and a 60% success in recanalizing totally occluded arteries [11]. The average stenosis decreased from 88.7% for atherosclerosis and 89% for aortoarteritis, to 15.5% and 8.3% following percutaneous angioplasty without neurological complications and with good long-term symptomatic relief (3–120 months) [11].

A prospective analytical study of 29 patients having undergone carotid angioplasty for severe symptomatic ipsilateral carotid stenosis by NASCET criteria was recently reported by Schoser et al. [12]. Neurological and ultrasonographic follow-up (mean of 33 months) revealed that 78% of patients suffered no further neurological sequelae, 10% suffered a single episode of ipsilateral transient ischemia or amaurosis fugax and 7% suffered recurrent episodes, with no patient suffering a stroke. Fifty percent (50%) of treated vessels remained with normal ultrasound (<50% stenosis), 40% with mild stenosis (50–70%), and 10% with severe stenosis (>70%). These findings suggest that angioplasty alone is satisfactory and can have sustained benefit even up to 6.5 years of follow-up [12] with an accepted percutaneous angioplasty risk profile (Table 3).

Angioplasty and Stenting
of the Extracranial Carotid Artery

Current State

Trials of stent-assisted versus simple percutaneous balloon angioplasty of the coronary circulation has consistently demonstrated a persistent benefit in event-free survival at one year and a lower rate of repeat angioplasty [13, 14]. The increased acceptance and reliance on stent placement in the coronary and peripheral vascular interventions has led to a similar trend in the treatment of supra-aortic cervical vessels including the carotid [15–17], subclavian [11], and vertebral arteries [18].

Recently, Yadav et al. reported their experience in balloon angioplasty and stenting of carotid restenosis in a series of 22 patients having previously undergone carotid endarterectomy [19]. They were able to successfully decrease the stenosis by 79±13% with a morbidity of 4% (a minor stroke in a single patient) and no restenosis (>50%) at 6 months follow-up. Given the high risk of re-operation on previous endarterectomized lesions which have been reported to suffer operative complication rates of 10.5% (Tables 4, 5) [20], balloon angioplasty and stenting is a promising approach (Table 3).

Vitek and Roubin reported having treated a total of 445 vessels in 404 patients using stent-assisted angioplasty using pre-dilatation, placement of stent, followed by stent dilatation [21]. Patients were pretreated with aspirin and ticlopidine and were not maintained under intravenous anticoagulation following the procedure, with same day and 23-hour discharges when possible. They reported on the treatment of 40 patients with contralateral carotid occlusion and 70 patients with post-endarterectomy restenosis. Overall technical success was 98%, with a 30-day mortality/morbidity and death of 1.9% (0.7% neurological and 1.2% systemic), 0.7% risk of major stroke and 5.8% minor stroke (Table 3). The authors determined their annual risk of minor stroke and showed a steady decline from 7.2% in 1994–95, to 4.4% and 2.2% in each successive year. The decrease in complication rate with experience illustrates the fact that stent-assisted angioplasty is still early. Nonetheless, stent-assisted balloon angioplasty appears to have short-term risk comparable to that reported for carotid endarterectomy. Six-month follow-up obtained in 80% of patients demonstrated stenosis greater than 50% in only 5% of patients and included 3.3% of cases due to collapse of the *Palmaz* balloon expandable stent [22] which was treated successfully in 3 patients (0.75%). Vitek et al. reported clinical follow-up in 95% of patients with 2 neurological deaths and one major and three minor strokes for a freedom of any stroke of 92% and freedom from disabling stroke or death of 98%, at two years.

Table 4. Sundt's classification system based on retrospective analysis of 3,111 consecutive endarterectomy patients [26]

Sundt' Class	Criteria for Classification	Combined Surgical Morbidity/(Mortality)
Class I	Neurologically stable, no major medical/angio-graphically defined risk, with unilateral/bilateral ulcerative-stenotic disease	0.9%
Class II	Neurologically stable, no major medical risks, with or without angiographic risks	1.7%
Class III	Neurologically stable, major medical risks, with or without angiographic risks	3.7% (1.3%)
Class IV	Neurologically unstable, with or without medical/angiographic risks	8.1% (2.9%)
Class V	Acute internal carotid artery occlusion, progressive neurological deficit within 6 hours of exam	Not included in study
Class VI	Recurrent symptomatic carotid stenosis	Not included in study

Table 5. Sundt's definition of medical, neurological and angiographic risk [26]

Risk	Definition
Medical	Coronary artery disease (angina, myocardial infarction <6 months, congestive heart failure), hypertension (>180/110 mmHg), severe peripheral vascular disease, chronic obstructive pulmonary disease, age>70 years, severely obese
Neurological	Neurological deficit within 24 hours, general cerebral ischemia, recent cerebrovascular accident (<7 days), frequent transient ischemic attacks.
Angiographic	Contralateral internal carotid artery occlusion, siphon stenosis, plaque>3 cm distally in internal carotid artery or >5 cm proximal in common carotid artery, bifurcation at C2 vertebra, short thick neck, and soft thrombus extending from an ulcerative lesion

Mathur et al. recently reported their analysis of multiple factors that portend a higher risk of complication in stent-assisted angioplasty of the carotid artery in 271 vessels involving 231 patients [23]. These patients constituted a high-risk subset suffering from coronary disease (71%), bilateral carotid disease (39%), and contralateral carotid occlusion (12%). The treated vessels had undergone previous endarterectomy (22%), contained ulcerated plaques (24%), or were calcified lesions (32%). Only 14% of these patients would have been eligible to undergo endarterectomy by NASCET criteria. The rate of minor stroke was 6.2% and that of major stroke 0.7% during the first 30 days after and including the procedure. Furthermore, the rate of any stroke for the NASCET eligible subset was 2.7% for the same time interval. Multivariate analysis demonstrated that advanced age, and long or multiple stenoses to be independent predictors of procedural-related stroke in carotid stent-assisted angioplasty [23]. These rates compare favorably with the risk of procedural stroke or death from endarterectomy in NASCET [24] which was 5.8% and in the Asymptomatic Carotid Artery Study (ACAS) [25] which was 2.3%, especially considering these high-risk patients [20], and rates of up to 18% in other high-risk subsets [20, 26]. In addition, they also compare favorably to the retrospective analysis of 3,111 carotid endarterectomies performed by Sundt et al. (Tables 4, 5) [20, 26] given that a large proportion of the patients undergoing stent-assisted angioplasty constitute Sundt Class III and IV [26].

Angioplasty-Induced Particulate Embolization

Ultrasound has been shown to be sufficiently sensitive to detect stenosis when compared to angiography in a series of 170 stent placements in 119 patients [27]. Robbin et al. [27] found that ultrasound did not fail to detect any significant stenosis and was promising in its ability to assess intra-stent intimal hyperplasia.

Angioplasty of atherosclerotic lesions has been reported to induce the release of multiple emboli including atheroma, cholesterol crystals, thrombus, and platelet aggregates [28–31]. Markus et al. monitored embolic signals using transcranial Doppler insonation of the ipsilateral middle cerebral artery in ten patients and detected emboli immediately after angioplasty in 9 out of 10 patients and in 8 out of 10 after catheter withdrawals from the artery [9]. The frequency decreased to 1 out of 5 patients at 4 hours, 1 out of 6 at 1 week and 1 out of 10 at 1 month [9]. Embolization of microparticles has also been demonstrated during open endarterectomy and has been shown to correlate with complex plaque morphology [32] and with clinical post-operative cerebral ischemia [33]. A direct contemporaneous analysis of 14 patients undergoing percutaneous angioplasty and 14 undergoing endarterectomy with shunt placement revealed that endarterectomy resulted in significantly greater total occlusion time (337 s vs. 26 s), but a lower count of microembolic signals (52 vs. 202 events) compared to angioplasty, although neither parameters were predictive of later neurologic events [30]. It is unclear whether stent placement concomitant with angioplasty may help decrease microemboli shower by trapping them under the metal interstices or whether primary stenting would decrease emboli compared to secondary stenting. The problem of distal embolization during balloon dilatation of atherosclerotic stenoses has engendered interest in various methods of protection. Distal protection using a specially designed triple-coaxial catheter has been described by Théron [34]. Distal embolic complications were found in 3 of 38 patients undergoing angioplasty without (8%) and in none of 136 undergoing angioplasty (0%) with distal protection [35]. A number of commercial devices are currently under development to provide distal protection as a means of decreasing the thromboembolic burden associated with angioplasty.

Complications Related to Angioplasty and Stenting

Although angioplasty and stent therapy has certain advantages when compared to the current standard of open surgery [36], it is also characterized by a set of unique complications to which the operator must acutely recognize both during the procedure and the subsequent inpatient recovery [37]. These can be segregated according to Dorros [37] to be related to *arterial access* including hematoma, retroperitoneal hemorrhage, pseudoaneurysm, arteriovenous fistula, arterial thrombosis, groin infection; related to *catheterization* including arterial dissection, embolism of air or thrombus, vessel perforation, tear or rupture; related to *contrast media*, including allergic reaction, hypotension, and acute renal failure; and related to *stent placement*, including pseudoaneurysm formation and stent infection and arteritis. Recent studies suggest that permanent neurological complications from diagnostic cerebral angiography is 0.8% in a consecutive series of 500 patients with no deaths [38]. In a recent meta-analysis, angiography-associated risk of combined and transient neurological complications ranged from 0.8% to 3.0% for patients undergoing the procedure for subarachnoid hemorrhage or for transient ischemic attack/stroke respectively. The rate of permanent neurological complication was found to be low at 0.07% for patients presenting with subarachnoid hemorrhage [39]. An excellent account of the multitude of technical complications relating to carotid stent-assisted angioplasty has recently been published by Théron et al. [40]. The authors eloquently described the type and mechanism of complications encountered, as well as precautionary measures needed for avoidance of such pitfalls including: 1) distal embolism into the internal carotid artery, 2) reflux of thrombus into an ophthalmic artery with a variant origin of the meningolacrimal branch of the middle meningeal artery and into a right vertebral artery via the right subclavian artery, both encountered during the thrombus flushing phase of protected angioplasty [35], 3) Internal carotid artery thrombosis from insufficient anticoagulation of a complex plaque, 4) internal carotid artery occlusion following deployment of a stent into a false lumen resulting from intimal dissection, 5) vasospasm during protective balloon use, 6) persistent thromboembolic events resulting from use of a low radial force variant of the *WallStent* leading to poor apposition of the stent mesh to the luminal lesion surface, and 7) carotid-cavernous fistula formation from inflation of the protective balloon after it had inadvertently migrated distally to the cavernous internal carotid artery as a result of over-aggressive flushing.

Future Trends

These complications make it clear that stent-assisted balloon angioplasty of the carotid artery may be a more technically complex procedure than other types of peripheral stenting procedures of the renal or iliac vessels. The endovascular approach presents certain advantages compared to open surgical procedures in its ability to reach areas of the carotid and vertebral artery which are not readily accessible by open techniques, such as the innominate artery, high cervical and petrous segments of the internal carotid artery [2]. A recent comparison of carotid stent-assisted angioplasty (107 patients) and endarterectomy (166 patients) by Jordan et al. [41] reported an early minor stroke rate of 6.6% for the former and 0.6% for the latter, and a combined major stroke/death rate of 2.8% for the former and 4.2% for the latter. These findings suggest promising results for stent-assisted angioplasty at its current stage [41] and bode well for its future, given the recent report of improved annual risk profile with accumulated technical experience even in the absence of distal protection [21].

However, an attempt at a randomized study in another institutional setting for 23 patients with symptomatic >70% stenosis resulted in a prohibitively high risk among the stent-assisted angioplasty group prompting an early halt of the trial in favor of endarterectomy [42]. The stent-assisted angioplasty procedure was performed by a radiologist specialized in peripheral interventional procedures, and it is unclear what led to the inordinately elevated rate of procedural-related stroke given the accumulating evidence from different centers pointing to significantly better results (Table 3) [15]. The consensus of experienced operators in the field suggests that extensive experience with carotid and cerebral angiography and with interventional procedures is one of the mandatory requisites to achieve a low technical complication rate [15, 40, 43]. In experienced hands, results from multiple centers (Table 3) suggest that carotid stent-assisted angioplasty may be an alternative to carotid endarterectomy in select patient subsets which are known to constitute very high risk for surgical complication (Tables 4, 5) [20, 26]. Future developments in carotid-specific stent design, angioplasty catheters, and methods of distal protection, coupled with long-term clinical and radiological follow-up will ultimately determine the role of stent-assisted angioplasty compared to surgical endarterectomy [36, 43]. There is currently an ongoing randomized trial of carotid and vertebral stent-assisted angioplasty and open surgery (CAVATAS) [44, 45], and future randomized prospective studies should shed light on the debate and provide the needed scientific data for appropriate decision-making in various patient subsets.

Protocol for Carotid Angioplasty and Stenting

The current patients undergoing balloon angioplasty and stent deployment at UCSF Medical Center mostly belong to Sundt's classes III to VI and include patients with atherosclerosis as well as dissection who have failed maximal medical therapy. In the carotid territory, high-risk patients such as patients with multiple advanced medical problems, contralateral occluded carotid artery with no collateral flow, high cervical and petrous lesions or low common carotid lesions, which are not readily accessible by surgery. Lesions treated in the posterior circulation include subclavian stenosis, vertebral artery origin stenosis, extracranial and intracranial vertebral stenosis and dissection [18, 46].

Technique

The patient initially undergoes a complete angiographic evaluation, including selective catheterization, using a high-quality digital subtraction unit to determine the location of the lesion, the degree of stenosis, the adequacy of collateral blood supply to the affected territory, the presence of any anatomic variant or aberrant anomaly. Following the study, the patient undergoes measurement of a baseline activated clotting time (ACT) and receives an initial weight-based (70 units/kg) intravenous bolus of heparin followed by a post-heparin ACT determination to achieve an ACT value equal or greater than 2.5 times the baseline value (>250 s). The patient then receives either an hourly dose equal to half the initial bolus or is placed on a heparin drip of 15–20 U/kg/h. Patients are administered enteric-coated aspirin (325 mg qd) and either ticlopidine (Ticlid 250 mg bid) or clopidogrel (Plavix 75 mg qd) starting one to two days prior to the procedure. Following the procedure, the patient is kept on daily aspirin indefinitely and on ticlopidine or clopidogrel for six weeks. The role of glycoprotein IIb/IIIa inhibitors, which have been shown to decrease mortality and morbidity in a number of coronary stent studies [47], remains to be defined in carotid and vertebral angioplasty and stenting.

During the procedure of cervical carotid angioplasty patients undergo placement of external cutaneous pacing leads and are constantly monitored by a transcutaneous pacer/defibrillator device in case of severe bradycardia or asystole from carotid body stimulation during angioplasty. In addition, patients are administered atropine 0.5–1 mg intravenously or an appropriate dose of glycopyrrolate prior to balloon dilatation of the carotid artery to decrease any parasympathetic discharge. The patients are well hydrated during the procedure which is tailored to the specific patient and their cardiac status. The procedure consists of placing a 7–9 Fr sheath (*Avanti*, Cordis Endovascular) depending on the type of stent to be used (7 Fr for low-profile balloon-mounted coronary stent catheter such as the *GFX* (Arterial Vascular Engineering, Santa Rosa, CA, USA), or *Multi-Link* (Guidant, Santa Clara, CA, USA) designs, or 8–9 Fr in the case of the *Smart Stent* (Johnson and Johnson, New Brunswick, NJ, USA) or *WallStent* (Schneider, Plymouth, MN, USA) designs. In the case of a complex, severely stenosed lesion, or in a high-cervical or intracranial location, a 2.3 French microcatheter (Rapid Transit, Cordis Endovascular Systems, Miami Lakes, FL) is used coaxially over an 0.014 inch microguidewire (Transend 14, Scimed Inc., MN).

After crossing the lesion using the microcatheter with meticulous care, a 300 cm long 0.014 inch exchange microguidewire (Stabilizer, Cordis Endovascular) is passed through the microcatheter and placed in the cavernous segment of the internal carotid artery or in the posterior cerebral artery, and the microcatheter is then withdrawn. With the exchange guidewire in place, primary or secondary stent-assisted angioplasty is performed. In case of secondary stent placement, a low-profile angioplasty balloon catheter is used to cross and pre-dilate the lesion. Once the stenosis has been pre-dilated, the stent is deployed, and a high-pressure non-compliant angioplasty balloon is then used to post-dilate the stent in order to firmly embed it into the plaque. In the case of less complicated and more proximal lesions, an 0.035 inch guidewire may be used as an exchange guidewire to cross the lesion, bypassing the need for microcatheterization (Fig. 1).

Stent Designs

The current experience with extracranial carotid atherosclerosis [15] involves the use of the *WallStent* or Palmaz stainless steel stents primarily, neither of which are specifically designed for use in the carotid artery, and more recently the SMART stent

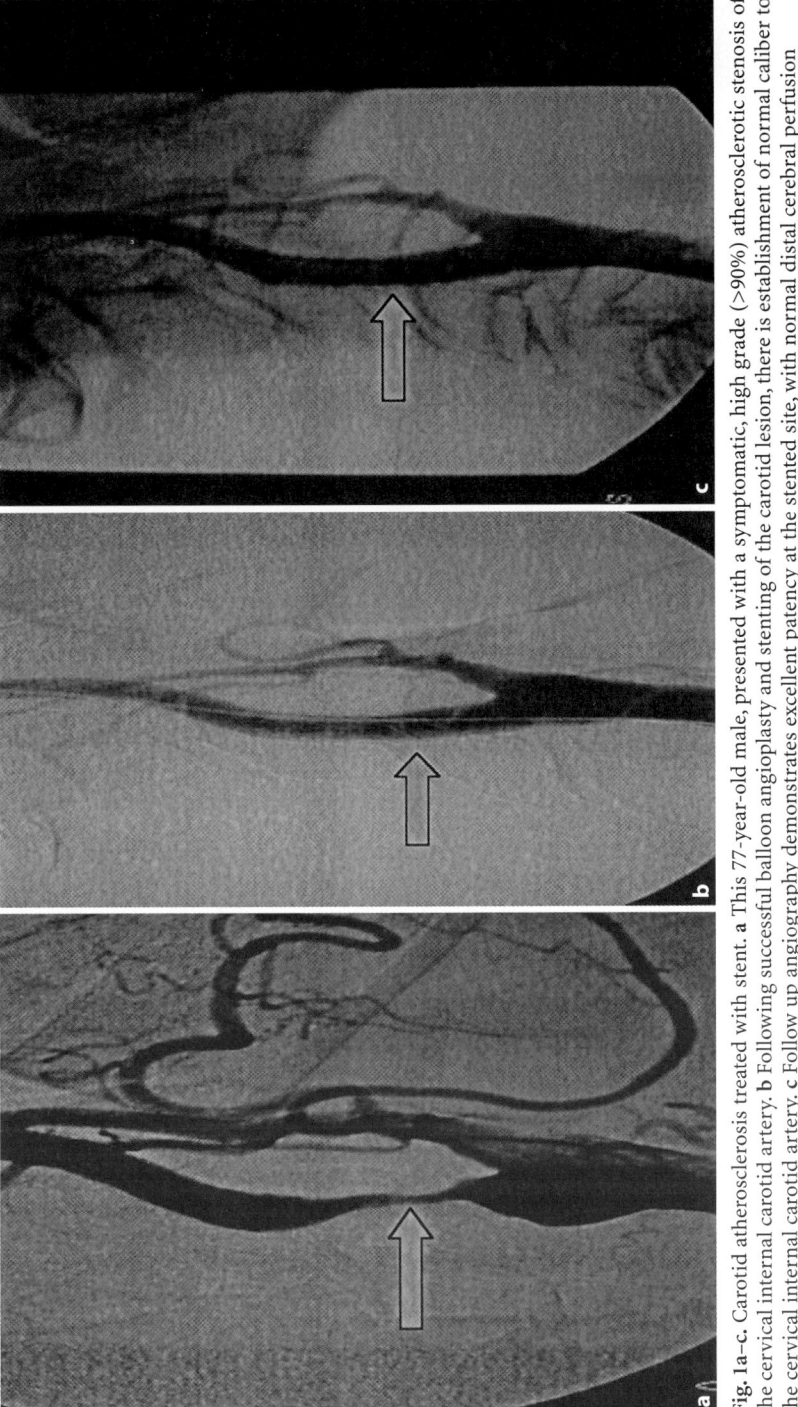

Fig. 1a–c. Carotid atherosclerosis treated with stent. **a** This 77-year-old male, presented with a symptomatic, high grade (>90%) atherosclerotic stenosis of the cervical internal carotid artery. **b** Following successful balloon angioplasty and stenting of the carotid lesion, there is establishment of normal caliber to the cervical internal carotid artery. **c** Follow up angiography demonstrates excellent patency at the stented site, with normal distal cerebral perfusion

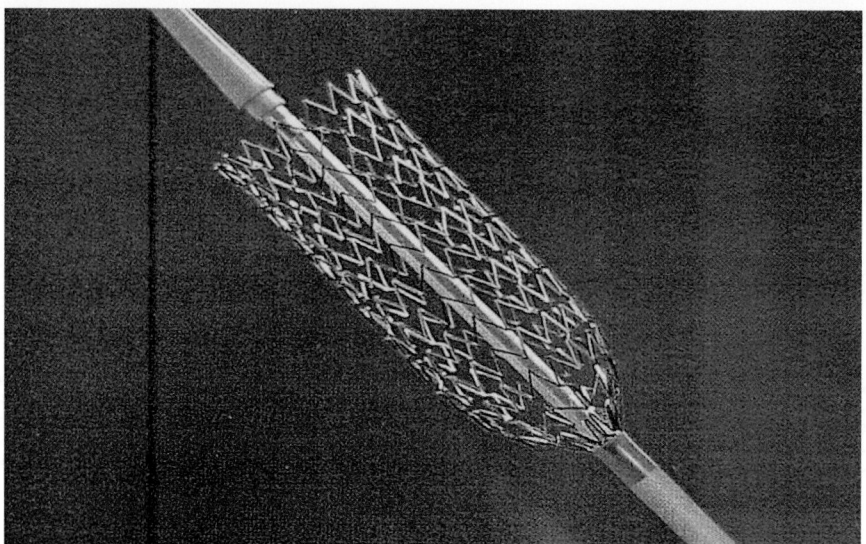

Fig. 2. Cordis nitinol SMART stent used for carotid artery stenting

which is a nitinol stent design (Fig. 2). The *Palmaz* stent is balloon-mounted, provides greater radial force, has less metal surface area coverage with larger and fewer interstices and is non-compliant. The *WallStent* is a self-expandable design with significant lower radial force, and with a greater metal surface area coverage with finer and more numerous interstices. A problem detected with the *Palmaz* non-compliant type of stent is that of external stent compression which may result in compression and narrowing [22]. This has been treated by repeat angioplasty but appears to be a fundamental problem with non-compliant stents used in the cervical region. In the case of the *WallStent*, its compliant design and the consequently lower radial force can be a hindrance in severely calcified lesions. In such lesions, poor embedding of the stent into the vessel wall may lead to focal regions of flow stasis and thrombus predilection [40]. Stent design is an active area with imminent new products some of which have been specifically designed for use in the carotid artery territory.

Intracranial Angioplasty and Stenting for Treatment of Atherosclerotic Lesions

Percutaneous angioplasty of the intracranial vessel has been used by a number of groups in a preliminary fashion to treat intracranial atherosclerosis in patients who have previously failed maximal medical therapy. Terada reported treatment of 12 lesions with greater than 70% stenosis in patients with clinical symptoms consistent of transient ischemic attack despite maximal medical therapy [48]. The angioplasty was performed in the distal vertebral and basilar arteries using a balloon with a 2.0–3.5 mm diameter inflated to 6 atm. The overall stenosis decreased from 84% to 44%; 8 patients had no complications, 2 suffered intimal dissection with subsequent small-size infarcts, and 2 sustained thromboembolism with consequent transient ischemic attack [48]. Long-term follow-up in 11 patients surviving beyond 6 months showed persistent freedom from symptoms in 10 patients and recurrent transient ischemia in 1 patient (Fig. 3).

A recent development has been the treatment of intracranial atherosclerotic stenoses of the carotid and vertebral arteries with stent placement following or concurrently with angioplasty [49]. This treatment is reserved for lesions that are symptomatic despite maximal medical management including oral anti-platelet and anticoagulant treatment. In the carotid artery, stent placement has been performed or reported in the intracranial petrous [50–52], cavernous, and proximal supraclinoid segment [53]. In the posterior circulation, stents have been deployed along the entire course of the extracranial vertebral artery, in the intracranial V4 segment, and in the mid-segment of the basilar artery [49, 53]. Compromise of median and paramedian perforator vessels by physical occlusion remains a limiting factor which may preclude the use of mid-basilar stent placement except as a last resort. Intimal dissection is not unexpected following plaque rupture by balloon angioplasty, and is anticipated to heal over time. Stent placement can be used as a bailout measure for treatment of a flow-limiting angioplasty-induced intimal dissection. Intracranial stent-assisted angioplasty decreases the incidence of vessel recoil following conventional angioplasty. We are currently treating focal high-grade intracranial atherosclerotic lesions using primary stent-assisted angioplasty with second-generation low-profile balloon-premounted coronary stents (*GFX*, AVE; *GR-2*, Cook; *MultiLink*, Guidant). The significantly improved mechanical properties of this new generation of stent catheters has enabled the safe navigation of the vessels at the base of the skull, and in certain cases inside the intracranial circulation [49] (Fig. 4). We have performed 12 such procedures in the intracranial vertebral and intracranial carotid artery. Treatment of severe stenoses in the intracranial vessels entails a significantly greater risk of complications because of the delicate vascular structure and the lack of media and muscular layers. Typical complications may include intimal dissection, vessel rupture, acute vessel thrombosis, and reperfusion injury [54]. We currently limit our treatment of intracranial atherosclerotic lesions to patients who have failed maximal medical therapy and are left with no options short of high-risk surgical bypass or revascularization procedures. As with all emerging indications, we advocate very close clinical and angiographic follow-up in order to better define the appropriate indications and drawbacks of this therapy in the future.

Intracranial Angioplasty and Stenting as an Adjunct for Thrombolysis of Acute Vessel Occlusion

Angioplasty of the cerebral arteries for acute occlusion has been reported to be of benefit in treatment of acute middle cerebral artery occlusion following a failed thrombolysis attempt [55]. The underlying mechanism remains unclear. It is possible that angioplasty may treat an underlying stenotic lesion. It is hypothesized that the increased flow resulting from the caliber improvement by the dilatation may increase the endogenous production of endothelial nitric oxide and prostacyclin, both of which have vasodilatory and platelet-inhibitory effects [56, 57],

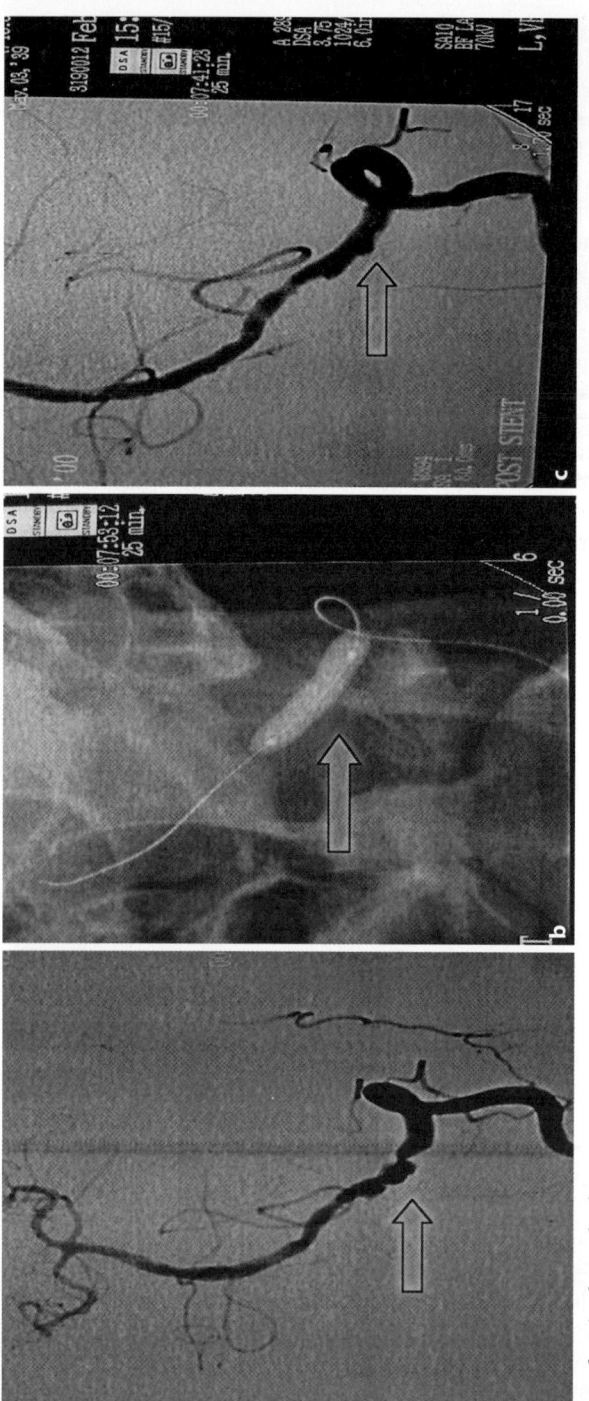

Fig. 3a–b. Distal vertebral artery stenosis treated with stenting. **a** This a 61-year-old man, presented with posterior fossa ischemia, and has a high grade (>80%) stenosis of the distal left vertebral artery, as it enters the skull base. The right vertebral artery is occluded. **b** Balloon angioplasty and stenting of the distal vertebral artery stenosis. **c** Following successful stent deployment, there is return to normal luminal diameter of the lesion, with improved blood flow to the posterior cerebral circulation

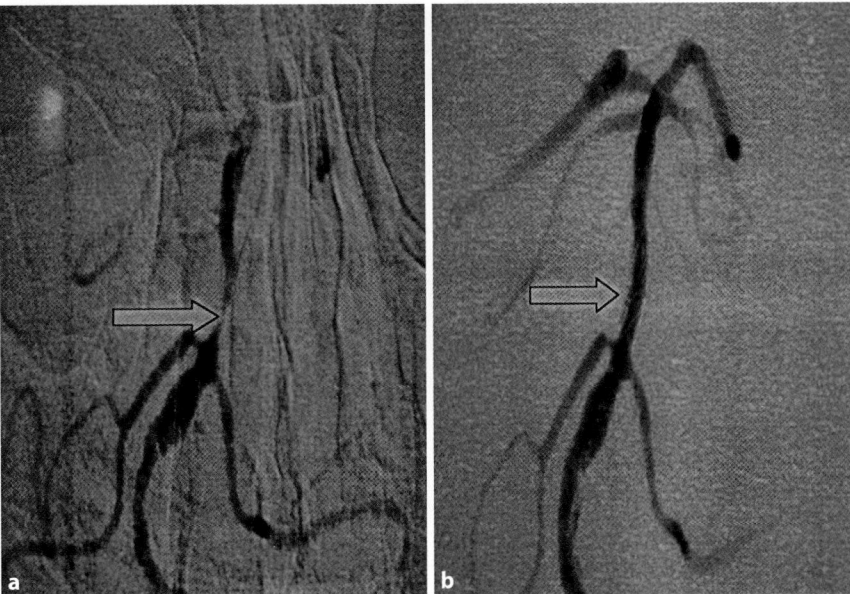

Fig. 4a,b. Intracranial basilar artery stenosis treated with stenting. **a** This 66-year-old female presented with severe posterior cerebral ischemic symptoms from a high grade (>90%) stenosis of the mid-basilar artery, and had failed maximal medical therapy with coumadin and antiplatelet medications. **b** Following successful angioplasty with stent placement across the mid-basilar stenosis, there is a return to normal vessel caliber, with improved blood flow to the distal basilar and posterior cerebral arteries

and increase the release and production of t-PA [58]. A host of endothelial-derived factors and cytokines have been shown to be regulated by prevailing flow and associated shear stress conditions [59]. The contribution of platelet aggregation to restenosis following successful thrombolysis has been recently confirmed by successful treatment of this condition using the glycoprotein IIb/IIIa inhibitor abciximab [60]. We reported a case of recalcitrant basilar thrombosis despite thrombolysis and angioplasty which responded to intracranial mid-basilar stent deployment [49]. A similar benefit of angioplasty when combined with suboptimal thrombolysis was also demonstrated in three cases of intracranial vertebrobasilar occlusion [61], and in four cases by Yokote et al. [62]. A preliminary report recently confirmed the merit of a similar approach in 11 out of 68 patients who had failed thrombolysis using superselective intraluminal urokinase [63].

Stent Deployment for Treatment of Cerebral Aneurysms and Extracranial Cervical Pseudoaneurysms

Stents have become increasingly useful for the treatment of wide-necked intracranial aneurysms and extracranial pseudoaneurysms. A stent has been deployed in the basilar artery across the wide-neck of a mid-basilar aneurysm to serve as an endovascular scaffold with subsequent placement of a microcatheter between the interstices of the stent [64]. Guglielmi detachable coils (GDC) were then deployed within the otherwise untreatable aneurysm because the stent precluded herniation of the coils within the parent vessel lumen. Such stent-assisted coil embolization of aneurysms has since been reported for the treatment of carotid [65] and vertebral aneurysms [66, 67] and has also been used successfully in the treatment of a petrous internal carotid dissecting pseudoaneurysm [68]. There have also been numerous reports on the effect of stent deployment on alteration of intra-aneurysmal hemodynamics with eventual thrombosis even in the absence of coil embolization [69, 70]. Future advances in stent technology including a lower-profile design with greater flexibility and specifically tailored strut porosity for intracranial use is expected to expand the use of stents in treatment of aneurysms.

Percutaneous Balloon Angioplasty for Treatment of Intracranial Vasospasm

Cerebral vasospasm following subarachnoid hemorrhage is a leading source of delayed cerebral ischemia following intracranial aneurysmal rupture and is the single most important cause of death and disability for survivors [71–73]. Angioplasty of intracranial arteries for the treatment of vasospasm following subarachnoid hemorrhage is a useful technique for treatment of cerebral hypoperfusion unresponsive to maximal hypertensive, hypervolemic and hemodilutional therapy (triple-H therapy) [74–76]. The angioplasty is performed while the patient is anticoagulated and utilizes a specifically designed low-profile compliant balloon mounted on an atraumatic flexible catheter. The balloon catheter is deployed via a guide catheter positioned in the extracranial internal carotid or vertebral artery. Upon deployment within the intracranial vessel to be treated, typically the intradural portion of supraclinoid internal carotid artery, the balloon is gently inflated under digital roadmap technique with a dilute mixture of radio-opaque contrast material in short durations to enable intermittent cerebral perfusion. More distally, the M1 segment of the middle cerebral artery is the most commonly treated vessel. On rare occasions, and in particular when one of the anterior cerebral arteries is dominant, the A1 segment is amenable to angioplasty as well. A recent study by Elliott et al. indicates that there is a longer-lasting benefit with mechanical balloon angioplasty than with intraluminal infusion of papaverine [74]. Intracranial vasospasm was assessed by using transcranial Doppler (TCD) measurement pre- and post-treatment in 101 vessel segments treated with angioplasty alone and 24 vessel segments treated with superselective intraluminal infusion of papaverine alone. Papaverine-treated vessels showed an average decrease in TCD velocity of 20% on post-procedure day 1, which by post-procedure day 2 was no longer significantly different from pre-treatment velocities. In contrast, vessels treated with angioplasty showed a 45% lower mean TCD velocity which remained sustained on post-procedure day 2. Eskridge demonstrated a similar long-lasting effect by angiographic, clinical and TCD velocity criteria, with only 1 out of 170 treated vessel segments requiring repeat angioplasty [75]. Balloon-dilatation of intracranial vessel segments using a compliant microballoon catheter has established its efficacy and relative safety in the treatment of subarachnoid hemorrhage-related intracranial vasospasm which has failed maximal hypertensive, hypervolemic, and hemodilutional therapy.

Angioplasty and Stenting for Treatment of Intracranial Venous Hypertension

Venous hypertensive disease can result from either stenosis or thrombosis of the dural sinuses of the internal jugular vein. Angioplasty of the transverse sinus has been reported to decrease intracranial venous draining pressure [77]. Based on experience in peripheral interventional procedures, stents have a higher risk of thrombosis when placed in the venous than in the arterial circulation. This higher thrombotic [78] tendency in the venous system may be the result of the lower flow velocity and lower shear stress for the same reasons described previously. Stent placement in the venous circulation has mainly consisted of treatment of stenosis in dialysis fistula, axillary-subclavian thrombosis and fresh venous thrombus [79]. We have successfully deployed a stent following recanalization of an occipital sinus in a patient suffering from pan-sinus cerebral thrombosis with excellent patency at 3 months angiographic follow-up [80]. A stent has similarly been deployed in the left internal jugular vein of a patient with post-traumatic bilateral internal jugular vein thrombosis. This procedure resulted in a measured decrease in both intracranial pressure and sigmoid sinus with resumption of venous drainage and maintained patency at 6 months. Although venous-side stenting for intracranial hypertension has provided clinical relief in a number of reported cases, it remains a procedure of last resort at the present time, also requiring oral anticoagulation with coumadin to decrease the likelihood of re-thrombosis [81]. Accumulation of future clinical experience and follow-up will help define the guidelines and limitations of such therapy.

Conclusion

Advances in endovascular techniques are making it possible to treat increasingly complex vascular lesions involving both the extracranial and intracranial arterial and venous aspects of the cerebral vasculature in an effort to combat ischemia and treat cerebral infarction. Angioplasty and stenting in the extracranial carotid artery is becoming a viable alternative to surgical carotid endarterectomy in certain subsets of very high-risk patients. Long-term clinical and angiographic follow-up, as well as randomized prospective trials will determine the role of percutaneous angioplasty with stenting in the treatment of carotid stenosis. The role of angioplasty has become more clearly established in the treatment of intracranial vasospasm from subarachnoid hemorrhage. Further experience will help determine the role of percutaneous angioplasty and stent deployment in the treatment of lesions that have no current surgical alternative such as intracranial atherosclerosis, cerebral venous hypertension, and carotid and vertebral dissection.

References

1. American Heart Association. 1999 Heart and Stroke Statistical Update. In:. Dallas, Tex.: American Heart Association; 1999.
2. Higashida RT, Tsai FY, Halbach VV, et al. Transluminal angioplasty, thrombolysis, and stenting for extracranial and intracranial vascular disease. J. Interven. Cardiol. 1996;9:245–255.
3. Dotter CT, Judkins MP. Transluminal treatment of arteriosclerotic obstruction: description of a new technique and a preliminary report of its application. Circulation 1964;30:654–670.
4. Gruntzig A. Transluminal dilatation of coronary-artery stenosis [letter]. Lancet 1978;1 (8058):263.
5. Kerber CW, Cromwell LD, Loehden OL. Catheter dilatation of proximal carotid stenosis during distal bifurcation endarterectomy. AJNR Am J Neuroradiol 1980;1(4):348–349.
6. Kachel R. Results of balloon angioplasty in the carotid arteries [see comments]. J Endovasc Surg 1996;3(1):22–30.
7. Higashida RT, Tsai FY, Halbach VV, et al. Cerebral percutaneous transluminal angioplasty. Heart Dis Stroke 1993;2(6):497–502.
8. Higashida RT, Tsai FY, Halbach VV, et al. Transluminal angioplasty for atherosclerotic disease of the vertebral and basilar arteries. J Neurosurg 1993;78(2):192–198.
9. Markus HS, Clifton A, Buckenham T, et al. Carotid angioplasty. Detection of embolic signals during and after the procedure. Stroke 1994;25(12):2403–2406.
10. Crawley F, Clifton A, Markus H, et al. Delayed improvement in carotid artery diameter after carotid angioplasty. Stroke 1997;28(3):574–579.
11. Tyagi S, Verma PK, Gambhir DS, et al. Early and long-term results of subclavian angioplasty in aortoarteritis (Takayasu disease): comparison with atherosclerosis. Cardiovasc Intervent Radiol 1998;21(3):219–224.
12. Schoser BG, Becker VU, Eckert B, et al. Clinical and ultrasonic long-term results of percutaneous transluminal carotid angioplasty. A prospective follow-up of 30 carotid angioplasties. Cerebrovasc Dis 1998;8(1):38–41.
13. Macaya C, Serruys PW, Ruygrok P, et al. Continued benefit of coronary stenting versus balloon angioplasty: one- year clinical follow-up of Benestent trial. Benestent Study Group. J Am Coll Cardiol 1996;27(2):255–261.
14. Serruys PW, van Hout B, Bonnier H, et al. Randomised comparison of implantation of heparin-coated stents with balloon angioplasty in selected patients with coronary artery disease (Benestent II). Lancet 1998;352(9129):673–681.
15. Wholey MH, Wholey M, Bergeron P, et al. Current global status of carotid artery stent placement. Cathet Cardiovasc Diagn 1998;44(1):1–6.
16. Yadav JS, Roubin GS, Iyer S, et al. Elective stenting of the extracranial carotid arteries. Circulation 1997;95(2):376–381.
17. Iyer SS, Roubin GS, Yadav S, et al. Elective Carotid Stenting. J Endovasc Surg 1996;3:42–62.
18. Storey GS, Marks MP, Dake M, et al. Vertebral artery stenting following percutaneous transluminal angioplasty. Technical note. J Neurosurg 1996;84(5):883–887.
19. Yadav JS, Roubin GS, King P, et al. Angioplasty and stenting for restenosis after carotid endarterectomy. Initial experience. Stroke 1996;27(11):2075–2079.
20. Piepgras DG, Sundt TM, Jr., Marsh WR, et al. Recurrent carotid stenosis. Results and complications of 57 operations. Ann Surg 1986;203(2):205–213.
21. Vitek J, Roubin G, Iyer S. Immediate and Late Outcome Of Carotid Angioplasty With Stenting. Joint Section Meeting, AANS/CNS/ASITN (Nashville) 1999(43, P1).
22. Mathur A, Dorros G, Iyer SS, et al. Palmaz stent compression in patients following carotid artery stenting. Cathet Cardiovasc Diagn 1997;41(2):137–140.
23. Mathur A, Roubin GS, Iyer SS, et al. Predictors of stroke complicating carotid artery stenting. Circulation 1998;97(13):1239–1245.
24. Beneficial effect of carotid endarterectomy in symptomatic patients with high-grade carotid stenosis. North American Symptomatic Carotid Endarterectomy Trial Collaborators. N Engl J Med 1991;325(7):445–453.

25. Endarterectomy for asymptomatic carotid artery stenosis. Executive Committee for the Asymptomatic Carotid Atherosclerosis Study [see comments]. Jama 1995;273(18):1421–1428.

26. Sundt TMJ, Meyer FB, Piepgras DG, et al. Risk factors and operative results. In: Meyer FB, editor. Sundt's Occlusive Cerebrovascular Disease. 2nd ed. Philadelphia, PA.: W.B. Saunders; 1994. p. 241–247.

27. Robbin ML, Lockhart ME, Weber TM, et al. Carotid artery stents: early and intermediate follow-up with Doppler US. Radiology 1997;205(3):749–756.

28. Théron J. Cerebral protection during carotid angioplasty [letter; comment]. J Endovasc Surg 1996;3(4):484–486.

29. Muller M, Behnke S, Walter P, et al. Microembolic signals and intraoperative stroke in carotid endarterectomy. Acta Neurol Scand 1998;97(2):110–117.

30. Crawley F, Clifton A, Buckenham T, et al. Comparison of hemodynamic cerebral ischemia and microembolic signals detected during carotid endarterectomy and carotid angioplasty. Stroke 1997;28(12):2460–2464.

31. Bladin CF, Bingham L, Grigg L, et al. Transcranial Doppler detection of microemboli during percutaneous transluminal coronary angioplasty. Stroke 1998;29(11):2367–2370.

32. Gaunt ME, Brown L, Hartshorne T, et al. Unstable carotid plaques: preoperative identification and association with intraoperative embolisation detected by transcranial Doppler. Eur J Vasc Endovasc Surg 1996;11(1):78–82.

33. Levi CR, O'Malley HM, Fell G, et al. Transcranial Doppler detected cerebral microembolism following carotid endarterectomy. High microembolic signal loads predict postoperative cerebral ischaemia. Brain 1997;120(Pt 4):621–629.

34. Théron J, Courtheoux P, Alachkar F, et al. New triple coaxial catheter system for carotid angioplasty with cerebral protection. AJNR Am J Neuroradiol 1990;11(5):869–74; discussion 75–77.

35. Théron JG, Payelle GG, Coskun O, et al. Carotid artery stenosis: treatment with protected balloon angioplasty and stent placement [see comments]. Radiology 1996;201(3):627–636.

36. Zarins CK. Carotid endarterectomy: the gold standard [see comments]. J Endovasc Surg 1996;3(1):10–5.

37. Dorros G. Complications associated with extracranial carotid artery interventions. J Endovasc Surg 1996;3(2):166–170.

38. Komiyama M, Yamanaka K, Nishikawa M, et al. Prospective analysis of complications of catheter cerebral angiography in the digital subtraction angiography and magnetic resonance era. Neurol Med Chir (Tokyo) 1998;38(9):534–539; discussion 9–40.

39. Cloft HJ, Joseph GJ, Dion JE. Risk of cerebral angiography in patients with subarachnoid hemorrhage, cerebral aneurysm, and arteriovenous malformation: a meta-analysis. Stroke 1999;30(2):317–320.

40. Théron J, Guimaraens L, Oguzman C, et al. Complications of carotid angioplasty and stenting. Neurosurgical Focus 1998;5((6)):4.

41. Jordan WD, Jr., Voellinger DC, Fisher WS, et al. A comparison of carotid angioplasty with stenting versus endarterectomy with regional anesthesia. J Vasc Surg 1998;28(3):397–402.

42. Naylor AR, Bolia A, Abbott RJ, et al. Randomized study of carotid angioplasty and stenting versus carotid endarterectomy: a stopped trial. J Vasc Surg 1998;28(2):326–334.

43. Dorros G. Carotid arterial obliterative disease: should endovascular revascularization (stent supported angioplasty) today supplant carotid endarterectomy? J Interven Cardiol 1996;9(3):193–196.

44. Sivaguru A, Venables GS, Beard JD, et al. European carotid angioplasty trial [see comments]. J Endovasc Surg 1996;3(1):16–20.

45. Naylor AR, London NJ, Bell PR. Carotid and Vertebral Artery Transluminal Angioplasty Study [letter; comment]. Lancet 1997;349(9061):1324–1325.

46. Feldman RL, Rubin JJ, Kuykendall RC. Use of coronary Palmaz-Schatz stent in the percutaneous treatment of vertebral artery stenoses. Cathet Cardiovasc Diagn 1996;38(3):312–315.

47. Tcheng JE. Glycoprotein IIb/IIIa receptor inhibitors: putting the EPIC, IMPACT II, RESTORE, and EPILOG trials into perspective. Am J Cardiol 1996;78(3 A):35–40.

48. Terada T, Higashida RT, Halbach VV, et al. Transluminal angioplasty for arteriosclerotic disease of the distal vertebral and basilar arteries. J Neurol Neurosurg Psychiatry 1996;60(4):377–381.
49. Phatouros CC, Higashida RT, Malek AM, et al. Endovascular stenting of an acutely thrombosed basilar artery: technical case report and review of the literature. Neurosurgery 1999;44(3):667–673.
50. Dorros G, Cohn JM, Palmer LE. Stent deployment resolves a petrous carotid artery angioplasty dissection. AJNR Am J Neuroradiol 1998;19(2):392–394.
51. Feldman RL, Trigg L, Gaudier J, et al. Use of coronary Palmaz-Schatz stent in the percutaneous treatment of an intracranial carotid artery stenosis. Cathet Cardiovasc Diagn 1996;38(3):316–319.
52. Mencken GS, Wholey MH, Eles GR. Use of coronary artery stents in the treatment of internal carotid artery stenosis at the base of the skull. Cathet Cardiovasc Diagn 1998;45(4):434–438.
53. Bernard JD, Vang MC, Williams JS. Intracranial Primary Stent-Assisted Angioplasty: A Case Series. Joint Section Meeting, AANS/CNS/ASITN (Nashville) 1999:44, p2.
54. Schoser BG, Heesen C, Eckert B, et al. Cerebral hyperperfusion injury after percutaneous transluminal angioplasty of extracranial arteries. J Neurol 1997;244(2):101–104.
55. Ueda T, Sakaki S, Nochide I, et al. Angioplasty after intra-arterial thrombolysis for acute occlusion of intracranial arteries. Stroke 1998;29(12):2568–2574.
56. Berthiaume F, Frangos JA. Flow-induced prostacyclin production is mediated by a pertussis toxin- sensitive G protein. FEBS Lett 1992;308(3):277–279.
57. Tsao PS, Lewis NP, Alpert S, et al. Exposure to shear stress alters endothelial adhesiveness. Role of nitric oxide. Circulation 1995;92:3513–3519.
58. Diamond SL, Eskin SG, McIntire LV. Fluid flow stimulates tissue plasminogen activator secretion by cultured human endothelial cells. Science 1989;243:1483–1485.
59. Malek AM, Izumo S. Molecular aspects of signal transduction of shear stress in the endothelial cell [editorial]. J Hypertens 1994;12:989–999.
60. Wallace RC, Furlan AJ, Moliterno DJ, et al. Basilar artery rethrombosis: successful treatment with platelet glycoprotein IIB/IIIA receptor inhibitor. AJNR Am J Neuroradiol 1997;18(7):1257–1260.
61. Nakayama T, Tanaka K, Kaneko M, et al. Thrombolysis and angioplasty for acute occlusion of intracranial vertebrobasilar arteries. Report of three cases. J Neurosurg 1998;88(5):919–922.
62. Yokote H, Terada T, Ryujin K, et al. Percutaneous transluminal angioplasty for intracranial arteriosclerotic lesions. Neuroradiology 1998;40(9):590–596.
63. Budzik R, Farkas J, Schwamm LH, et al. Intra-arterial balloon assisted thrombolysis for acute stroke. Joint Section Meeting, AANS/CNS/ASITN (Nashville) 1999:53, A10.
64. Higashida RT, Smith W, Gress D, et al. Intravascular stent and endovascular coil placement for a ruptured fusiform aneurysm of the basilar artery. Case report and review of the literature. J Neurosurg 1997;87(6):944–949.
65. Perez-Cruet MJ, Patwardhan RV, Mawad ME, et al. Treatment of dissecting pseudoaneurysm of the cervical internal carotid artery using a wall stent and detachable coils: case report. Neurosurgery 1997;40(3):622–625; discussion 5–6.
66. Sekhon LH, Morgan MK, Sorby W, et al. Combined endovascular stent implantation and endosaccular coil placement for the treatment of a wide-necked vertebral artery aneurysm: technical case report [see comments]. Neurosurgery 1998;43(2):380–383; discussion 4.
67. Lylyk P, Ceratto R, Hurvitz D, et al. Treatment of a vertebral dissecting aneurysm with stents and coils: technical case report. Neurosurgery 1998;43(2):385–388.
68. Mericle RA, Lanzino G, Wakhloo AK, et al. Stenting and secondary coiling of intracranial internal carotid artery aneurysm: technical case report. Neurosurgery 1998;43(5):1229–1234.
69. Lieber BB, Stancampiano AP, Wakhloo AK. Alteration of hemodynamics in aneurysm models by stenting: influence of stent porosity. Ann Biomed Eng 1997;25(3):460–469.
70. Wakhloo AK, Lanzino G, Lieber BB, et al. Stents for intracranial aneurysms: the beginning of a new endovascular era? Neurosurgery 1998;43(2):377–379.
71. Awad IA, Carter LP, Spetzler RF, et al. Clinical vasospasm after subarachnoid hemorrhage: response to hypervolemic hemodilution and arterial hypertension. Stroke 1987;18(2):365–372.

72. Origitano TC, Wascher TM, Reichman OH, et al. Sustained increased cerebral blood flow with prophylactic hypertensive hypervolemic hemodilution ("triple-H" therapy) after subarachnoid hemorrhage. Neurosurgery 1990;27(5):729–739; discussion 39–40.

73. Higashida RT, Halbach VV, Cahan LD, et al. Transluminal angioplasty for treatment of intracranial arterial vasospasm. J Neurosurg 1989;71:648–653.

74. Elliott JP, Newell DW, Lam DJ, et al. Comparison of balloon angioplasty and papaverine infusion for the treatment of vasospasm following aneurysmal subarachnoid hemorrhage. J Neurosurg 1998;88(2):277–284.

75. Eskridge JM, McAuliffe W, Song JK, et al. Balloon angioplasty for the treatment of vasospasm: results of first 50 cases. Neurosurgery 1998;42(3):510–516; discussion 6–7.

76. Higashida RT, Halbach VV, Dowd CF, et al. Intravascular balloon dilatation therapy for intracranial arterial vasospasm: patient selection, technique, and clinical results. Neurosurg Rev 1992;15(2):89–95.

77. Marks MP, Dake MD, Steinberg GK, et al. Stent placement for arterial and venous cerebrovascular disease: preliminary experience. Radiology 1994;191(2):441–446.

78. Malek AM, Izumo S. Control of endothelial cell gene expression by flow. J Biomech 1995;28(12):1515–1528.

79. Rutherford RB. Primary subclavian-axillary vein thrombosis: the relative roles of thrombolysis, percutaneous angioplasty, stents, and surgery. Semin Vasc Surg 1998;11(2):91–95.

80. Malek AM, Higashida RT, Balousek PA, et al. Endovascular recanalization with balloon angioplasty and stenting of an occluded occipital sinus for treatment of intracranial venous hypertension: technical case report. Neurosurgery 1999;44;4:890–901.

81. Duke BJ, Ryu RK, Brega KE, et al. Traumatic bilateral jugular vein thrombosis: case report and review of the literature. Neurosurgery 1997;41(3):680–683.

82. Mathias K. Stent placement in supra-aortic artery disease. In: Lieberman DD, editor. Stents. State of the art and future developments. Morin Heights, Canada: Polyscience Publication; 1995. p. 87–92.

83. Diethrich EB, Ndiaye M, Reid DB. Stenting in the carotid artery: initial experience in 110 patients. J Endovasc Surg 1996;3(1):42–62.

84. Vozzi CR, Rodriguez AO, Paolantonio D, et al. Extracranial carotid angioplasty and stenting. Initial results and short-term follow-up. Tex Heart Inst J 1997;24(3):167–172.

85. Henry M, Amor M, Masson I, et al. Angioplasty and stenting of the extracranial carotid arteries. J Endovasc Surg 1998;5(4):293–304.

Therapeutic Moderate Hypothermia and Fever

D.W. Marion

Introduction

Trauma, subarachnoid hemorrhage (SAH), cerebrovascular occlusive disease, and spontaneous intracranial hemorrhage all can cause significant brain injury. It is increasingly clear that two distinct phases of injury result in the ultimate neurologic dysfunction suffered by the patient. The first phase involves direct physical damage to the brain tissue, either from the percussive effects of trauma to the head, or compression and tearing of the brain tissue from an enlarging blood clot. The second phase, often called secondary brain injury, is due to a variety of metabolic and physiologic processes initiated by regional cerebral ischemia. These processes include breakdown of the blood-brain barrier, disruption of cerebral autoregulatory mechanisms, the accumulation of toxic extracellular levels of excitatory amino acids and free radicles, the cellular inflammatory response, and regional hyperthermia. Ultimately, the result of secondary injury is cytotoxic and vasogenic edema, elevated intracranial pressure, and cell death.

A mismatch of blood flow and metabolism is a likely underlying abnormality responsible for secondary brain injury, though it is clear that both abnormal hypermetabolism as well as ischemia itself is worsened in the face of hypothermia [25]. In rodent ischemia models, hyperthermia (39°C) superimposed on transient ischemia leads to a ten-fold increase in the number of ischemic neurons and a significant increase in calpain activation and spectrin degradation [2, 5]. Hyperthermia occurring even at 24 hours after transient ischemia leads to a significant increase in the number of ischemic neurons in selectively vulnerable brain-injured regions [12, 23].

In patients with spontaneous intracerebral hemorrhage, Swartz, et al. have documented a significant association between the duration of fever (>37.5°C) and poor outcomes for 196 patients surviving for the first 72 hours after their hemorrhage [21]. A significant increase in morbidity and mortality associated with fever after a patient has suffered a stroke was found in a metaanalysis of 3,790 patients. Finally, prevention of fever in 20 patients with middle cerebral artery infarcts has been shown to provide better control of critically elevated intracranial pressure and better than expected outcomes. The clinical studies of the use of therapeutic moderate hypothermia for the treatment of brain injury may have found benefit of this treatment not only because of a lower than normal temperature during the early period after injury, but also by assuring that hyperthermia was avoided in that group.

Therapeutic Moderate Hypothermia for the Treatment of Severe TBI

The intentional cooling of patients with severe TBI as a therapeutic option was first reported by Temple Fay in the 1930's. During the next 20 years or so, others also reported its use for TBI patients and all of these investigators suggested a possible benefit, though none of the studies were prospective randomized clinical trials [19]. In the late 1980's there was a resurgence of interest in this treatment when it was demonstrated that cooling to as little at 32°C might be effective [2–8, 10, 16, 17, 24, 26, 27]. This was an important observation since it was clear that cooling below 30° C was associated with an increased risk for cardiac arrhythmias [14]. During the last 10 years, numerous clinical studies have been conducted investigating the efficacy of therapeutic moderate hypothermia for severe TBI [18, 22]. Those studies found a 20–30% reduction in cerebral blood flow, possible decrease in cerebral blood volume, increase in tissue pO_2 and preservation of ATP stores with the use of this treatment. In addition, seven clinical studies of patients with TBI and one study of patients with stroke have found a significant reduction of intracranial pressure with the use of hypothermia to as little as 34°C [1, 13]. The clinical studies also have found that hypothermia causes a significant suppression of interleukin 1-β (IL-1β) and glutamate in the ventricular cerebral spinal fluid [7]. A prospective randomized trial of 82 patients with severe TBI published in 1997 found a two-fold increase in the number of patients achieving mild or no disability at six months after injury if they were cooled to 32–33°C for 24 hours after injury as compared to a similar group of TBI patients kept normothermic [18].

Deep Brain Temperature Often is Higher Than Body Temperature

Using an external ventricular drainage catheter that contained a microthermistor, the direct measurement of deep brain temperature was studied in eight patients with severe TBI for five days to determine how well rectal and bladder temperatures correlate with brain temperatures. Based on some 30,000 minute-by-minute observations, we found a frequent disparity between rectal or bladder and brain temperatures, which ranged from .1 to as high as 2°C difference. Differences were greatest when the rectal or bladder temperatures were above 38°C. On several occasions we recorded rectal temperatures of 38 or 39°C while the deep brain temperature was 40 to 41°C. These findings have led us to change our protocol in the neurotrauma ICU. In the past, we began treatment for fever when rectal temperatures exceeded 38.5°C. Currently, we begin treatment of fever when rectal temperature exceeds 37.5°C in order to be sure that we are adequately treating presumed higher brain temperatures.

Fever in the Neurosurgical Intensive Care Unit

It has long been the impression of neurosurgeons that fever is very common in critically ill neurosurgical patients. Febrile episodes may occur as the result of pulmonary problems such as atelectasis or pneumonia, urinary tract infections, or deep venous thrombosis. Fever in a neurosurgical patient also can be the result of hypothalamic dysfunction or SAH, either of which can cause an increase in IL-1ß levels [7]. It also is well known that the longer the patient resides in the ICU, the more likely they will have one or more febrile episodes.

In order to prospectively quantify the occurrence of fever we studied 428 consecutive patients admitted to our neurovascular or neurotrauma ICU's from January through June of 1997 [15]. Thirty-four percent of these had cerebrovascular accidents, 13% had aneurysmal SAH, and 32% had TBI as their primary diagnoses. Rectal temperatures were obtained every 2 to 4 hours and a febrile episode was defined as a rectal temperature that exceeded 38.5°C. Febrile episodes (temperatures >38.5°C) were aggressively managed in our ICU's with the use of external cooling blankets, acetaminophen, and in particularly refractory cases, nasogastric ice water lavage. In this study, we found that 46.7% of the patients had at least one febrile episode, and there were a total of 946 febrile episodes recorded for the population as a whole. There was no apparent correlation with diagnoses, though there was a very strong correlation with length of stay in the ICU. Thus, those patients staying less than 24 hours had only a 15.5% incidence of febrile episodes, while those hospitalized for greater than 14 days had a 92.6% incidence. It was clear from this study that fever is an even more common problem than we had anticipated despite aggressive conventional methods of fever management.

Benefits of Intravascular Fever Management

Conventional treatment for fever in the ICU can be described as "reactive". That is, the patient is hospitalized in the ICU and rectal or bladder temperatures are monitored. When the temperature exceeds a predefined threshold, the nurse begins standard treatment for the fever. This may involve administration of acetaminophen either orally or rectally. In addition, one or more cooling blankets may be applied over the torso and abdomen. This treatment, however, may take 30 minutes to an hour or so to have maximum benefit. There is controversy, however, about the possibility of such external cooling causing the patient to shiver and the shivering contributing to an increase in body temperature. In addition, the beneficial effects of cooling blankets takes time. When fever is particularly refractory, internal lavage of the stomach is often used with ice-saline solution. This, however, requires the primary nurse to stand by the bedside for extended periods of time manually infusing and draining the saline solution from the nasogastric tube. In addition to the relative "labor intensive" aspects of this treatment, it can be seen from our study of 428 patients that these methods are often not effective in preventing fever.

An alternative to these techniques may be intravascular cooling. We recently completed a phase-one trial using intravascular cooling technology in 20 patients with SAH, intracerebral hemorrhage, TBI, and stroke. The patients were followed for seven days after the onset of their disease. Ten of the patients had intravascular cooling with a CoolGard™ (Alsius Corporation, Irvine, California) cooling catheter and 10 had their fever controlled with the conventional methods described above. That study revealed that those patients whose temperature was controlled with the intravascular device had a fever less than half of the time of a similar group of patients treated without the intravascular device. There were no significant complications associated with the use of the intravascular venous catheter and the management of fever was significantly less labor intensive from a nursing standpoint.

Conclusions

Fever above 38°C that occurs in patients with acute neurosurgical diseases appears to worsen secondary brain injury and presumably ultimate neurologic outcomes. Laboratory investigations are quite clear regarding the adverse effects of fever in terms not only of functional outcomes but also histologic and neurochemical injury. Several preliminary clinical studies also suggest worsened neurologic outcome in patients who are febrile compared to those who are not. Unfortunately, however, a large prospective study of 428 patients with acute neurosurgical diseases has shown that fever is extraordinarily common during the first seven days after SAH, stroke and TBI. The ability to eliminate fever in most of these patients during the first five to seven days after their injury would seem desirable. Based on a phase-one trial, it appears that intravascular cooling is a promising new method for avoiding fever in the neurosurgical ICU.

References

1. Azzimindi G, Bassein L, Nonino F, et al: Fever in acute stroke worsens prognosis: a prospective study. Stroke 26:2043–2050, 1995.
2. Buki A, Koizumi H, Povlishock JT: Moderate posttraumatic hypothermia decreases early calpain-mediated proteolysis and concomitant cytoskeletal compromise in traumatic axonal injury. Exp.Neurol 159:319–328, 1999.
3. Busto R, Dietrich WD, Globus MY, et al: Postischemic moderate hypothermia inhibits CA1 hippocampal ischemic neuronal injury. J Cereb Blood Flow Metab 9:S266, 1989.
4. Castillo, J, Martinez F, Leira R, et al: Mortality and morbidity of acute cerebral infarction related to temperature and basal analytical parameters. Cerebrovascular Disease 4:56–71, 1994.
5. Chatzipanteli K, Alonso OF, Kraydieh S, et al: Importance of posttraumatic hypothermia and hyperthermia on the inflammatory response after fluid percussion brain injury: biochemical and immunocytochemical studies. J Cereb Blood Flow Metab 20(3):531–542, 2000.
6. Chatzipanteli K, Wada K, Busto R, et al: Effects of moderate hypothermia on constitutive and inducible nitric oxide syntase activities after traumatic brain injury in the rat. J Neurochem. 72:2047–2052, 1999.
7. DeKosky ST, Miller PD, Styren S, et al: Interleukin-1B elevation in CSF following head injury in humans is attenuated by hypothermia. J Neurotrauma 11:106, 1994(Abstract).
8. Dempsey RJ, Combs DJ, Maley EM, et al: Moderate hypothermia reduces postischemic edema development and leukotriene production. Neurosurg 21:177–181, 1987.
9. Dietrich WD, Alonso O, Busto R, et al: Post-traumatic brain hypothermia reduces histopatho-

logical damage following concussive brain injury in the rat. Acta Neuropathol 87:250–258, 1994.

10. Globus MY, Alonso O, Dietrich WD, et al: Glutamate release and free radical production following brain injury: effects of posttraumatic hypothermia. J.Neurochem. 65:1704–1711, 1995.

11. Hajat C, Hajat S, Sharma P: Effects of poststroke pyrexia on stroke outcome: a meta-analysis of studies in patients. Stroke 31(2):410–414, 2000.

12. Hindfelt B: The prognostic significance of subfebrility and fever in ischemic cerebral infarction. Acta Neurol Scand 53:72–79, 1976.

13. Hindman BJ, Todd MM, Gelb AW, et al: Mild hypothermia as a protective therapy during intracranial aneurysm surgery: A randomized prospective pilot trial. Neurosurg 44:23–33, 1999.

14. Johansson T, Lisander B, Ivarsson I: Mild hypothermia does not increase blood loss during total hip arthroplasty. Acta Anaesthesiol. Scand 43:1005–1010, 1999.

15. Kilpatrick MM, Lowry DW, Firlik AD, et al: Uncontrolled hyperthermia in the neurosurgical intensive care unit. Neurosurgery 2000 (In Press).

16. Kim SH, Stezoski SW, Safar P, et al: Hypothermia, but not 100% oxygen breathing, prolongs survival time during lethal uncontrolled hemorrhagic shock in rats. J Trauma 44: 485–491, 1998.

17. Koizumi H, Povlishock JT: Posttraumatic hypothermia in the treatment of axonal damage in an animal model of traumatic axonal injury. J Neurosurg. 89:303–309, 1998.

18. Marion DW, Penrod LE, Kelsey SF, et al: Treatment of traumatic brain injury with moderate hypothermia. N Engl J Med 336: 540–546, 1997.

19. Rosomoff JL, Shulman K, Raynor R, et al: Experimental brain injury and delayed hypothermia. Surg Gynecol Obstet 110:27–32, 1960.

20. Schwab S, Schwarz S, Spranger M, et al: Moderate hypothermia in the treatment of patients with severe middle cerebral artery infarction. Stroke 29:2461–2466, 1998.

21. Schwarz S, Hafner K, Aschoff A, et al: Incidence and prognostic significance of fever following intracerebral hemorrhage. Neurology 54:354–361, 2000.

22. Shiozaki T, Sugimoto H, Taneda M, et al: Effect of mild hypothermia on uncontrollable intracranial hypoertension after severe head injury. J Neurosurg 79:363–368, 1995.

23. Shum-Tim D, Nagashima M, Shinoka T, et al: Postischemic hyperthermia exacerbates neurologic injury after deep hypothermid circulatory arrest. J Thorac Cardiovasc Surg 116:780–792, 1998.

24. Smith SL, Hall ED: Mild pre- and posttraumatic hypothermia attenuates blood-brain barrier damage following controlled cortical impact injury in the rat. J Neurotrauma 13:1–9, 1996.

25. Sternau LL, Globus MYT, Dietrich WD, et al: Ischemia-induced neurotransmitter release: effects of mild intraischemic hyperthermia, in Globus MYT, Dietrich WD (eds): The role of neurotransmitters in brain injury. New York, Plenum press:33–38, 1992.

26. Suehiro E, Fujisawa H, Ito H, et al: Brain temperature modifies glutamate neurotoxicity in vivo. J Neurotrauma 16:285–297, 1999.

27. Yager JY, Asselin J: The effect of pre hypoxic-ischemic (HI) hypo and hyperthermia on brain damage in the immature rat. Brain Res Dev Brain Res 117:139–143, 1999.

Cerebral Hemodynamics and Stroke Risk in Patients with Complete Carotid Artery Occlusion: Is There a Role for Cerebral Revascularization?

R.L. Grubb, Jr, and W.J. Powers

Patients with complete carotid artery occlusion comprise approximately 15% of those with carotid territory transient ischemic attacks or infarction [1–3]. Prevention of subsequent stroke in patients with carotid artery occlusion remains a difficult challenge. The overall risk of subsequent stroke is 7% per year and the risk of stroke ipsilateral to the occluded carotid artery is 5.9% per year [4]. These risks persist in the face of platelet inhibitory drugs and anticoagulants [5]. The importance of hemodynamic factors in the prognosis of carotid occlusion and the role of surgical re-vascularization in the treatment of these patients has been a subject of controversy for many years. The technique of extracranial-intracranial (EC/IC) arterial bypass surgery was developed in the late 1960's and applied to patients with carotid occlusion in an attempt to prevent subsequent stroke by improving the hemodynamic status of the cerebral circulation distal to the occluded vessel. The results of an international multicenter randomized trial to determine the efficacy of EC/IC arterial bypass for the prevention of subsequent stroke was reported in 1985. Among 808 patients with symptomatic carotid occlusion who were randomized, no benefit of superficial temporal artery – middle cerebral artery (STA-MCA) bypass surgery could be demonstrated [6]. Based on the results of this trial, EC/IC bypass was generally abandoned as a treatment for symptomatic carotid artery occlusion. This trial has, however, been criticized for failing to identify and separately analyze the subgroup of patients with hemodynamic compromise in whom surgical revascularization might be more beneficial [7–10]. At the time that this trial was conducted, there was no reliable and proven method for identifying a subgroup of patients in whom cerebral hemodynamic factors were of primary pathophysiologic importance. In addition, STA-MCA bypass has been criticized for not providing adequate augmentation of blood flow to restore cerebral hemodynamics to normal. This has led to the development of other surgical revascularization strategies based on the promise that hemodynamic factors are important [11]. The relative importance of hemodynamic and embolic factors in these patients remains unclear [12–14]. These patients may suffer stroke from hemodynamic insufficiency distal to the carotid occlusion or from emboli arising from several sources including the stump of the occluded internal carotid artery in the neck, the tail of the stagnation thrombus that forms distal to the occlusion, or the contralateral carotid artery. This distinction is of more than just academic interest since treatment with antithrombotic drugs such as aspirin or warfarin is unlikely to prevent hemodynamic stroke. Surgical revascularization procedures have the potential to improve regional cerebral perfusion pressure (CPP) and regional cerebral blood flow (rCBF) and prevent hemodynamic infarction. Since these patients are at risk for both hemodynamic and embolic stroke, a better understanding of the relationship between cerebral hemodynamics and stroke risk is critical for the proper design of studies to evaluate both medical and surgical therapies to prevent stroke. Therapeutic trials are most effective when restricted to those patients who will benefit. This approach improves statistical power, decreases the likelihood that benefits in small subgroups will be overlooked and permits more specific applications of the results to clinical practice. Trials of anticoagulant and platelet inhibitory drugs should ideally exclude patients with hemodynamically mediated cerebral ischemia. Consideration of hemodynamic factors is, perhaps, even more important in the proper design of trials of surgical therapy for cerebrovascular disease. Superficial temporal artery-middle cerebral artery (STA-MCA) bypass surgery was developed to improve CBF in patients with complete carotid occlusion or intracranial carotid stenosis not amenable to conventional extracranial endarterectomy. Since this surgery is unlikely to provide protection from embolic stroke, its efficacy in preventing stroke should be greatest in those patients in whom hemodynamic factors are important in the pathogenesis of cerebral infarction. Thus, a better understanding of the importance of cerebral hemodynamics is critical in determining future research directions into improved methods for stroke prevention.

Assessment of Cerebral Hemodynamics

The development of modern imaging techniques has made it possible to indirectly assess the hemodynamic status of the human cerebral circulation in vivo. A variety of different imaging techniques have been used for the assessment of cerebral hemodynamic status. However, these methods are not interchangeable. They rely on different physiologic mechanisms by which the presence of hemodynamic compromise is inferred. Measurements of CBF alone are inadequate for this purpose. They cannot distinguish reduced CBF caused by the hemodynamic effects of arterial occlusive disease from compensatory physiological reductions in CBF caused by the reduced metabolic demands of damaged tissue. It has been necessary, therefore, to rely on indirect assessments based upon the compensatory responses made by the brain to progressive reductions in CPP. When CPP is normal (Stage 0), CBF is closely matched to the resting metabolic rate of the tissue. As a consequence of this resting balance between flow and metabolism, the oxygen extraction fraction (OEF) of the brain shows little regional variation. Moderate reductions in CPP have little effect on CBF. Vasodilation of arterioles reduces cerebrovascular resistance, thus maintaining a constant CBF (Stage I). This phenomenon is known as cerebrovascular autoregulation. As a consequence of arteriolar vasodilation, the intravascular cerebral blood volume (CBV) is often elevated, although this has been an inconsistent finding. With more severe reductions in CPP, the capacity for compensatory vasodilation is exceeded and autoregulation fails. CBF begins to decline but a progressive increase in OEF now maintains cerebral oxygen metabolism and brain function (Stage II) [15–17]. This more severe form of cerebral hemodynamic failure has also been termed "misery perfusion" [18].

Two basic approaches have been used to assess regional cerebral hemodynamics in humans. The first approach is based on detecting Stage I autoregulatory vasodilation by either measuring CBF and CBV or by determining if there is reduced responsiveness of CBF to a vasodilatory stimulus. A variety of vasodilatory stimuli have been used to make the paired measurements of cerebral perfusion needed for evaluating the vasodilatory response including hypercapnia, acetazolamide and physiologic tasks such as hand movement [5, 13, 15, 19]. Normally each of these vasodilatory stimuli will produce a robust increase in CBF. Failure of this augmentation is interpreted as evidence of pre-existing autoregulatory vasodilation (Stage I hemodynamic compromise). Although this is a logical interpretation, certain difficulties arise. There is not always a good correspondence between the CBF response to different vasodilatory stimuli in the same individual indicating that the mechanisms are different and may be related t o factors other that autoregulatory vasodilation [19–21].

The second approach is based on detecting more severe Stage II hemodynamic failure by measuring increases in regional OEF [15, 17]. As opposed to the use of CBV measurements or vasodilatory stimuli, interpretation of increased OEF does not require any inferences about hemodynamic status since it is the direct measurement of the pathophysiological response. Measurement of OEF currently is only possible with positron emission tomography (PET). While MR pulse sequences sensitive to the amount of deoxyhemoglobin (blood oxygen level dependent or BOLD) in venous blood are commonly used to identify changes in regional blood flow with brain activation, their application to static measurements of brain oxygenation has proven more difficult [22–24]. The signal contribution from non-vascular tissue and the effect of variation in CBV currently precludes the use of BOLD sequences for quantitative measurement OEF at this time, although research in this area is being actively pursued [25–29]. The correlation between the CBF response to vasodilatory agents and increased OEF has been somewhat variable and inconsistent. [21, 30–35]. One attempt to substitute the measurement of CBF reactivity to acetazolamide for PET measurements of OEF was based on criteria derived from a comparison of paired studies in 14 subjects [33]. However, in a subsequent prospective study of 105 patients, the PET-derived acetazolamide-CBF criteria for increased OEF failed to predict subsequent stroke [36], a result very different from the three studies in which OEF was measured directly [5, 37, 38]. It is not possible at this time to identify a non-PET method for assessing OEF that has sufficient proven sensitivity and specificity for a substitute method.

Cerebral Hemodynamics and Stroke Risk

Multiple different methodologies have used to assess the impact of cerebral hemodynamics on the pathogenesis and treatment of stroke (Table 1) [13, 14]. In many of these reports follow-up information about patients studied with these techniques has been limited and insufficient to allow for any definitive conclu-

Table 1. Cerebral hemodynamics and stroke risk

	Study Design	No. of Patients	Follow-Up (Months)	Technique	Cerebral Vasoreactivity (No. of Patients) (Ipsilateral Annual Stroke Risk)		
					Normal	Moderate Impairment	Severe Impairment
Powers – 1989 [45]	Retrospective	30	12	PET CBV/CBF & OEF	9 11%	21 0	
Hasegawa – 1992 [46]	Prospective	51	18.5	SPECT CBF Acetazolamide	31 0	20 0	
Kleiser – 1992 [41]	Prospective	*85	38	Transcranial Doppler CO_2 Reactivity	48 0	26 7%	11 24%
Widder – 1994 [44]	Prospective	*86(111)	[a]19 [b]31.7	Transcranial Doppler CO_2	[b](48) 1%	[b](37) 1%	[a](26) 8%
Yonas – 1993 [39]	Retrospective	*41	24	Xenon-CT CBF Acetazolamide	25 0	16 16%	
Webster – 1995 [40]	Retrospective	*64	19.6	Xenon-CT CBF Acetazolamide	26 0	38 13%	
Yamauchi – 1996 [37]	Prospective	40	12	PET OEF	33 6%		7 57%
Yamauchi – 1999 [38]	Prospective	40	60	PET OEF	33 13%		7 11%
Yokota – 1998 [36]	Prospective	105	32.5	SPECT CBF Acetazolamide	50 4%	55 4%	
Grubb – 1998 [5]	Prospective	*81	31.5	PET OEF	42 3%		39 13%

* Only ICA occlusion patients. ( ) No. of cerebral hemispheres.

sions to be made. Stage I hemodynamic compromise was found to have an increased stroke risk in four studies and three studies did not find an association. Yonas and co-workers tested cerebrovascular reserve in patients with atherosclerotic occlusive carotid artery disease by paired CBF measurements obtained with the stable Xenon-CT scanning method, with the cerebral vasodilatory agent acetazolamide given intravenously 20 minutes prior to the second study [39]. 41 of the 68 patients in the study had internal carotid artery occlusion. The patients were placed in one of two groups based on the vascular territory found to have the lowest cerebral vasoreactivity and a relatively low baseline CBF. This categorization was done retrospectively based on assessment of the characteristics of the patients who went on to develop a stroke. The first group (n=27) had baseline blood flow values >45 ml · 100 g^{-1} · min^{-1} or cerebrovascular reserves ≥5%. The second group (n=41) had initial blood flow values <45 ml · 100 g^{-1} · min^{-1} and cerebrovascular reserves <5%. Sixty-eight patients with either carotid artery stenosis of ≥70% or carotid artery occlusion were followed for a mean of 24 months. There were two contralateral strokes in the first group and eight ipsilateral strokes in the second group (12.6 times greater chance of stroke). None of the 25 patients with internal carotid artery occlusion in the first group had an ipsilateral stroke, whereas 5 of 16 patients with internal carotid artery occlusion in the second group suffered a subsequent ipsilateral stroke (31% stroke risk). These authors subsequently added 27 patients for an analysis of 95 patients with either stenosis of ≤70% or carotid artery occlusion [40]. The patients were followed for a mean of 19.6 months. In the second group with the more severe impairment of cerebral vasoreactivity, 8 of 38 patients with occlusion of the internal carotid artery had a subsequent ipsilateral stroke (21% stroke risk). These patients were classified into two groups based only on a paradoxical response of CBF to the cerebral vasodilatory agent acetazolamide, different criteria than those used in the first study. Another longitudinal study tested the cerebrovascular reserve capacity in 85 patients with internal carotid artery occlusion using transcranial Doppler sonography [41]. There were 81 angiographically proven unilateral and four bilateral ICA occlusions in the study group. At the time of entry into the study, 46 patients were asymptomatic on the ipsilateral side of the ICA occlusion, 13 had presented with reversible symptoms, and 26 had had a minor stroke. 2 patients had a TIA and 8 had a stroke contralateral to the ICA occlusion. Middle cerebral artery (MCA) blood flow velocity and end-tidal PCO$_2$ were monitored during steady states of normocapnia, hypercapnia induced by breathing 5% CO$_2$ in 95% O$_2$, and hypocapnia produced by voluntary hyperventilation. The results of CO$_2$ reactivity studies were classified into three categories. Sufficient CO$_2$ reactivity was defined as an increase of MCA blood flow velocity of 10% during hypercapnia and a decrease of 10% during hypocapnia; diminished cerebrovascular reactivity was characterized by a marked decrease or lack of increase in flow velocity during hypercapnia with a normal response to hypocapnia; and exhausted CO$_2$ reactivity was defined by a marked decrease or lack of change in blood flow velocity during hypercapnia combined with a diminished response during hypocapnia. The patients were followed for a mean of 38 (±15 SD) months. A total of 8 patients had an ipsilateral stroke and 8 patients had an ipsilateral TIA or prolonged reversible ischemic neurologic deficit (PRIND) during the follow-up period. There were four contralateral strokes and one contralateral TIA, which occurred in conjunction with progression of an ICA stenosis on the same side in three cases. In the group with sufficient cerebrovascular reserve, 4 of 48 patients had an ipsilateral TIA or PRIND, but no patient had a stroke. 6 of 26 patients with diminished CO_2 reactivity had an ipsilateral ischemic event [three (12%) strokes, three TIAs, and 3 patients had a contralateral event (two strokes, one TIA). In the group with exhausted cerebrovascular reserve capacity, 5 of 11 patients (45%) had an ipsilateral stroke and 1 patient had an ipsilateral TIA. 2 patients had a contralateral hemisphere stroke. During the follow-up period, 10 patients died of noncerebral causes. In this study a significant correlation was found between diminished CO_2 reactivity of the cerebral circulation and ischemic events ipsilateral to an internal carotid artery occlusion. There was no significant relationship between patients with and without a history of neurological symptoms at the time the ICA occlusion was discovered. This is puzzling since the prognosis of asymptomatic carotid occlusion is relatively benign [42, 43]. The increased risk of contralateral stroke in the patients with a diminished or exhausted CO_2 reactivity suggests that the two groups were not matched with the normal CO_2 reactivity group for other stroke risk factors, and this may explain the differences observed. These same authors later reported 86 patients with carotid artery occlusion who were followed for variable periods of time [44]. A stroke ipsilateral to an occluded internal carotid artery occurred in 3 of 26 patients with an exhausted CO_2 reactivity, corresponding to an annual stroke rate of 8% (mean follow-up time of 19 months). The annual stroke rate in patients with exhausted CO_2 reactivity was much lower in this study, compared to the group of patients previously reported by these investigators. In 37 patients with diminished CO_2 reactivity and 48 patients with sufficient CO_2 reactivity, only 1 patient in each group developed an ipsilateral stroke (mean follow-up time of 31.7 months). There are a number of potential problems with the interpretation of the results of these two studies. The criteria for selecting patients in the second study were not given. In the first study, 46 of 85 patients were asymptomatic. In the second study, the number of asymptomatic patients was not given. The 86 patients in the second study were selected from 452 patients with ICA occlusion studied with transcranial Doppler cerebrovascular resistance studies. The dates of data collection in the two studies overlap and the impact of this on the results of the two studies was not given.

A small longitudinal retrospective study followed 30 medically treated patients with a mixture of cerebrovascular lesions including carotid artery occlusion and intracranial stenoses for one year [45]. PET measurements of the CBV/CBF ratio and OEF were carried out in these patients. In 21 patients with increased CBV/CBF ratios distal to a stenotic or occluded artery, no ipsilateral ischemic strokes occurred during the one-year follow-up period. One of nine patients with normal cerebral hemodynamics had an ipsilateral ischemic stroke during the follow-up period.

Another small prospective study followed 51 patients for 1 1/2 years [46]. There was a mixture of asymptomatic and symptomatic carotid artery and intracranial artery stenoses of 75% or greater and occlusions in these patients. Each patient had a SPECT study of cerebral perfusion using I-123 IMP and measurement of cerebrovascular reactivity using acetazolamide. Impaired cerebrovascular reactivity was defined as changes in relative blood flow lower then the 95% confidence limit for normals. Twenty patients had impaired cerebrovascular reactivity. No patient had a stroke during the follow-up period.

The largest and most methodologically sound study that did not demonstrate a relationship between Stage I impairment of cerebral hemodynamics and the risk of subsequent stroke was a prospective study reported by Yokota and co-workers [36]. 105 patients with evidence of ischemic cerebrovascular events, minimal infarct on a CT scan, and unilateral occlusion or severe stenosis (>75% in diameter) of the ICA or proximal MCA confirmed by cerebral angiography were entered into the study. Risk factors for stroke at entry were recorded and included in the final data analysis. The primary endpoint was stroke occurrence. The median follow-up period in the study was 32.5 months. Each patient had a SPECT study of cerebral perfusion using I-123 IMP and measurement of cerebrovascular reactivity using acetazolamide. Based on the local cerebral perfusion reactivity to acetazolamide, the patients were divided into two groups, those with normal cerebrovascular reactivity and those with impaired cerebrovascular reactivity. 55 patients had an abnormal cerebral vasoreactivity response to acetazolamide and 50 patients had a normal response. There was no significant difference in the stroke risk factors between the two groups, except the group with an abnormal response to acetazolamide had a higher systolic blood pressure at entry into the study. The sites of the vascular lesions were comparable between the two groups. During the follow-up period, 13 patients had a stroke, 11 died, 16 had surgical cerebral revascularization procedures (9 EC/IC bypasses and 7 carotid endarterectomies), and 11 were lost to follow-up. 8 of the 13 patients with subsequent stroke had stenosis of the ICA or MCA at entry into the study. There was no significant difference in the rate of subsequent stroke in the two groups during the period of follow-up. When stroke occurrence and death were combined, the two groups again had no significant difference. Follow-up SPECT studies with acetazolamide testing showed that cerebrovascular reactivity became normal at an average of 2 years in 11 of 24 patients with initially impaired response to acetazolamide. There are a number of potential problems in this study. The SPECT cerebral perfusion measurements were qualitative, and there is a possibility that the measurements of cerebrovascular reactivity in this study failed to differentiate a group of patients with severe impairment of cerebral hemodynamics. The patients in the study had a variety of extracranial and intracranial cerebrovascular lesions and included only a small number of patients with ICA occlusion. A relatively large number of patients were censored from the study because of subsequent cerebrovascular surgery and a significant number of patients were lost to follow-up. Since the criteria used for separating patients into those with normal and abnormal cerebrovascular reactivity were based on a previous study which demonstrated complete agreement with PET measurements of OEF [33], the negative results of this study are puzzling in light of two PET studies which demonstrated a strong association between increased OEF and the subsequent risk of stroke (see below).

A positive association of stage II cerebral hemodynamic compromise and stroke risk has been found by two groups. In these studies the finding of increased OEF increased the subsequent risk for ipsilateral stroke.

A small longitudinal study performed PET measurements of rCBF, rCBV, rOEF, and rCMRO$_2$ in 40 patients with symptomatic occlusion or intracranial stenosis of the internal carotid or middle cerebral arterial system treated medically [37]. 6 patients had TIAs and 34 patients had minor infarctions. The intervals between the most recent cerebral ischemic event and the PET studies was one to 55 months, with 17 of the 40 patients studied 30 to 90 days following the most recent cerebrovascular event. All patients were treated with antiplatelet therapy. All patients were followed for at least 12 months. During the period in which these patients were studied, 12 other symptomatic patients with internal carotid artery or middle cerebral artery occlusive disease also underwent PET studies, but were excluded from the study because of subsequent vascular reconstructive surgery. 7 patients had a STA-MCA anastomosis and 5 patients had a carotid endarterectomy. Patients were divided into two categories based on the absolute mean hemispheric value of oxygen extraction in the symptomatic cerebral hemisphere: patients with normal OEF and those with increased OEF. At one year following the PET studies, 5 of 7 patients with increased OEF had developed a stroke, 4 strokes were ipsilateral and 1 was contralateral. 4 of 33 patients with normal OEF had developed a stroke. 2 strokes were ipsilateral and 2 were contralateral. In patients with increased OEF, 3 of 4 ipsilateral strokes were watershed infarctions corresponding to an area of increased rOEF. All the patients with a stroke in the follow-up period had had a minor stroke at entry into the study. After the first year of follow-up, 1 ipsilateral stroke and 1 contralateral stroke occurred, with both of these strokes occurring in patients with normal OEF.

In a subsequent study by these authors, a five year follow-up of these 40 patients was reported [38]. In this study, increased OEF was evaluated in two ways: based on absolute OEF values and based on left cerebral hemisphere to right cerebral hemisphere ratios. Based on absolute OEF values in the symptomatic cerebral hemisphere, 7 patients had increased OEF values and 33 had normal OEF values. During the five-year follow-up period, there were 11 total and 9 ipsilateral ischemic strokes. In the data analysis using absolute values of OEF, ischemic strokes occurred in 5 of 7 patients with increased OEF and 6 of 33 patients with normal OEF. There were 4 ipsilateral ischemic strokes in the increased OEF group and 5 ipsilateral ischemic strokes in the normal OEF group. All the strokes in patients with increased OEF occurred within one year. When the data was analyzed using OEF asymmetry based on left-to-right cerebral hemisphere OEF ratios, ischemic strokes occurred in 6 of 14 patients with increased OEF and 5 of 26 patients with normal OEF. There were 5 ipsilateral ischemic strokes in patients with increased OEF and 4 ipsilateral ischemic strokes in patients with normal OEF.

The strongest evidence to an association of cerebral hemodynamic impairment and stroke has been provided by the St. Louis Carotid Occlusion Study (STL-COS) [5]. This was a blinded, prospective study to test the hypothesis that Stage II hemodynamic failure (increased oxygen extraction) in the cerebral hemisphere distal to complete carotid artery occlusion was an independent predictor of the subsequent risk of stroke in symptomatic medically treated patients. Inclusion criteria were occlusion of one or both common or internal carotid arteries demonstrated by contrast angiography or MR angiography in patients with transient ischemic neurological deficits (including transient monocular blindness) or mild to moderate neurological deficits (stroke) in the territory of the occluded carotid artery. Patients who had undergone ipsilateral external carotid endarterectomy (CEA) or contralateral CEA prior to PET were eligible whether or not they had had recurrent symptoms. Any subsequent cerebrovascular surgery after the initial PET caused the patient to be censored from the study at the time of surgery. Just prior to PET, each subject underwent neurological evaluation including detailed questioning regarding any symptoms. Focal ischemic symptoms in the territory of the occluded carotid artery were categorized as cerebral TIA (<24 hours duration), cerebral infarct (>24 hours duration), or retinal event (any duration) and as single or recurrent episodes. Time from most recent symptom was recorded. Pertinent medical records, CT scans, and angiograms were reviewed. The following baseline risk factors were specifically determined: age, gender, hypertension, previous myocardial infarction, diabetes mellitus, smoking, alcohol consumption, and parental death from stroke. The degree of contralateral carotid stenosis and collateral arterial circulation to the ipsilateral middle cerebral artery (MCA) was determined from arteriograms if available. Blood samples were collected for determination of hemoglobin, fasting lipid levels (triglyceride, HDL-cholesterol, LDL-cholesterol) and fibrinogen levels. A non-contrast CT scan of the brain was performed if a CT had not been done as part of usual clinical care sufficiently long after an ischemic event to permit accurate definition of infarct location. This CT was used only to determine the site of tissue infarction so as to exclude these regions from subsequent PET analysis (see below).

PET measurements of CBF, CBV, $CMRO_2$, and OEF were carried out. Regional OEF was measured by the method of Mintun et al using $H_2^{15}O$, $C^{15}O$, and $O^{15}O$ [47, 48]. For each subject, 7 spherical regions of interest 19 mm in diameter were placed in the cortical territory of the middle cerebral artery in each hemisphere using stereotactic coordinates [49, 50]. Any regions in well-demarcated areas of reduced oxygen metabolism, which corresponded to areas of infarction by CT or MRI and their homologous contralateral regions, were excluded. The mean OEF for each MCA territory was calculated from the remaining regions and a left/right MCA OEF ratio was calculated. The maximum and minimum ratios from 18 normal control subjects were used to define the normal range. A separate range of normal for $H_2^{15}O/O^{15}O$ images was determined. Patients with left/right OEF ratios outside the normal range were categorized as having Stage II hemodynamic compromise in the hemisphere with higher OEF. These categorizations were made without knowledge of the side of the carotid occlusion or of the clinical course of the patients since the initial PET study. No information regarding the PET results was provided to the patients, treating physicians or the investigator responsible for determining endpoints.

The primary endpoint was subsequent ischemic stroke defined clinically as a neurological deficit of presumed ischemic cerebrovascular cause lasting greater than 24 hours in any cerebrovascular territory. Secondary endpoints were ipsilateral ischemic stroke and death. All living patients were followed for the duration of the study.

Subjects were divided into two groups: those with Stage II hemodynamic compromise and those with normal (symmetric) OEF. Comparison of 17 baseline risk factors and subsequent medical treatment between the two groups was performed with unpaired t-tests and Chi square analysis. Bonferroni adjusted p values of .05/18 = .003 were used as the criterion of statistical significance. The primary analysis compared the two groups with respect to the length of time before reaching the primary endpoint by means of the Mantel-Cox log rank statistic and Kaplan-Meier survival curves. A value of p<.05 was used as the criterion of statistical significance. Secondary endpoints were analyzed in a similar manner. No interim analysis was planned or performed. The Cox proportional hazards model was used to test nineteen candidate predictor variables in a univariate analysis. This included seventeen baseline variables, PET categorization of Stage II hemodynamic compromise, and subsequent medical treatment. All variables except medical treatment were treated as time-constant variables whereas medical treatment was treated as a time-dependent variable. All variables with p<0.05 in the univariate analysis were included in a subsequent multivariate analysis. Both forward and backward stepwise selections based on maximum partial likelihood estimates were used. Those variables that remained significant at p<.05 in the multivariate analysis were included in the final model.

81 patients successfully underwent initial data collection and PET measurements and were enrolled in the study. 39 patients had Stage II hemodynamic failure (increased OEF) in one hemisphere and 42 did not. In all 39 patients with Stage II hemodynamic failure, the hemisphere with increased OEF was ipsilateral to the occluded carotid. There were no subjects with bilateral carotid occlusion. There were no significant differences between the two groups in baseline risk factors or subsequent medical treatment. Arteriographic collateral circulation did not permit distinction between the two groups. Three subjects who underwent contralateral carotid endarterectomy prior to occurrence of ipsilateral ischemic stroke were censored after being followed for 13 months, 29 months, and 29 months respectively. Two had not reached any endpoint and one had experienced a vertebrobasilar stroke. A fourth patient who had experienced an ipsilateral stroke underwent subsequent endarterectomy and was censored at 13 months.

Mean follow-up duration of the patients was 31.5 months. 15 total and 13 ipsilateral ischemic strokes occurred during the follow-up period. There were no hemorrhages. In the 39 stage II subjects, 12 total and 11 ipsilateral strokes occurred. In the 42 subjects with normal OEF, there were 3 total and 2 ipsilateral strokes. The Kaplan-Meier estimates for the risk of subsequent stroke at one and two years are given in Table 2. The risk of all stroke and ipsilateral ischemic stroke in symptomatic Stage II subjects was significantly higher than in those with normal OEF (p=.005 and p=.004 respectively). 12 deaths occurred during the follow-up period. 10 deaths were due to non-stroke causes and 2 deaths resulted from large cerebral infarctions ipsilateral to a symptomatic occluded internal carotid artery. Both stroke-related deaths occurred in patients with increased OEF. There were 6 deaths in each group. No significant difference in the risk of death was demonstrated (p=.942). In the univariate analysis of the relationship to outcome of patient characteristics and subsequent medical treatment, only younger age and Stage II hemodynamic failure were significant predictors of both all stroke and ipsilateral ischemic stroke. Both variables remained significant in the multivariate analysis. The age adjusted relative risk conferred by Stage II hemodynam-

Table 2. Stroke risk for symptomatic patients [5]

	Total Patients (81)	Increased OEF (39)	Normal OEF (42)
All Stroke			
1 year	7.7%	13.2%	2.4%
2 years	19.0%	29.2%	9.0%
Ipsilateral Stroke			
1 year	6.4%	10.6%	2.4%
2 years	15.8%	26.5%	5.3%

Event rates were derived from Kaplan-Meier estimates of survival. The number of patients in each group is given in parenthesis.

ic failure was 6.0 (95% CI 1.7–21.6) for all stroke and 7.3 (95% CI 1.6–33.4) for ipsilateral ischemic stroke.

This study demonstrated that Stage II hemodynamic failure (increased oxygen extraction) distal to a symptomatic occluded carotid artery is an independent predictor of subsequent ischemic stroke. The study was prospective, blinded and addressed the possible effect of treatment and other risk factors for stroke. The rates for stroke and ipsilateral ischemic stroke in the total group of 81 symptomatic patients were similar to those reported by others and the risk factor profile was typical for patients with carotid artery disease [4, 6, 51].

Cerebral Hemodynamics and Extracranial Intracranial Arterial Bypass Surgery

Multiple studies with PET have demonstrated postoperative improvement of cerebral hemodynamics by STA-MCA bypass surgery [18, 52–58]. In patients with Stage II hemodynamic failure (increased oxygen extraction), EC/IC bypass surgery will return hemispheric OEF ratios to normal [52–55]. Improvement in impaired cerebral vasoreactivity to CO_2 or acetazolamide following EC/IC bypass for atherosclerotic occlusive cerebrovascular disease has been demonstrated [10, 59–63]. In most of these patients resting rCBF showed little change, although some patients with low resting rCBF demonstrated improvement in blood flow in the affected cerebral hemisphere following surgery. EC/IC bypass has been recommended for symptomatic patients with appropriate cerebrovascular lesions in whom impaired cerebral vasomotor reactivity to acetazolamide or CO_2 testing is demonstrated [10, 40, 64]. All of these studies were retrospective analyses of surgical patients. No prospective study of patients with occlusion of the internal carotid artery and impaired cerebral vasoreactivity to CO_2 or acetazolamide or increased oxygen extraction randomized to medical treatment or EC/IC bypass, with other risk factors for stroke controlled, has been carried out. Thus the long-term benefit of using impaired cerebral hemodynamics in the selection of patients for EC/IC bypass to prevent stroke remains unproven at this time.

The results of medical treatment of Stage II patients in the SLCOS were poor and comparable to those reported for medically treated patients with symptomatic severe carotid stenosis [51]. Surgical procedures that improve cerebral hemodynamics, such as extracranial-intracranial (EC/IC) arterial bypass surgery, would be a logical treatment for these patients. However, in the absence of an empiric trial, it cannot be assumed that the stroke risk in operated patients would be equal to that in patients with normal OEF or that the morbidity and mortality due to surgery would be outweighed by any subsequent reduction in stroke risk. The large, multicenter randomized trial of EC/IC bypass surgery conducted from 1977 to 1985 showed no benefit of surgery in preventing subsequent stroke [6]. At the time that this trial was conducted, there was no reliable and proven method for identifying a subgroup of patients in whom cerebral hemodynamic factors were of primary pathophysiologic importance. It is now established that such a subgroup can be identified and, furthermore, that they are at high risk for subsequent stroke when treated medically. Based on the finding of the STLCOS, it is appropriate to perform a new trial of EC/IC bypass surgery restricted to patients with symptomatic carotid occlusion and Stage II (increased OEF) impairment of cerebral hemodynamics.

Carotid Occlusion Surgery Study (COSS)

Before proposing a clinical trial based on using PET to select patients with symptomatic carotid occlusion for EC/IC bypass, a thorough examination of cost-effectiveness is necessary [65]. Cost-effectiveness analysis also allows investigation on cost and quality-adjusted survival of the impact of different variables – such as the effect of using more or less specific PET screening thresholds to identify surgical candidates. A Markov chain model was created to compare the costs and effectiveness of (1) medical treatment alone to (2) screening with PET followed by EC/IC bypass (if OEF was elevated) in patients with symptomatic carotid occlusion. The incremental costs per incremental quality adjusted life year (QALY) gained were calculated.

The cohort used in this analysis consisted of a high-risk group of 45 patients with recent (<120 days) symptoms of cerebral hemispheric ischemia identified by retrospective subgroup analysis from the STLCOS. In the medical treatment cohort the stroke outcomes for each patient from the STLCOS for the first two years of the model was used. After the first two years, the annual rate of any stroke was estimated as 3% per year. This estimate was based on interpolation of the Kaplan-Meier stroke-free survival curves for the medically treated patients in the EC/IC bypass trial (from months 24 through 60) [6]. There is evidence that severe hemodynamic impairment may spontaneously improve over time [36, 44, 66].

In the PET-screening strategy, patients identified with normal OEF received medical therapy. Two-year stroke outcomes for each of these patients were based on the two-year stroke outcomes in the STLCOS for patients with normal OEF. A literature-based estimate of 3% per year was used after the first two years. Patients identified with increased OEF underwent EC/IC bypass. The 30-day probabilities of perioperative stroke and death were from the EC/IC Bypass Trial (11.1% and 1.1%, respectively) [6]. The rates of stroke after the perioperative period were estimated from the Kaplan-Meier stroke-free survival curves for the surgical patients in the EC/IC bypass trial: 7% for months 2 through 12, 5% for year 2, and 3% for each following year. The rates of stroke-related and non stroke-related death were the same as the medically treated groups.

The utility of stroke-free current health was estimated as 0.90 [67–69]. The utility for stroke was based on the severity of the 10 nonfatal ipsilateral strokes observed in the relevant 45-member cohort in the STLCOS. Six of these strokes received the 0.76 utility of minor stroke because their post-stroke Barthel score was at least 95. The remaining 4 strokes were assigned the utility of 0.39 for moderate to severe strokes [68]. A base-case utility of 0.61 was used as a weighted average utility for the 6 minor and 4 major nonfatal strokes observed in the STLCOS.

The medical component of the Consumer Price Index was used to adjust all costs to 1998 dollars (Bureau of Labor Statistics web site, http://stats.bls.gov/cpi-home.htm). The Medicare reimbursement, including physician fees, for a fluoro-deoxyglucose (FDG) PET examination of the lung for pulmonary nodules was used as an estimate the cost of a screening PET study (General American/Medicare B, June 1998). There are no data for the cost of an oxygen-15 PET study. Because EC/IC bypass is no longer routinely performed or reimbursed by Medicare, its cost was estimated as the cost of clipping an asymptomatic, unruptured intracranial aneurysm [70]. Both procedures require a craniotomy and an operative microscope. Estimates of acute and long-term stroke care costs were obtained from the relevant literature [71–74]. Costs due to lost wages were not included, as they are difficult to estimate and small in this population [71].

In the base-case analysis, the count-based OEF threshold determined a priori from the range of normal values was used. In addition, different OEF thresholds were evaluated to identify the optimal one in terms of cost-effectiveness. Sensitivity analyses were performed to determine which variables had the greatest effect on the cost-effectiveness estimates and to determine a range of plausible cost-effectiveness estimates.

With medical therapy alone, 14 strokes (12 ipsilateral and 2 contralateral) occurred in the cohort of 45 patients within the first two years. PET screening, using the base-case OEF threshold, identified 9 patients with normal OEF and 36 patients with increased OEF. These 36 patients underwent EC/IC bypass so that only 8 strokes occurred within the first two years. This two-part strategy yielded 256 QALYs over 10 years, a gain of 22.8 versus medical therapy alone. The cost was $19,600 per QALY gained versus medical therapy.

In the secondary analysis of OEF threshold, a more specific OEF threshold that cost less and was nearly as effective as the base case was found. Screening with this OEF threshold identified 18 surgical candidates, (as compared to 36 with the base case) including 9 of the 12 patients who would have had a stroke during the first two years with medical therapy alone. Treated medically, these 18 patients had a two-year ipsilateral stroke risk of 50% compared with the remaining 27 patients with low OEF who had a two-year ipsilateral stroke risk of 12%. A total of 8.5 ipsilateral strokes were incurred during the first 2 years with this more specific screening strategy. This more specific threshold yielded a total of 256 QALYs over 10 years, a gain of 22.2 compared to medical therapy alone. However, screening with this threshold lost 0.6 QALYs compared to the base-case OEF threshold. The total cost was less than either medical therapy alone or the base-case two-step

PET-screening strategy. Therefore, the more specific OEF threshold dominated medical therapy alone because it was less expensive and yielded more QALYs. The incremental cost per incremental QALY gained (0.6 QALYs) for the slightly more effective base-case threshold compared to the more specific threshold (the marginal cost-effectiveness) was $800,000.

Sensitivity testing demonstrated that the results were most sensitive to the perioperative stroke rate and the stroke risk reduction conferred by EC/IC bypass. Despite the sensitivity of the model to the perioperative and post-operative stroke rates, screening with the more specific OEF threshold (followed by surgery for those with high OEF) remained cost-effective even with estimates of these two rates 50% higher than in the EC/IC Bypass Trial [6]. This result is not surprising given the high risk of stroke in the medically treated patients who have high OEF. The cost of PET had little effect on the results of the model. It was more that offset by reducing the number of operations (thus reducing the attendant risk and expense) performed on patients at low risk for subsequent stroke.

Based on this analysis, screening of patients with carotid occlusion who have had hemispheric symptoms within 120 days and then proceeding to EC/IC bypass would prolong quality-adjusted survival when compared to medical therapy alone, if the perioperative morbidity and mortality and subsequent rate of stroke after surgery in patients are similar to the rates observed in the EC/IC Bypass Trial. This strategy would also be cost effective. In the base-case analysis, using an a priori OEF threshold, the two-step strategy cost $19,600 per QALY gained compared to medical therapy alone. This cost per QALY is considered to be highly cost-effective [75]. A more specific (post hoc) OEF threshold resulted in costs less than medical treatment and still improved quality-adjusted survival. The more specific threshold was only slightly less effective (22.2 rather than 22.8 QALYs gained over 10 years) than the base-case OEF threshold and a lot less expensive.

Why does this analysis suggest that EC/IC bypass may be effective in reducing stroke in patients with symptomatic carotid occlusion when the EC/IC Bypass Trial, a large, prospective, and randomized trial of EC/IC bypass versus aspirin in similar patients, failed to demonstrate a benefit with surgery? In the EC/IC Bypass Trial, the risk for ipsilateral stroke at two years was approximately 14% in the medical patients and was not outweighed by the 12% perioperative mortality and the subsequent 6% stroke rate in the surgical patients [6]. The STLCOS has demonstrated that there are a subgroup group of patients with increased OEF who have a two-year ipsilateral stroke risk of 26.5% [5]. Using a combination of two additional clinical criteria (hemispheric symptoms within 120 days) and a more specific OEF threshold derived from cost-effectiveness analysis, a high risk group of 45 patients was identified who had an overall risk of ipsilateral stroke at two years in this group of patients of 50%. (Table 3)

Applying these retrospectively derived criteria for high risk to the entire sample of 81 patients from STLCOS divides them into 63/81 who did well on medical therapy with a two-year ipsilateral stroke rate of only 5.4% and 18/81 with increased OEF who had a two-year risk of ipsilateral stroke of 50%.

If it is assumed that the surgical morbidity and mortality of clinically high risk patients with increased OEF is the same 12.2% as in the EC/IC Bypass Trial and that the two-year post perioperative ipsilateral stroke rate in these patients is the

Table 3. Risk of ipsilateral stroke in 45 patients with clinical high risk due to hemispheric symptoms within 120 days

Ipsilateral Stroke	All Clinical High Risk Subjects (45)	Specific OEF Threshold Met (18)	Normal OEF (27)
1 year	11%	22%	3.7%
2 years	27%	50%	12%

Table 4. Comparison of risks of ipsilateral stroke in patients at high risk (specific OEF threshold met, hemispheric symptoms within 120 days) and remaining patients at low risk for all 81 patients in STLCOS

Ipsilateral Stroke	Total Sample (81)	High Risk (18)	Low Risk (63)
1 year	7.7%	22%	1.6%
2 years	19.0%	50%	5.4%

same 12% as those with normal OEF to start with (Table 4), (the same estimates used in the cost effectiveness analysis), a relative risk reduction of 50% is anticipated based on a two year ipsilateral stroke rate in the non-operated group of 50% vs the operated group of 24.2%. Even including those low risk patients with retinal events and symptoms older than 120 days, the two-year ipsilateral stroke rate is 26.5% for non-operated patients and 17.5% (12.2% surgical morbidity and mortality plus post surgical stroke rate of 5.3% equal to that of clinically comparable patients with normal OEF from STLCOS – Table 2). This represents a 33% relative risk reduction for surgery. It must be remembered that while the existence of a subgroup of patients with carotid occlusion with a two-year ipsilateral risk of 26.5% was demonstrated by a blinded prospective study, the extraordinarily high-risk subgroup with a 2-year ipsilateral stroke risk of 50% was identified by retrospective subgroup analysis and should be confirmed prospectively. Furthermore, although the estimate of the surgical morbidity is conservative in that it includes "trifling symptoms" and does not correct for the 3.4% occurrence of similar events in the medical group, these patients with high OEF may be at higher risk for surgical complication due to their poor collateral circulation [6].

These results support a trial of PET screening followed by EC/IC bypass in carefully selected patients with symptomatic carotid occlusion. Would this trial be a reasonable expense of limited research dollars? Approximately 730,000 first-ever or recurrent strokes occur each year in the United States [76]. Up to 15% of patients presenting with carotid territory stroke are found to have carotid occlusion [1–3]. This is approximately the same percentage who have stroke due to intracranial disease [77]. Many of these patients would not be surgical candidates, however. A possibly more accurate estimate of the number of patients who would ultimately undergo EC/IC bypass may be generated from the number of patients who undergo carotid endarterectomy for symptomatic stenosis. Approximately

100,000 carotid endarterectomies were performed in 1994, 75,000 in Medicare beneficiaries [77]. 108,000 Medicare beneficiaries with high grade carotid stenosis underwent carotid endarterectomy in 1996 [78]. Assuming a similar number of patients covered by other third party payers as in 1994, approximately 130,000 patients underwent carotid endarterectomy for high grade stenosis in 1996. Half of these patients were likely to have been symptomatic [79]. Therefore, there were roughly 65,000 carotid endarterectomies performed in 1996 for symptomatic carotid stenosis. There is approximately one patient with carotid occlusion for every 4 patients with severe carotid stenosis presenting with TIA [80]. This proportion may be higher in patients presenting with stroke. If there is one operable patient with carotid occlusion for every 4 patients with operable symptomatic carotid stenosis, then approximately 16,000 patients per year with symptomatic carotid occlusion could undergo screening with PET. The number with increased OEF who would be eligible go on to EC/IC bypass is likely somewhere between 20–40% (18/81 total from STLCOS versus 18/45 with recent cerebral symptoms) depending in the fraction with hemispheric symptoms within 120 days.

Is PET the right technology to identify these patients? There are other methodologies for assessing cerebral hemodynamics. However at this time, the scientific data linking test result to stroke risk is strongest for PET. We have demonstrated by cost-effectiveness analysis that the cost of PET is not an issue. It is more than offset by reducing the number of operations (thus reducing the attendant risk and expense) performed on patients at low risk for subsequent stroke. Another issue is availability. There are approximately 70 clinical PET facilities in the United States (Institute for Clinical PET web site, 1999, http://www.icppet.org). There is at least one scanner in most major cities. PET screening for increased OEF in patients with symptomatic carotid occlusion does not need to be done on an emergent or inpatient basis and therefore could be accomplished using existing facilities as regional referral centers at a projected rate of approximately 223 patients per year at each existing facility. Regional centers of expertise would be advantageous for the performance of such specialized surgery as well. The measurement of oxygen extraction requires the administration of oxygen-15 labeled radiopharmaceuticals (oxygen-15 labeled water and oxygen-15 labeled oxygen), which are not currently used in many PET centers. The equipment required for their synthesis would have to be installed if a need for it can be demonstrated.

We believe at this time that the most appropriate course of action to plan a trial based on the use of PET rather than other modalities. There are no good data to suggest that other modalities are superior to PET in identifying patients with carotid occlusion who are at high risk for subsequent stroke due to hemodynamic factors and who may be helped by surgical improvement of hemodynamics. If a trial based on PET does not show a benefit, there is no reason to go further and this issue can be laid to rest once and for all. If the trial is positive, then further studies comparing other modalities to PET can be performed. The sensitivity and specificity versus the PET criteria used in this study can be determined and the effectiveness and cost of substituting other modalities for PET can then be calculated.

EC/IC bypass will be cost effective in patients with symptomatic carotid occlusion who have increased OEF identified by PET under the following conditions:

(1) if the perioperative and post operative stroke rates are similar to those reported in the EC/IC Bypass Trial and (2) The stroke rate in medically treated patients are similar to those from the STLCOS. A third outstanding practical issue regards the feasibility of enrolling sufficient subjects in a trial. Enrollment is difficult to predict for a surgical procedure that is no longer being done regularly. During the STLCOS approximately 60% of the referred patients declined to participate. Possibly this percentage would go down if treatment was offered.

At this juncture the logical next step would seem to be to perform a pilot trial to settle these three outstanding issues. Sample size calculations indicate that this strategy has significant drawbacks. In order to obtain an accurate estimate of the surgical morbidity and mortality, it would be necessary to study several hundred patients (Table 5). On the other hand, it may take only a small number of patients in each group to complete the trial if the retrospective data from STLCOS turns out to be accurate. As discussed above, two-year ipsilateral strokes rate in the non-operated group of .50 vs the operated group of .242 or a 50% relative risk reduction is anticipated. The sample size necessary to achieve 80% power with a 5% false positive rate (two-tail) is 54 patients per group based on chi square distribution. We have also calculated a maximum sample size based on the two year ipsilateral stroke rates prospectively determined from the entire St. Louis Carotid Occlusion sample. The stroke risk at two years is .265 for non-operated patients and .175 for operated patients. The sample size necessary for achieve 80% power with a 5% false positive rate (two-tail) is 332 patients per group. Thus there is a possibility that a sample size of less that 300 patients per group would be sufficient to complete a definitive trial. These numbers would be barely adequate to estimate accurately the surgical morbidity and mortality in a pilot trial.

In the COSS trial, which is currently being organized, it has been elected to use an innovative experimental design which will allow the acquisition of data on these three issues as the trial progresses and use the information to make further decisions regarding the feasibility and advisability of continuing the trial. If the surgical morbidity is unsatisfactory at any time, the entire trial may be stopped. The initial sample size will be based on the conservative value of 332 patients per group. At the conclusion of the pilot phase of the trial when 200 patients (100 in each group) have been followed for two years, the sample size will be recalculated based on the actual ipsilateral stroke rate in the non-operated group and a futility analysis based on the newly calculated sample size will be performed. The NINDS PSMB will then decide whether to extend recruitment to achieve a sample size necessary to test the primary hypothesis with 80% power and 5% false posi-

Table 5. 95% Confidence intervals for observed surgical morbidity and mortality of 6–20% in cohorts of 100, 200 or 300 patients (normal approximations of binomial probabilities)

	6%	8%	10%	12%	14%	16%	18%	20%
n=100	±5	±5	±6	±6	±7	±7	±8	±8
n=200	±3	±4	±4	±5	±5	±5	±5	±6
n=300	±3	±3	±3	±4	±4	±4	±4	±5

tive rate (two-tail). If the sample size is too large for recruitment performance, the trial can be stopped. If futility analysis indicates that the trial is unlikely to show a benefit of surgery, the trial can be stopped.

This approach has several major advantages over a sequential strategy in which a pilot trial is first performed to determine safety and feasibility and to confirm the high stroke risk in the unoperated group. Such a strategy requires a hiatus between the pilot and definitive trial and the subjects enrolled in the pilot trial cannot be included in the definitive trial. With the proposed strategy, information regarding surgical morbidity and mortality and recruitment success can be gathered just as from a pilot trial. Most importantly, if the stroke rate in the non-operated patients is as high as projected and the necessary sample size is achieved early, this strategy permits early stopping of the trial independent of the results in the surgical group with subsequent analysis at the at the $p=.05$ level. At the same time it also permits interim analyses based on comparison of the two groups employing more conventional stopping at the stringent levels required to adjust for the multiplicity of comparisons.

References

1. Balow J, Alter M, Resch JA. Cerebral thromboembolism. A clinical appraisal of 100 cases. Neurology 1966; 16:559–564.
2. Pessin MS, Duncan GW, Mohr JP, et al. Clinical and angiographic features of carotid transient ischemic attacks. N Engl J Med 1977; 296:358–362.
3. Thiele BL, Young JV, Chikos PM, et al. Correlation of arteriographic findings and symptoms in cerebrovascular disease. Neurology 1980; 30:1041–1046.
4. Hankey GJ, Warlow CP. Prognosis of symptomatic carotid occlusion-an overview. Cerebrovasc Dis 1991; 1:245–256.
5. Grubb RL Jr, Derdeyn CP, Fritsch SM, et al. Importance of hemodynamic factors in the prognosis of symptomatic carotid occlusion. JAMA 1998; 280:1055–1060.
6. EC/IC Bypass Study Group. Failure of extracranial-intracranial arterial bypass to reduce the risk of ischemic stroke. N Engl J Med 1985; 313:1191–1200.
7. Day AL, Rhoton AL, Jr., Little JR. The extracranial-intracranial bypass study. Surg Neurol 1986; 26:222–226.
8. Awad, IA, Spetzler, RA: Extracranial-intracranial bypass surgery: a critical analysis in light of the International Cooperative Study. Neurosurgery 1986, 19:655–664.
9. Yonas H, Pindzola RR. Effect of Acetazolamide Reactivity and Long-term Outcome in Patients with Major Cerebral Artery Occlusive Diseases. Stroke 1998; 29:1742–1744.
10. Schmiedek P, Piepgras A, Leinsinger G, et al. Improvement of cerebrovascular reserve capacity by EC–IC arterial bypass in patients with ICA occlusion and hemodynamic cerebral ischemia. J Neurosurg 1994; 81:236–244.
11. Diaz FG, Ausman JI, Mehta B, et al. Acute cerebral revascularization. J Neurosurg 1985; 63:200–209.
12. Barnett HJM. Hemodynamic cerebral ischemia – An appeal for systematic data gathering prior to a new EC/IC trial. Stroke 1997; 28:1857–1860.
13. Klijn CJM, Kappelle LJ, Tulleken CAF, et al. Symptomatic carotid artery occlusion: A reappraisal of hemodynamic factors. Stroke 1997; 28:2084–2093.
14. Derdeyn CP, Grubb RL, Jr, Powers WJ. Cerebral hemodynamic impairment. Neurology 1999; 53:251–259.
15. Powers WJ. Cerebral hemodynamics in ischemic cerebrovascular disease. Ann Neurol 1991; 29:231–240.

16. Gibbs JM, Wise RJS, Leenders KL, et al. Evaluation of cerebral perfusion reserve in patients with carotid-artery occlusion. Lancet 1984; 1:310–314.

17. Grubb, RL, Jr, Powers, WJ. Role of cerebral hemodynamics in ischemic atherosclerotic cerebrovascular disease. Neurosurg Quart 1993; 3:83–102.

18. Baron JC, Bousser MG, Rey A, et al. Reversal of focal "misery-perfusion syndrome" by extra-intracranial arterial bypass in hemodynamic cerebral ischemia. A case study with ^{15}O positron emission tomography. Stroke 1981; 12:454–459.

19. Inao S, Tadokoro M, Nishino M, et al. Neural activation of the brain with hemodynamic insufficiency. J Cereb Blood Flow Metab 1998; 18:960–967.

20. Kazumata K, Tanaka N, Ishikawa T, et al. Dissociation of vasoreactivity to acetazolamide and hypercapnia. Comparative study in patients with chronic occlusive major cerebral artery disease. Stroke 1996; 27:2052–2058.

21. Hasegawa Y, Minematsu K, Matsuoka H, et al. CBF Responses to Acetazolamide and CO_2 for the Prediction of Hemodynamic Failure: A PET Study. Stroke 1997; 28:242

22. Ogawa S, Lee TM, Kay AR, et al. Brain magnetic resonance imaging with contrast dependent on blood oxygenation. Prc Natl Acad Sci 1990; 87:9868–9872.

23. Ogawa S, Menon RS, Tank DW, et al. Functional brain mapping by blood oxygenation level-dependent contrast magnetic resonance imaging. Biophysical J. 1993; 64:803–812.

24. Kwong K, Belliveau JW, Chesler DA, et al. Dynamic magnetic resonance imaging of human brain activity during primary sensory stimulation. Proc Natl Acad Sci USA 1992; 89:5675–5679.

25. Lin W, Paczynski RP, Celik A, et al. Experimental hypoxemic hypoxia: Effects of variation in hematocrit on MR T2* weighted brain images. J Cereb Blood Flow Metab 1998; 18:1018–1021.

26. Lin W, Paczynski RP, Celik A, et al. Effects of acute normovolemic hemodiulation on T2*-weighted images of rat brain. Magn Res Med 1998; 40:857–864.

27. Lin W, Celik A, Paczynski RP, et al. Quantitative MRI in experimental hypercapnia: Improvement in the relationship between changes in brain R2* and the oxygen saturation of venous blood after correction for changes in the cerebral blood volume. J Cereb Blood Flow Metab 1999; 19:853–862.

28. Jezzard P, Heineman F, Taylor J, et al. Comparison of EPI gradient-echo contrast changes in cat brain caused by respiratory changes with direct simultaneous evaluation of cerebral oxygenation via a cranial window. NMR in Biomed 1994; 7:35–44.

29. Kennan RP, Scanley BE, Gore JC. Physiological basis for BOLD MR signal changes due to hypoxia/hyperoxia: Separation of blood volume and magnetic susceptbility effects. Magn Res Med 1997; 37:353–356.

30. Hayashida K, Hirose Y, Tanaka Y, et al. Stratification of severity by cerebral blood flow, oxygen metabolism and acetazolamide reactivity in patients with cerebrovascular disease. Recent Advances in Biomedical Imaging 1997; 113–119.

31. Herold S, Brozovic M, Path FRC, et al. Measurement of regional cerebral blood flow, blood volume and oxygen metabolism in patients with sickle cell disease using positron emission tomography. Stroke 1986; 17:692–698.

32. Kanno I, Uemura K, Higano S, et al. Oxygen extraction fraction at maximally vasodilated tissue in the ischemic brain estimated from the regional CO_2 responsiveness measured by positron emission tomography. J Cereb Blood Flow Metab 1988; 8:227–235.

33. Hirano T, Minematsu K, Hasegawa Y, et al. Acetazolamide reactivity on 123I-IMP single photon emission computed tomography in patients with major cerebral artery occlusive disease: correlation with positron emission tomography parameters. J Cereb Blood Flow Metab 1994; 14:763–770.

34. Nariai T, Suzuki R, Hirakawa K, et al. Vascular reserve in chronic cerebral ischemia measured by the acetazolamide challenge test: Comparison with positron emission tomography. AJNR Am J Neuroradiol 1995; 16:563–570.

35. Sugimori H, Ibayashi S, Fujii K, et al. Can transcranial Doppler really detect reduced cerebral perfusion states? Stroke 1995; 26:2053–2060.

36. Yokota C, Hasegawa Y, Minematsu K, et al. Effect of acetazolamide reactivity and long-term outcome in patients with major cerebral artery occlusive diseases. Stroke 1998; 29:640–644.

37. Yamaguchi H, Fukuyama Y, Nagahama Y, et al. Evidence of misery perfusion and risk for recurrent stroke in major cerebral arterial occlusive diseases from PET. J Neurol Neurosurg Psychiatry 1996; 61:18–25.

38. Yamauchi H, Fukuyama H, Nagahama Y, et al. Significance of increased oxygen extraction fraction in five-year prognosis of major cerebral arterial occlusive diseases. J Nucl Med 1999; 40:1992–1998.

39. Yonas H, Smith HA, Durham SR, et al. Increased stroke risk predicted by compromised CBF reactivity. J Neurosurg 1993; 79:483–489.

40. Webster MW, Makaroun MS, Steed DL, et al. Compromised cerebral blood flow reactivity is a predictor of stroke in patients with symptomatic carotid artery occlusive disease. J Vasc Surg 1995; 21:338–345.

41. Kleiser B, Widder B. Course of carotid artery occlusions with impaired cerebrovascular reactivity. Stroke 1992;23:171–174.

42. Bornstein NM, Norris JW. Benign outcome of carotid occlusion. Neurology 1989; 39:6–8.

43. Powers, WJ, Derdeyn CP, Frtisch SM, et al. Benign prognosis of never-symptomatic carotid occlusion. Neurology 2000; 54:878–882.

44. Widder B, Kleiser B, Krapf H. Course of cerebrovascular reactivity in patients with carotid artery occlusions. Stroke 1994; 25:1963–1967.

45. Powers WJ, Tempel LW, Grubb RL, Jr. Influence of cerebral hemodynamics on stroke risk: One year follow-up of 30 medically treated patients. Ann Neurol 1989; 25:325–330

46. Hasegawa Y, Yamaguchi T, Tsuchiya T, et al. Sequential change of hemodynamic reserve in patients with major cerebral artery occlusions or severe stenosis. Neuroradiology 1992; 34:15–21.

47. Mintun MA, Raichle ME, Martin WRW, et al. Brain oxygen utilization measured with O–15 radiotracers and positron emission tomography. J Nucl Med 1984; 25:177–187.

48. Videen TO, Perlmutter JS, Herscovitch P, et al. Brain blood volume, blood flow, and oxygen utilization measured with O–15 radiotracers and positron emission tomography: revised metabolic computations. J Cereb Blood Flow Metab 1987; 7:513–516.

49. Powers WJ, Press GA, Grubb RL Jr, et al. The effect of hemodynamically significant carotid artery disease on the hemodynamic status of the cerebral circulation. Ann Intern Med 1987; 106:27–34.

50. Powers WJ, Grubb RL, Jr, Darriet D, et al. Cerebral blood flow and cerebral metabolic rate of oxygen requirements for cerebral function and viability in humans. J Cereb Blood Flow Metab 1985; 5:600–608.

51. North American Symptomatic Carotid Endarterectomy Trial Collaborators: Beneficial effect of carotid endarterectomy in symptomatic patients with high–grade stenosis. N Engl J Med 1991; 325:445–453.

52. Powers WJ, Martin WR, Herscovitch P, et al. Extracranial–intracranial bypass surgery: hemodynamic and metabolic effects. Neurology 1984; 34:1168–1174.

53. Grubb RL, Jr. Management of the patient with carotid occlusion and a single ischemic event. Clin Neurosurg 1986; 33:251–260.

54. Samson Y, Baron JC, Rousser MG, et al. Effects of extra-intracranial arterial bypass on cerebral blood flow and oxygen metabolism in humans. Stroke 16:609–616, 1985.

55. Gibbs JM, Wise RJ, Thomas DJ, et al. Cerebral haemodynamic changes after extracranial-intracranial bypass surgery. J Neurol Neurosurg Psychiatry 1987; 50:140–150.

56. Baron JC, Rey A, Guillard A, et al. Non–invasive tomographic imaging of cerebral blood flow (CBF) and oxygen extraction fraction (OEF) in superficial temporal artery to middle cerebral artery (STA–MCA) anastomosis, in Meyer JS, Lechner H, Reivich M, Ott EO (eds): Cerebral Vascular Disease. Amsterdam, Excerpta Medica, 1981, pp 58–64.

57. Leblanc R, Tyler JL, Mohr G, et al. Hemodynamic and metabolic effects of cerebral revascularization. J Neurosurg 1987; 66:529–535.

58. Kawamura S, Sayama I, Yasui N, et al. Haemodynamic and metabolic changes following extra–intracranial bypass surgery. Acta Neurochir 1994; 126:135–139.

59. Bishop CCR, Burnarel KG, Brown M, et al. Reduced response of cerebral blood flow to hypercapnia: restoration by extracranial–intracranial bypass. Brit J Surg 1987; 74:802–804.

60. Vorstrup S, Brun B, Lassen NA. Evaluation of the cerebral vasodilatory capacity by the acetazolamide test before EC–IC bypass surgery in patients with occlusion of the internal carotid artery. Stroke 1986; 17:1291–1298.

61. Batjer H, Devous MD, Purdy PD, et al. Improvement in regional cerebral blood flow and cerebral vasoreactivity after extracranial–intracranial arterial bypass. Neurosurgery 1988; 22:913–919.

62. Karnik R, Valentin A, Ammerer HP, et al. Evaluation of vasomotor reactivity by transcranial Doppler and acetazolamide test before and after extracranial-intracranial bypass in patients with internal carotid artery occlusions. Stroke 23:812–817, 1992.

63. Anderson DE, McLane MP, Reichman OH, et al. Improved cerebral blood flow and CO_2 reactivity after microvascular anastomosis in patients at high risk for recurrent stroke. Neurosurgery 1992; 31:26–34.

64. Widder B, Kornhuber HH. Extra–intracranial bypass surgery in carotid artery occlusions: who benefits? Neurol Psychiat Brain Res 1994; 2:126–131.

65. Hornberger J, Wrone E. When to base clinical policies on observational versus randomized trial data. Ann Int Med 1997; 127:697–703.

66. Derdeyn CP, Yundt KD, Videen T, et al. Temporal stability of hemodynamic stage in patients with carotid occlusion. J Neurosurg 1998; 88:196A-197 A.

67. Fryback DG, Dasbach EJ, Klein R, et al. The Beaver Dame Health Outcomes Study: Initial catalog of health-state quality factors. Med Decis Mak 1993; 13:89–102.

68. Gage BF, Cardinalli AB, Owens DK. The effect of stroke and stroke prophylaxis with aspirin or warfarin on quality of life. Arch Int Med 1996; 156:1829–1836.

69. Mark DB, Hlatky MA, Califf RM, et al. Cost effectiveness of thrombolytic therapy with tissue plasminogen activator as compared with streptokinase for acute myocardial infarction. N Engl J Med 1995; 332:1418–1424.

70. King JT, Glick HA, Mason TJ, et al. Elective surgery for asymptomatic, unrupture, intracranial aneurysms: a cost effectiveness analysis. Journal of Neursurgery 1995; 83:403–412.

71. Hartunian N, Smart C, Thompson M. The incidence and economic costs of cancer, motor vehicle injuries, coronary heart disease, and stroke: a comparative analysis. American Journal of Public Health 1980; 70:1249–1260.

72. Smurawaska LT, Alexandrov AV, Blandin CF, et al. Cost of acute stroke care in Toronto,Canada. Stroke 1994; 25:1628–1631.

73. Taylor TN, Davis PH, Torner JC, et al. Lifetime cost of stroke in the United States. Stroke 1996; 27:1459–1466.

74. Thorngren M, Westling B. Utilization of health care resources after stroke. A population based study of 258 hospitalized cases followed during the first year. Acta Neurol Scand 1991; 84:303–310.

75. Kupersmith J, Holmes-Rovner M, Hogan A, et al. Cost-effectivenss analysis in heart disease, Part III: Ishemia, congestive heart failure, and arrhythmias. Prog Cardiovasc Dis 1995; 37:(5)307–346.

76. Broderick JP, Brott T, Kothari R, et al. The Greater Cincinnati/Northern Kentucky Stroke Study: preliminary first-ever and total incidence rates of stroke among blacks. Stroke 1998; 29:415–421.

77. Sacco RL, Kargman DE, Gu Q, et al. Race-Ethnicity and determinants of intracranial atherosclerotic cerebral infarction. Stroke 1995; 26:14–20.

78. Hsi DC, Moscoe LM, Kurshat WM. Epidemiology of carotid endarterectomy among Medicare beneficiaries: 1985–1996 update. Stroke 1998; 29:346–350.

79. Karp HR, Flanders WD, Shipp CC, et al. Carotid endarterectomy among Medicare beneficiaries: a statewide evaluation of appropriateness and outcome. Stroke 1998; 29:46–52.

80. Bogousslavsky J, Hachinski VC, Boughner DR, et al. Cardiac and arterial lesions in transient ischemic attacks. Arch Neurol 1986; 43:223–228.

Subject Index

Printing: Mercedes-Druck, Berlin
Binding: Stürtz AG, Würzburg